Management for Hospital Doctors

Management for Hospital Doctors

Maurice Burrows MB, BCh, BAO, FRCA
*Formerly Chairman, Wirral Hospital NHS Trust, Wirral; Chairman CCHMS of BMA and
President of the Association of Anaesthetists, UK*

Roger Dyson BA, PhD
*Professor and Director of the Clinical Management Unit,
Centre for Health Planning and Management, University of Keele*

Peter Jackson FRCOG
*Information Advisor to Huddersfield NHS Trust; Consultant Obstetrician and Gynaecologist,
Huddersfield Royal Infirmary, Huddersfield*

Hugh Saxton MB, BS, FRCP, FRCR
Formerly Clinical Director of Radiology and Chairman of Management Board, Guy's Hospital, London

Foreword by Kenneth C. Calman MD, PhD, FRCS (Glas Ed),
FRCP (Lond Ed), FRCGP, FRCR, FFPHM, FRSE
The Government's Chief Medical Officer, Department of Health

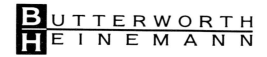

Butterworth-Heinemann Ltd
Linacre House, Jordan Hill, Oxford OX2 8DP

𝓡 A member of the Reed Elsevier group

OXFORD LONDON BOSTON
MUNICH NEW DELHI SINGAPORE SYDNEY
TOKYO TORONTO WELLINGTON

First published 1994

British Library Cataloguing in Publication Data
A catalogue record for this book is
available from the British Library

Library of Congress Cataloguing in Publication Data
A catalogue record for this book is available
from the Library of Congress

ISBN 0 7506 0880 3

Printed and bound in Great Britain by Bath Press Ltd, Avon

Contents

Foreword

Doctors have always been involved in management. General and private practitioners have run their own businesses, public health doctors and those working in investigative services have always had a heavy managerial workload, and in addition, right across the board, doctors have had to manage themselves, manage their time and manage their staff. What has changed to increase the prominence of medical management?

Two important forces were at work in the 1980s: first, the increasing realization that there will always be a relative scarcity of resources compared with expectations and second, improvements in specialty and patient costing. These led to pressure for ever-increasing precision in decision making, and recognition that effective management requires collaborative relationships between doctors and managers.

In response, the Department of Health's Resource Management Programme set out the principles of delegated management, which have evolved in many hospitals into clinical directorate arrangements; and specified the necessary management information systems – capable of providing timely, accurate costed data about patients' treatment.

The culture change of explicit involvement in strategic, operational and financial management for doctors revealed substantial educational and training needs, to which this book responds. Many of the contributors come from the innovators of delegated management in the NHS, indeed most of the Resource Management pilot sites are represented. The book provides practical insights into the realities of management in most clinical specialties. It also emphasizes how critical for effective health care is collaboration between the clinicians and the managers.

The doctors of tomorrow will be involved in management in ever more sophisticated roles. Those who serve as medical directors of trusts or as clinical directors will continue to require a substantial understanding of management theory and to develop and refine their management skills. This book covers a variety of aspects of management and will be of value for both of these groups of doctors for regular reference. However, it will also be an important resource for a wider range of consultants and for doctors in training heading for consultant posts. They will identify with many of the issues and examples in the book as matching with the tasks they are called upon to do in their professional lives.

Kenneth C. Calman

Preface

Most textbooks are written with a specific readership in mind. This book is no exception since it aims to meet the needs of a consultant who finds that he or she is expected to take on management responsibilities with little previous training or experience. It draws quite largely on the experiences of those who have been in this situation as well as on the knowledge of established experts in fields such as management, computing, finance and so forth. Naturally many decisions have had to be made as to what to include and leave out. Our broad aim has been to cover mainly those matters which touch on the day-to-day work of a hospital doctor involved in management. Some subjects which we have included are, admittedly, background information but will, we believe, give a perspective against which to view everyday issues. As a result there are matters of more general interest, such as the funding and organization of health care systems in other countries, for which we have to refer the reader to appropriate works.*

The reader will find that some points and even some topics are mentioned in more than one section. This is not due to lapses in editing. It is because we do not expect the book to be read from cover to cover: rather we see it as one into which readers will dip selectively and, we hope, repeatedly as they pursue different aspects of management. In this situation we see advantages in reinforcing those messages which are common to the experience of doctors who have been involved in management.

We must in all this rely on our readers to tell us if there are topics we should have covered or covered more fully. Equally we would like to know if any sections appear unnecessary even as background information. The involvement of doctors in management is, we believe, here to stay: we would like, in future editions, to cater as well as we can to the needs of successive doctors who take on these important responsibilities. There is, after all, no reason why audit should be confined to medicine and not applied to its textbooks. In the meantime we wish our readers well in their new responsibilities.

Maurice Burrows
Roger Dyson
Peter Jackson
Hugh Saxton

---

* An excellent introduction to this subject is: Ham, C., Robinson, R. and Benzeval, M. (1990) *Health Check. Health Care Reforms in an International Context*. King's Fund Institute, London.

Contributors

Mark R. Baker MD, MB BS, MRCP, FFCM
Director of Research and Development, Yorkshire Regional Health Authority, Harrogate
Barry Barber MA, PhD, FBCS, FInstP, CEng, CPhys
Principal Consultant, Security and Data Protection Programme Manager, NHS Information Management Centre, Birmingham
Alison Brunsdon BA(Hons)
Assistant Regional Personnel Manager, Trent Regional Health Authority, Sheffield
Nigel Brunsdon MBA
Director of Human Resources, Derby City General Hospital Trust, Derbyshire
Robert W. Buckland MB, ChB, FFARCS
Consultant Anaesthetist, Royal Hampshire County Hospital, Winchester
Sheila Bullas
Director, Health Strategies
Frank Burns
Chief Executive, Wirral Hospital Trust, Wirral
Maurice Burrows MB, BCh, BAO, FRCA
Formerly Chairman, Wirral Hospital NHS Trust, Wirral; Chairman CCHMS of BMA and President of the Association of Anaesthetists, UK
Sandra Carnall
Projects Director, Projects Directorate, Guy's Hospital, London
Cyril Chantler MA, MD, FRCP, LIHSM
Children Nationwide Professor of Paediatric Nephrology and Principal, United Medical and Dental Schools of Guy's and St Thomas's Hospitals, London
Patrick Cryne ACMA
Managing Partner, KPMG Health Systems, Manchester
Roger Dyson BA, PhD
Professor and Director of the Clinical Management Unit, Centre for Health Planning and Management, University of Keele
Brian Edwards CBE, FHSM, CBIM
Regional Chief Executive, West Midlands Regional Health Authority, Birmingham
Paul Eldridge PhD, FRCPath
Clinical Director of Pathology, Department of Clinical Chemistry, Lewisham Hospital, London
Howard Glennerster
Professor of Social Administration, Department of Social Policy and Administration, London School of Economics, London
Robin Gourlay MA, DipIET, FIPM, CintMC
Consultant in Health Care Management, Seminar Designs, Winchester
Roy Griffiths MA, BCL(Oxon)
Deputy Chairman, NHS Policy Board, London
Mark Harrison MA, FRCS
Consultant Urological Surgeon and Divisional Director of Surgery, Royal Hampshire County Hospital, Winchester
John Hassard BA, PhD
Professor of Organizational Behaviour, Department of Management, University of Keele and formerly Fellow in Organizational Behaviour, London Business School, London

Elizabeth Hunter Johnson MA
Citizen's Charter Unit, NHS management executive and formerly Head of NHS Trust Finance Team, NHSME, Department of Health, London
Peter Jackson FRCOG
Information Advisor to Huddersfield NHS Trust; Consultant Obstetrician and Gynaecologist, Huddersfield Royal Infirmary, Huddersfield
Barbara Jones RGN, RM
Director of Nursing and Midwifery Services, Queen Charlotte's and Chelsea Hospital, London
James D. Laird MB, FRCR, FFRRCSI
Consultant Radiologist, Royal Victoria Hospital, Belfast
Kenneth Lee BSc(Econ), MA
Professor and Director, Centre for Health Planning and Management, University of Keele
Karin Lowson BA(Econ), MSc (Health Econ), IPEA
Director of Information, Bradford Community NHS Trust, Yorkshire
G. C. McGarrity
Deputy Chief Executive, Wirral Hospital Trust, Clatterbridge Hospital, Wirral
Keith McLean
Regional General Manager, Yorkshire Regional Health Authority, Harrogate
Rafeek Mahmood DPM, FRCPsych
Consultant Psychiatrist/Psychotherapist, Clinical Director (Psychiatry), Executive Director, Wirral Hospital Trust, Wirral
David Mathias MB, BS, FRCS
Consultant ENT Surgeon, Freeman Hospital, Newcastle-upon-Tyne
Alan Maynard Professor of Economics and Director of the Centre for Health Economics, University of York
John Meecham MD, MB, ChB, FRCP, DCH, DRCOG
Medical Director and Consultant Physician, Wirral Hospital Trust, Arrowe Park Hospital, Wirral
Ann Naylor MB, BS, FRCA
Director of Anaesthesia and Allied Services, Basildon and Thurrock General Hospitals Trust, Essex
Ron Parker MB, ChB, FRCS
Consultant Surgeon and Chairman of Surgical Division, Walsgrave General Hospital, Coventry
Calum R. Paton MA, MPP, DPhil
Professor of Health Policy, Centre for Health Planning and Management, University of Keele
Hazel Penny
Business Manager, Medical Directorate, Huddersfield Royal Infirmary, Huddersfield
Rob Peters FCCA
Director of Finance and Information, South Essex Health Authority, Essex
Malcolm J. Prowle BSc, MA, FCCA, IPFA
Management Consultant and Associate of the School of Advanced Urban Studies, University of Bristol
Max Rendall FRCS
Formerly Clinical Superintendent and Consultant Surgeon, Guy's Hospital, London
John Rogers
Formerly Regional Director of Personnel, Trent Regional Health Authority, Sheffield
David Russell
Director of Performance Management, Yorkshire Regional Health Authority
Hugh Saxton MB, BS, FRCP, FRCR
Formerly Clinical Director of Radiology and Chairman of Management Board, Guy's Hospital, London
Charles D. Shaw PhD, MBBS, FHSM, FFCM
Director, Bristol Clinical Audit Unit, University of Bristol

John Stuart MD, FRCP, FRCPath
Head of Department of Haematology, Medical School, The University of Birmingham
David A. Walker MD, FRCP
Consultant Geriatrician, St Luke's Hospital, Huddersfield and Chairman of Medical Directorate, Huddersfield Royal Infirmary, Huddersfield
Peter D. Wright MD, FRCS
Consultant Surgeon and Medical Director, Freeman Hospital, Newcastle-upon-Tyne

Section 1

Doctors in management –
three personal perspectives

Introduction – should doctors be involved in management?

Peter Jackson

'Doctors to be managers' – so ran the headline in the *Times* in June 1984 following the government's acceptance of the Griffiths Report on the management of the NHS. How much of an outcry would there have been if the reverse had been recommended – 'Managers to be doctors'? However, with the changes that have occurred since 1984, doctors, especially hospital doctors, have been drawn more and more into management roles. Many doctors remain hostile to this idea or are, at best, apathetic. Others question whether it is right for clinicians to take on a new responsibility when it involves developing new skills.

It is, therefore, appropriate that the first chapter in this book should tackle this issue. First a practising clinician, Hugh Saxton, puts the practical arguments from the doctor's viewpoint, showing why some hospital consultants should have a part-time involvement in general management. Then a health economist, Roger Dyson, sets out the historical background and points out that doctors have often been managers in some ways and now have an even more significant part to play in the management of resources. Finally Cyril Chantler, a clinician and academic, looks at the issues from a standpoint which is rooted both in hospital practice and in the wider fields of NHS management. In their different ways, all three sections support the arguments for 'Doctors to be managers'.

1.1 Personal perspective 1

Hugh Saxton

Leading doctors is a bit like herding cats (Bennis, 1992).

Doctors are best placed to shift the emphasis of the managerial enquiry from its pre-occupation with resources and costs to health outcome or patient satisfaction. For this reason alone medical participation in management is imperative. By ensuring that resources are devoted optimally to serve the interests of patients, doctors will find that their own clinical freedom is maximised (Hoffenberg, 1987).

These two quotations summarize both the problem of getting doctors to take management issues seriously and the reasons why they should do so. It should be stated at the outset that taking management seriously does not mean doing so full-time. This book therefore does not aim to make doctors into managers. The doctors who wish to follow that path will probably seek full-time training, perhaps via an MBA. Our purpose is to encourage and help the great majority of hospital doctors who will need to know enough about management to make them useful and effective contributors when they are dealing with management issues. If they are effective in that part of their time, there will be less sense of strain, less waste of time and so more time for their clinical role.

The traditional attitude of the NHS doctor to management is rooted in the past and its origins are explored in more detail by Roger Dyson in the following chapter. The pattern was set when 'honoraries' became the first NHS consultants, using hospital facilities but with a base outside the hospital. Most hospital consultants now being appointed do have an office but this symbol of fuller commitment to their hospital may not always be matched by a sense of responsibility for the way the hospital, or their part of it, is run. It is therefore worth exploring in more detail why some doctors should be involved, for part of their time, in management and why, cultural reasons apart, so many resist this.

1 *They are best placed to make resource decisions.* No one can escape the current and future limitations on resources. In this environment, optimizing resources is the most effective way to ensure that resources are used to best advantage. Doctors must be at the centre in such decision-making: otherwise they will find themselves in the easy but unworthy position of letting someone else make the decisions and then complaining about what has happened.

2 *They should have something to offer.* This is not true of all hospital doctors: there are some very capable clinicians who should not be given managerial responsibility. But many others can offer leadership, the ability to motivate, a passion for the work being undertaken and an understanding of how to build a team who will work together.

3 *Continuity: a 30-year perspective.* Hospital consultants mostly work in the same institution for some 30 years. Career managers, especially the high-flyers, seldom stay for more than 5. Thus the doctor has an involvement of a different sort and that long-term view should be reflected in discussions of management problems.

4 *They have an independence not shared by career managers.* This may change, but today a consultant who disagrees with, say, a health authority or trust's decision is not in the position of its paid managers. He or she is therefore freer to express contrary points of view, which may be an important aspect of the democratic debate.

5 *They may take their clinical colleagues with them.* Once a doctor is convinced of the rightness – or perhaps the inevitability – of a particular course of action he or she is likely to be the most persuasive voice in altering the views of his or her clinical colleagues.

6 *If they don't manage, somebody else usually will.* This point returns to the earlier comment about the 'easy way out', inherent in avoiding responsibility while criticizing the decisions that are made. It is however not always true that if doctors don't manage someone will. If the issue or area is one in which hospital managers do not have an interest there may be no effective management input even when it is needed. Take a matter like the handling and storage of medical notes. It requires firm management, clear rules and self-discipline by all involved. The poor availability of medical records in many hospitals is because no one is willing to

manage this, when management would mean being tough with medical colleagues.

7 *They will learn from and teach their colleagues in management.* An open-minded interaction with colleagues in management, finance and other disciplines gives an illuminating perspective of the problems and complexities inherent in running a modern hospital. It can also make a doctor aware of the ability and dedication of colleagues in many other disciplines.

At the same time those in the management field learn more of the medical/nursing perspective. This is particularly true for business managers working in clinical directorates. They usually come to identify closely with the directorate's work and when this happens the 'them-and-us' barrier between managers and the wider medical profession is broken. The generation of managers now working in clinical directorates will have a more relaxed and understanding but also a more clear-eyed view of the medical and nursing professions.

8 *They can see through shrouds.* It is often extremely difficult for a lay manager to judge the validity of some 'patients-will-die' utterances by consultants. Other doctors will usually know only too well when such statements are exaggerated. On the other hand they will give credibility and support to those cases which are genuine.

Why some doctors resist management

Faced with these arguments it might seem hard for doctors to resist the pressure to take on some management responsibility. However there are a number of reasons, some good, some less admirable, why doctors may decline. The reasons are perhaps best expressed in the words they might use.

1 *'I haven't the time'.* This may or may not be valid. Reorganization of timetables; selected delegation of work; a long-term part-time locum; improved secretarial support and similar strategies may yield enough time for those who are willing to make the effort. No one else can know.

2 *'I'm not trained for it'.* This clearly is true, but it is also true that many have the capability to learn. Those who discuss the issues of being a clinical director in Section 8 are united in believing that clinical directors should have the support of their colleagues. This is important not only for the reason that lack of support will undermine all that the clinical director is trying to do, but also because it would imply that colleagues felt that he or she lacked certain essential qualities. The issue of training is discussed below but experience indicates that doctors do grow into such roles and many become very effective part-time managers.

3 *'I'm too involved in private practice'.* Involvement in private practice is a further reason why time may not be easy to find but there are positive aspects of private practice. As Roger Dyson points out in Section 1.2, private practice itself makes demands on management capabilities. It certainly requires good time management. And it can also make doctors aware of constraints on resources, whether those of the patient or the insurance company.

4 *'It's not my scene'.* A genuine aversion to management may spring from awareness that the individual concerned has no intrinsic ability in management. However some who express these feelings later turn out to be able and interested, so such comments should not be taken as the end of the argument.

5 *'I couldn't do the best for my patients'.* When a doctor talks about clinical freedom it can mean anything from the proper wish to be able to do whatever is genuinely best for the patient through to a wish to be left alone by managers or indeed by other doctors. For some, clinical freedom still means holding on to outdated practices in investigation or treatment. Such 'freedoms' are indefensible and are likely to be exposed by audit programmes. In fact, as Williams (1988) has pointed out, clinical freedom is to some extent a myth. Moreover in the present environment the surest way to achieve a measure of freedom within inevitable resource constraints is to take responsibility for management of those resources (Hoffenberg, 1987). This at least gives the ability to use resources in the most positive way. Most doctors now see that when resources are restricted, unfettered clinical freedom applied to the management of one patient simply means that resources will not be available for other patients. It is, of course, right to maintain pressure for more resources but this is best done by those who can show that they are already using resources effectively.

6 *'I might get out of touch'.* This, like finding the time, can be a major problem. To begin with anyone who takes on a significant management role will find him or herself involved in a great deal of paper work, both reading papers and writing letters. This is in itself time-consuming and can limit the time available for reading medical journals. In addition, if a significant amount of the working week is involved in management – say more than two sessions – it begins to reduce the involvement in clinical work and may even necessitate long-term cover. This in turn can lead to loss of familiarity in some parts of one's clinical work and so to problems on re-entry, further discussed below. Those who decide on a major involvement in management may find it even harder to re-enter clinical practice both because they have lost some of their clinical skills and perhaps because of changes in practice during their period of absence.

Some solutions

If some management responsibility is accepted it needs to be taken seriously and the time used efficiently. Hospital managers can have a major part to play in ensuring that doctors who take on management roles do not find them unduly irksome. The aspects which are important are:

1 *Managerial support.* This means a business manager, either part-time or whole-time. A good business manager will take issues and work through them so that the clinician uses his or her time to define issues, indicate approaches and make decisions when issues have been worked out. The partnership of management often includes a nursing manager or professional manager, e.g. radiographer, and within such a triumvirate roles and responsibilities must be clear and a mutually supportive attitude developed. It hardly needs adding that proper secretarial support must be available.

2 *Training (coaching).* Management courses abound both within the NHS and outside but many are poorly focused and irrelevant, doing little to help the medical manager to grow in certainty and confidence. Furthermore few consultants would wish to spend more than a week or two on management courses unless they were intending to change their careers completely. The value of courses should be to bring major issues into focus and to make individuals more clearly aware of their own strengths and weaknesses.

Beyond this there is a need for continuing support of a different kind. This has been called 'coaching' by the American management expert Mr Ben Heirs (personal communication). His point is that a coach is there to improve performance over an extended period; to comment constructively and encouragingly so that the person coached gains in confidence. This support, he suggests, is best given by someone outside the organization who has management expertise, e.g. a retired business person, who could be available for an hour or so once a month for a discussion of the major problems under review at the time. This approach should be seriously considered by those who want to see a new culture among doctors in the NHS. In time, perhaps, senior doctors will be able to provide similar coaching to those at the beginning of their management experience.

3 *Spreading the load.* Apart from the support given by a business manager it may be possible for individual clinical colleagues to take on part of the management responsibility in a particular field. This has the double advantage of reducing the pressure on a particular doctor and of spreading the management culture more widely.

4 *Efficient paper and committee work.* Career managers take for granted the need to read many letters and papers. Few are concerned to ensure that what is sent out is concise and well-written with the main issues clearly defined. In the same way committees are often poorly structured with debate on matters which are essentially only for information. Whenever possible, doctors should be presented with a minimum of papers, clearly written and with fully worked out issues. Doctors must exert continuing pressure to ensure that their managerial colleagues consider these matters more seriously. At an individual level the business manager, or personal assistant, may have a useful function in filtering and highlighting incoming mail and of reviewing the need for and structure of each regular committee. The points made by John Stuart on the value of short-term task forces (Section 8.6) are important in ensuring that committees are not held simply out of habit.

5 *Re-entry to clinical work.* There are two issues here:
   (a) *Reacquisition of skills.* Those who have been heavily involved in management may have given up part of their previous range of activities. The combined effect of reduced time for books and journals and a reduction in everyday practice may have impaired previously swift association patterns or manual skills. In this situation it may be that confidence has been diminished, if only to some extent. The re-entrant should plan for this, as for retirement, and may choose to spend extra time at refresher courses or in other appropriate ways.
   (b) *Problems with supporting colleagues.* If any kind of long-term medical support has been arranged for the doctor manager, his or her reappearance may create difficulties. The resumption of the earlier distribution of workload may be acceptable to both parties but this cannot be guaranteed. There is no simple answer here but the issues should be examined at the outset of the time as a manager. For example, it might be possible to find an extra part-time secretary who would increase the clinician's effectiveness and so allow him or her to maintain the clinical workload as well as being a part-time manager. Arranging for a senior registrar to 'act up' is another possibility. As with many management problems, the recognition of the problem in advance will often make the solution obvious.

Conclusion

This brief discussion introduces issues which are covered in more detail elsewhere in this book, particularly in Section 8. Doctors who are beginning to take on a management responsibility may find it helpful to read that section before they study the wider perspectives opened in other sections of this book.

References

Bennis, W. (1992) Quoted in Smith, R. Leadership and doctors. *British Medical Journal* **305**, 137–138.

Hoffenberg, R. (1987) *Clinical Freedom*. Nuffield Provincial Hospitals Trust, London.

Williams, A. (1987) Health economics: the end of clinical freedom? *British Medical Journal*, **297**, 1183–1186.

1.2 Personal perspective 2

Roger Dyson

In the traditional debate about the role of doctors in the management of the NHS there are always doctors and others who will question why doctors should be involved in management at all. The objective of this introduction is to respond to such questioning and to put forward some of the reasons why most doctors, both inside and outside the NHS, are inescapably involved in the management of the services they provide. Some of the propositions advanced in this introduction will be developed in more detail in subsequent chapters.

Medicine may not be the oldest profession but it is nevertheless one of that small inner circle of the great professions in any society. Those who practise law, whether as solicitors or barristers, have long been accustomed to managing their legal business. In the established religions of the world the organizational, as well as the spiritual, direction of the faith, has been largely in the hands of the ordained professionals. In large areas of medicine, even in the UK, doctors are fully used to directing and managing their clinical affairs in private practice, or through the independent-contractor status of general practitioners.

It is sometimes argued that doctors in the NHS are different because they are salaried employees of a public service and that this somehow absolves them from the organization and management of their clinical services. The best parallel to this would be the universities which are public institutions with salaried academics. Those academic staff, however, have almost total *de facto* governance and direction of their institutions, managing senates and being the principal influence on university councils. So in the nearest comparable model to the NHS (the universities), assumptions about the restrictive nature of salaried employment do not apply, and one is left to find other explanations for the view that salaried doctors should not be involved in NHS management; and given the examples of private practice and general practice, these explanations clearly do not lie in the nature of medicine itself.

A view that is attractive to some doctors is that in the NHS doctors are free to do things how and when they want, and that a group of underlings called administrators, nurses, etc., rush about seeing that everything is made possible. It may be a comfortable image to some, and it may once have been partly true, but no one in today's NHS can seriously believe that this describes the service.

To get nearer to answering the question about the role of doctors in management, it is necessary to look at the development of the NHS itself. For almost 30 years the NHS was free from anything but the mildest financial constraint and remained a service that was organized and run in small units by management committees of local worthies. A system of historic cost plus funding dominated the period, and doctors wishing to develop clinical services could in the main expect the funds to do so. This was the Golden Age that is still capable of bringing a dreamy, far-away look into the eye of an elderly consultant. But it is often conveniently forgotten that this was also the Golden Age of the medical superintendent in ex-municipal hospitals who organized and ran the hospital with the aid of a matron and a hospital secretary, the former to implement his clinical decisions and the latter to implement his administrative/business decisions. Those regimes were often disliked by doctors themselves because of their tutelage to the medical superintendent, but the medical role in managing and delivering this system is undeniable. Despite the element of caricature in this image, it is instantly recognizable to many doctors with working recollections of the 1950s and 1960s.

The 1970s were a decade of major change and the two most significant changes both had adverse effects for doctors. When the government of the day went technically bankrupt at the end of 1976 and called in the International Monetary Fund, the service began to experience, from 1977, a restriction in NHS funding relative to clinical demand for resources. In the first 5 or so years of that restriction, doctors comforted themselves with the view that it was a temporary phenomenon, but today it is recognized that all doctors working in the public sector of health care face a restriction of resources relative to the clinical opportunities available and that this imbalance of supply and demand will be a permanent feature of public health care – a position increasingly recognized to apply worldwide. The UK's difficulty with its economy in the late 1970s merely served to sharpen the emphasis upon a chronological turning point and the wider reasons for this imbalance of clinical resource and clinical opportunity are explored more deeply in the following chapters.

The second major change of the 1970s was not as instantly recognizable. The NHS had started to group its local hospital services as early as 1968 to make it easier to organize the provision of a growing number of major clinical and technological developments and this culminated in 1974, with a major reorganization which placed local resource allocation and direction far distant from the hospital at the level of a county or city area authority. Real decision-making about resources and management was, with these changes, taken away from the level at which senior doctors worked and placed within management structures to which doctors had little real access because their full-time work commitment was tied to hospitals and clinics. At the area authority only a community physician represented doctors on the management team, while at the district or operational level the three doctors on the team included only one senior hospital doctor whose post rotated among colleagues, very much on a part-time basis, whilst district management team colleagues were full-time and permanent, with the exception of the general practitioner member.

It is almost impossible to overstate the importance for doctors of the juxtaposition of the transfer of management responsibility outside the hospitals, at the same time as the start of resourcing restriction in the late 1970s. The medical role in the allocation of resources was organizationally diminished just at the time when resource decisions started to become quite critical for the relative development or decline of clinical services. In a number of cases, organizational change led to the virtual abdication through apathy of the medical profession from decision-making activities because of the difficulties of playing an effective role. On a wider basis, it has contributed to shaping the belief that doctors ought not the have a significant role in resource allocation and in the strategic management of the service.

Three professions dominate the NHS: medicine, nursing and administration, which includes the new breed of non-clinical managers. In the first age of the NHS there was a clear clinical, institutional and organizational hierarchy between them. Consultants had overall clinical responsibility for patients and nurses recognized that; hospital secretaries in the main deferred to medical superintendents and were often effectively managed by them.

Today the relationship between the three dominant professions is very different. The picture can be so different between institutions that any generalization would be wrong. Despite this, trends have emerged and administration has been strengthened by the experience of strategic management in the late 1970s, and by the more formal acquisition of managerial authority through the changes of the 1980s, particularly the introduction of general management. Whatever the intentions of Sir Roy Griffiths and others, the non-clinical administrators have come to dominate general management and chief executive positions and that seems likely to continue. For the nurses the development of a non-practising management hierarchy increased the aspirations of the profession and its self-assurance, and when that hierarchy was largely demolished in the mid 1980s, the NHS experienced the rapid development of a new clinical hierarchy in nursing and a much greater assertiveness in the profession that sought and is still seeking what it sees as a more equitable relationship with medicine. These changes in the relationships between the major professions further helped to reinforce the view among some doctors that they should not have that role in management that they would take for granted in their private practice or in general practice.

For behavioural scientists examining the power relationships between the professional tribes that make up the NHS, this analysis might seem to be complete, but it omits the main purpose of a health care service. It exists primarily to treat patients who attend clinics and hospitals because they believe they are ill and because they want to be made better. This is not to ignore the critical importance of preventive health care, but it is a recognition of how the bulk of health care resources will always have to be spent. Doctors are often told they are running an illness service as if that is an insult or a term of abuse. If it were not for the fact that people believe they are ill, wish to be made better and seek treatment, many of those who sneer at illness services would be having to find employment elsewhere.

Doctors are inescapably managers first and foremost because they are responsible for the clinical management of patients who come to them or are referred to them. For hospital doctors with admitting facilities, this personal responsibility for clinical management exists at three levels. They are responsible for the clinical management of the individual patient, from diagnosis through to treatment. They are also responsible for managing inpatient and/or outpatient waiting lists. This clinical management responsibility is a macroresponsibility for resource allocation within the NHS and the successful conduct of that management responsibility is crucial to the success and equity of the NHS. Doctors who claim that they are only concerned with getting the best possible treatment for the patient in front of them forget that another very important part of their task is to decide who gets treatment now and who waits – whose access to resources takes priority over someone else's.

The third level of clinical management, and now the most controversial, is the management and leadership of the multidisciplinary clinical team or network that focuses upon the care of the individual patient. Traditionally and at present doctors are responsible for seeking to ensure that treatment is both timely and appropriate to the patient's needs. As the multidisciplinary clinical team or network becomes larger and more complex, the organizational responsibility becomes that much greater for hospital inpatient and outpatient services. It is not universally accepted that this responsibility belongs to the hospital consultant and the issue is developed further in later chapters.

These three levels of clinical management are the responsibility of most doctors: the tasks are not denied by doctors but there is a reluctance to see them as *management*. Some doctors still confine the definition of management to the task of assembling those resources of staff, equipment, buildings, transport and supplies that make possible the treatment of patients at every level, i.e. to organize and manage the resources needed to provide clinical care. Yet the long-term scarcity of resources relative to demand makes efficiency essential in the delivery of good and effective clinical care, and this requires the coordination of clinical management and these wider resource management activities, because to achieve efficiency the latter needs to be directed and determined by the former. It is the recognition of this, aided by the current reforms of the NHS, that is drawing the medical profession back into a more effective and strategic role in determining the use and allocation of NHS resources.

The following chapters aim to provide a guide both to the broader concepts of management theory and their relevance to and application within the health care industry.

1.3 Personal perspective 3

Cyril Chantler

Doctors in different specialties, including clinical staff, have a contribution to make to the management of the NHS at all levels (see Section X.X). The purpose of this chapter is to discuss the role of a clinician contributing to the management of a clinical service. It is written particularly from the perspective of a clinical director in an acute hospital unit, but this experience will also be relevant to clinicians assuming managerial responsibility in primary health care or community services.

Why should clinicians be involved in management?

Most young people enter medical school because they wish to help the sick. This vocation is later defined more specifically, be it in active clinical practice, in hospital or in the community, in investigatory medicine, in scientific research, in public health medicine or in industry. There are an increasing number of doctors who are interested in full-time medical administration or management and who obtain further education to qualify them for these roles. Such individuals are appointed as medical directors or chief executive officers of hospitals abroad, or as general managers within the NHS. This role is separate from that of an active clinician who wishes to contribute to the management of the clinical service and it is the latter role that is the subject of this chapter.

Clinicians are rightly concerned about the potential conflict between their role as the advocate of individual patients' needs and a role as a medical manager. The reality is that it is now no longer possible in any health care system in the world to provide the resources to meet all the demands.

Rationing exists everywhere in terms of what is provided, to whom it is provided or when it is provided (Heginbotham, 1992). There is a fundamental difference between a cash-limited public hospital and a private hospital. Within the latter, the doctor is in effect a customer because she or he introduces the patient who pays the bill, either directly or through some third party. The manager of the hospital knows that unless the doctor is maintained as a customer, the organization will not be profitable. Strategies are necessary within such an organization for expenditure to be controlled and standards of medical care to be audited. Increasingly, the third-party payers within such systems are striving to influence the costs of care. This is particularly so in countries where government money is expended in the private sector where a requirement for regulation is paramount. In such systems the costs of regulation can sometimes exceed the costs of the money saved by the regulation (Woolhandler and Himmelstein, 1991). Often unnecessarily bureaucratic systems, such as peer review, accreditation, recertification, etc., are being introduced and an old established way of trying to cope with doctors who have only limited managerial accountability in private hospitals is to have a medical director as a salaried employee who is responsible for trying to influence the rest of the medical staff and act as a buffer between them and the hospital manager. Such an organization is very different from one which is cash-limited, such as an NHS hospital, where efficiency in the utilization of resources is an absolute requirement. Experience from other organizations and indeed now from within the NHS shows that maximum efficiency can only be achieved if all the staff in the organization work together and contribute to the management (Harvey Jones, 1988; Heirs, 1989).

General management in hospitals

In the UK general management as a concept was introduced into the NHS in 1983 by Sir Roy Griffiths who, when asked to examine management arrangements in British hospitals, simply could not understand the idea of all professionals managing themselves without regard to the overall efficiency and management strategy of the organization. It is important to emphasize that the intention was not to create a new professional group of managers but rather that individual doctors, administrators, nurses and those from other professions would contribute to the management of the service (Griffiths, 1983, 1992).

Clinical freedom

Anxieties are often expressed concerning a possible lack of clinical freedom. However, the exercise of clinical freedom requires the resources to implement plans for care. Thus, maximizing the efficiency of the organization will increase clinical freedom. There is also a need to recognize that, where cash limits and rationing exist, profligacy in the care of one patient will limit the freedom to provide care for another; thus a contribution to ensure the efficiency and effectiveness of the use of scarce resources becomes almost an ethical duty for a clinical practitioner.

Hampton, in 1983, concluded that clinical freedom was often a cloak for ignorance and in reality a myth, whilst a decade earlier, Cochrane, in his famous Rock Carling lecture, argued that in future clinicians would abandon the pursuit of what was almost certainly impossible and settle for reasonable probability in determining treatments (Cochrane, 1972). Given that cash is limited and choices have to be made, it is vital that they are clinically informed. Unfortunately, information concerning the efficiency (resource management) and effectiveness (clinical audit) of medical interventions and clinical care is woefully lacking and new treatments are introduced or sustained within the NHS without proper evaluation. This is not only harmful to patients, but extremely wasteful (Council for Science and Society, 1982).

Resource management and clinical audit

Clinical directors with their management teams have a responsibility to encourage all staff in their directorate to cooperate in both resource management and clinical audit and should also initiate studies to examine the efficiency and effectiveness of their practice. Such studies can be simple and inexpensive to carry out; we recently showed that urine that is crystal clear is unlikely to be infected and therefore does not need to be sent for laboratory examination unless there are strong clinical indications. Adopting this policy throughout Guy's Hospital would save about £100 000 (Rawal *et al.*, 1990).

The appointment of a director of research and development for the NHS is an important initiative (Peckham, 1991). Regional appointments have been made and it is likely that clinical audit and resource management initiatives at local level will increasingly be coordinated through a locally established health service research unit which will work with clinical directorates.

Models of clinical management

A number of different models for involving clinicians, not just doctors, in general management are in use (Disken *et al.*, 1990). Some are satisfactory, but some are inappropriate, either in structure or function, and can cause damage both to professional relationships and to the provision of care. Clinical directorates or clinical management teams should allow decision-making closer to service delivery and give all professional staff, including doctors, nurses and administrators working together, the responsibility for the quality of care provided and control over the use of resources necessary for service provision. Effective team work not only improves staff morale, but should provide a more efficient and effective service to the patient. Poorly organized or poorly functioning clinical directorates can be destructive (Rey, 1992). They can fail to exert any control over the quality or cost of service delivery and simply promote the individual professional interests of the management team. Power without responsibility and accountability is dangerous and in the context of clinical directorates can lead to general staff demoralization and uncoordinated clinical activity.

Any institution contemplating the introduction of general management with the involvement of clinicians needs to spend considerable time and effort in discussing the structure and functional relationships within the structure with all concerned, rather than concentrating initially on the introduction of information systems.

A useful analysis of the benefits of a clinically based management structure which is working well has been produced (Wraith and Casey, 1992). There is a need initially to understand the cultural climate of the hospital or unit concerned and determine what aspects of it inhibit team work and general management. These problems need to be confronted. There are certain principles that need to be considered when designing and introducing a new structure of management (Chantler, 1990).

Decentralization

To the extent that decentralization encourages decision-making at the appropriate level, it is to be commended. It is important that responsibility and authority are commensurate. There is a tendency for those who wish to assume authority to fail to understand that it involves both responsibility including financial responsibility and accountability within the management structure.

Difficult choices have to be made in the use of resources. Whilst broad areas of health service policy are set by government, commissioners, both district health authorities and fund-holding general practitioners will determine with and on behalf of a local population what services are to be provided. None the less, there is a vitally important role for the clinician working with individual patients to determine individual priorities and choice. Defined in this way, clinical freedom is important because we all expect our doctors and nurses to do the very best they can for us within the resources available when we are sick. The practice of medicine has become increasingly difficult and tensions arise as the gap widens between what can be provided and what doctors wish to provide, and patients' expectations. Operating within clear guidelines can serve to reduce this tension and to share this responsibility.

As a generalization, management can be divided into two parts: guidance or strategy and delivery or operational management. The role of a clinical director is very much as part of an operational management team. None the less, it is important that the director represents the corporate view of his or her management team and directorate within strategic discussions.

Thus, at Guy's Hospital clinical directors sat on the hospital management board, which was chaired by the medical director who was also a clinician. Advice which is given by those who carry responsibility and accountability is much more powerful than the advice given by the old medical advisory comittees, who increasingly found themselves operating as a Greek chorus, commenting on what was going on, but with increasingly less influence as cash limits were introduced into the NHS. It is therefore important that any management structure should be 'broad and flat' if the influence of clinical directors on strategic discussions is not to be removed. In my view, clinicians should resist the introduction of structures which are not compatible with these considerations or which simply involve them as a lead clinician in an advisory role separate from the management structure.

It is important to consider how patient services are delivered, where they are delivered and who is responsible for providing them. The clinical teams concerned should themselves carry responsibility, authority and accountability, as discussed above. In small hospitals this will be a matter for the directorate, but in larger hospitals further decentralization at a subdirectorate level may be necessary.

At Guy's Hospital in 1988 an experiment was carried out whereby the paediatric nephrology subdirectorate, based on one ward with associated outpatient facilities, was put under the joint management of the senior nurse and a paediatric nephrologist. The budget included all staff costs, including nursing, medical, secretarial etc., equipment, both capital and maintenance, drugs, and at that time the marginal costs of various investigations. The system was introduced at the end of the fourth month of the financial year, by which time the paediatric nephrology budget was overspent by £18 000. By the end of the year it was back in balance, four beds previously closed through inadequate resources had been reopened, and substantial sums had been spent on new equipment both for the wards and for introducing an office management system. An extra senior house officer had been recruited and paid for and a state enrolled nurse had been sent for further training, all paid for from the budget. This had been achieved by cutting expenditure by £60 000 per annum, largely by reorganizing – but not reducing – clinical activity so that fewer nursing staff were required.

The key point was to allow the ward sister full control over the skill mix and staffing levels on the ward. She abolished five staff nurse posts whilst recruiting an extra sister as a teaching sister. The remaining staff nurses were therefore better supported and were able to work more efficiently and an internal cover system was developed so that at busy times and on rotation nurses could be called in to provide extra help. The nursing budget was calculated simply by adding up the number of nursing hours available each week and accounting for those used at the end of each week. A simple algebraic formula allowed the extra costs of different grades of nurses, overtime, etc. to be computed, demonstrating that complicated information systems are not always necessary for sound financial management.

Professional and management accountability

It is important to separate professional and management accountability within the organizational structure. It is obviously undesirable and probably intolerable for professionals to be accountable in terms of their professional skills and responsibilities to others who come from different professional backgrounds. Management accountability is different and in a public service we should be accountable for the resources we use. Thus, in the system at Guy's Hospital it is possible for nurses to be accountable managerially to doctors and vice versa or to non-clinically qualified staff. Professional lines of accountability, however, remain so that nurses are all accountable professionally to the Chief Nurse of the hopsital. Her (as it happens) role is to manage nursing rather than nurses. Whilst it could be argued that such separation of professional and management accountability is unclear and confusing, in practice few problems have arisen in the 7 years since it was introduced and indeed similar systems exist in many industries where professional skills are paramount, such as British Steel (R. Scholey, personal communication).

Part-time commitment

Doctors involved in clinical management will wish to continue their clinical practice and indeed it is important that they should do so because it is their involvement in day-to-day clinical activity that provides them with the necessary knowledge and experience to inform their management role. There is also the question of leadership, which is likely to be more effective if staff know that the doctor is clinically involved. This means, however, that the clinical management team has to work as a team, sharing the work, the authority and the responsibility, though one individual (not necessarily the doctor) has to be the leader and be personally accountable. The system we introduced, which has now become widely utilized, involves a team comprising a doctor, a business manager who may be from an administrative, a finance or a nursing background, and a nurse manager; there are variations such as the nurse manager being in addition the business manager but provided with administrative assistance. The roles of each need to be carefully thought out, understood and written down, within a clear job description from which personal objectives can be developed. A useful check list for this is available (Wraith and Casey, 1992).

It is important for clinicians to take their management role seriously; to seek and listen to criticism and not to be too proud or dismissive to recognize the need for training in specific management skills. A short training course, so that the scope of the job and the environment in which it exists are understood before taking up responsibilities, may be useful and such courses are provided by a number of organizations such as The King's Fund in London or through membership of the British Association of Medical Managers.*

Further short courses may be useful to acquire or develop specific management skills such as negotiating skills, financial understanding, team work or personal skills. However, much can be learnt on the job given a sympathetic and effective chief executive, financial director, personnel director, etc.

*For information contact Dr Jenny Simpson, Chief Executive, BAMM, Barnes Hospital, Kingsway, Cheadle, Cheshire SK8 2NY. Tel: 061 491 4229; fax: 061 491 4254.

Information systems

A constant complaint by clinical managers is the inadequacy of the information systems available to them. Whilst accurate information is important, doctors do need to remember that many of the important clinical decisions they have to make are based on inadequate information or understanding. Management is no different and is not a precise science and never will be, given that it involves human behaviour. Doctors could be perhaps a little more understanding of and patient with the problems that non-medically qualified managers have to face whilst the latter in turn could perhaps try to be more understanding about the difficulties of clinical practice. Hospitals are extremely complicated and provide a management challenge which is probably greater than in any other organization. The information available is often late or inaccurate and it is difficult to set budgets, not least because the money available to the institution as a whole is usually not determined until well into the financial year. This, incidentally, is because the Treasury budgets year on year and has to do so because the economy is unpredictable. It is important to remember that 70–80% of the costs in the NHS is in salaries and wages and a tight control of staffing levels, which is possible with minimal information systems, is the most important component of budgetary control. Having said that, it is important that better information systems are introduced (Chantler, 1992). Large sums of money are currently being spent in the NHS to achieve this and some of this money is being wasted. Whilst it is impossible to be specific, as a general rule the first test of an information system is whether it will provide information which will improve the clinical service and whether it will be helpful to the users who have to provide the raw information to feed the system. If the latter point is not certain, then the quality of information introduced into the system will be flawed. Costing and activity information can usually be added on to a clinically based system and the various systems can be networked to provide the facts and figures required by central administration.

References

Chantler, C. (1990) Management reform in a London hospital. *In:* Carle, N. (ed) *Managing for Health Result*, pp 74–87. King Edward's Hospital, London.

Chantler, C. (1992) Management and information, *British Medical Journal*, **304**, 632–635.

Cochrane, A. L. (1972) *Effectiveness and Efficiency; Random Reflections of Health Services.* Nuffield Provincial Hospitals Trust.

Council for Science and Society (1982) *Expensive Medical Techniques*, pp 1–59. Council for Science and Society, 3/4 St Andrews Hill, London EC4V 5BY.

Disken, S., Dixon, M., Halpern, S. and Schockett, G. (1990) *Models of Clinical Management.* Institute of Health Services Management, London.

Griffiths, R. (1983) *The NHS Management Enquiry.* Department of Health and Social Security, London.

Griffiths, R. (1992) Seven years of progress – general management in the NHS. *Health Economics* **1**, 61–70.

Hampton, J. R. (1983) The end of clinical freedom. *British Medical Journal* **287**, 1237–1238.

Harvey Jones, J. (1988) *Making it Happen (Reflections on Leadership).* William Collins, Glasgow.

Heginbotham, C. (1992) Rationing. *British Medical Journal* **304**, 496–499.

Heirs, B. (1989) *The Professional Decision Thinker and the Art of Team Thinking Leadership.* Grafton, London.

Peckham, M. (1991) Research and development for the National Health Service. *Lancet* **338**, 367–371.

Rawal, K., Senguttuvan, T., Morris, M., Chantler, C. and Simons, N. (1990) Significance of crystal clear urine. *Lancet* **335**, **1228**.

Rey, C. (1992) Gang mentality. *Health Services Journal*, 26 March 31–33.

Woolhandler, S. and Himmelstein, D. U. (1991) The deteriorating administrative efficiency of the US health care system. *New England Journal of Medicine* **324**, 1253–1258.

Wraith, M. and Casey, A. (1992) *Implementing Based Management – Getting Organisational Change Underway.* Wraith-Casey 1–30, Droitwich, Worcestershire WR9 8LE.

Section 2

Managing health care

Health care management – theory and emerging practice

Kenneth Lee and Calum R. Paton

Introduction

It is important to establish, at the outset, a definition for health care management. In this chapter, it is taken to mean both a wide-ranging understanding of health policy and a practical approach to the achievement of policy objectives through the successful implementation of policy: in other words, management as common sense: the meeting of objectives, coherently organized.

Accordingly, a distinction can be made immediately between strategic management and operational management. Strategy deals with steering towards long-term or overall goals in furtherance of the mission of the organization. Operational management both takes a short time-scale as its focus, and tends to be task-oriented – albeit consistent with the strategic direction spelt out in the overall strategic plan. One can also distinguish between general management on the one hand and professional (or functional) management on the other hand: commonly the former is concerned with the management of the whole institution and the latter with, for example, medical management, nursing management, property management, catering management, and so forth.

Albeit that these distinctions are important in their own terms, it appears important also to state at the outset that management ought fully to involve people from different professional backgrounds. As well as overtly trained managers, doctors, nurses, finance people, general administrators, and others all ought to provide the raw material for the managers of tomorrow, whether they will be seen as managers within their own professional domains or as potential general managers. At the national level, politicians ought to be aware of the management agenda and bureaucrats ought to be imbued with management skills to add to the other skills they possess (political, diplomatic, organizational or technical).

It follows, therefore, that a key element of successful management is its ability to sustain management succession through management development. Training one's successor is the best means of ensuring good management in the future. Hence, management development ought to be part of an overall management strategy, so that the right people are located in the right places in the right systems (*structural* features of management), doing the right thing in the right way, and in the right relationships with other people (aspects of management *process*), to achieve the right results (the *outcomes* of the management system).

This chapter is structured as follows. It outlines the concepts relevant to health care management; the balance between national and local responsibilities; the move to general management in health care and its theoretical underpinnings; distinctions between policy, planning and management; the political environment and political structures surrounding the domain of strategic management in health care; the distinction between public administration and management; and political issues associated with the periodic rise and fall of interest in the strategic management in health care. The chapter concludes with a series of observations on the nature and role of management, with reference to health care in general and the 1990s in particular.

Concepts and trends in management

In any general text on health care management, it is first important to define one's terms. This section of the chapter serves that purpose, before addressing the emergence of general management in health care and its visibility at both national and local levels.

General management of a health care agency, such as a hospital complex, concerns the management of the whole organization with a view to achieving its strategic objectives. The strategic objectives in turn may be defined as the outputs (whether particular services, treatments or programmes) which help to achieve the overall aims of the enterprise. Aims, in other words, are the broadest level of achievement: achieving one's aims may be restated as achieving the desired outcomes, in line with the mission of the organization.

Examples of outcomes in health care are: a better health status of the population as a whole or for targeted groups within the population; more 'consumer-friendly' health services; and/or greater equality in health status. The achievement of strategic objectives may be considered to be the achievement of outputs (such as the construction of appropriate facilities, the attainment of specified standards of service or operation of appropriate services) which have been analysed as contributing to, or as likely to contribute to, the desired outcomes.

Functional management is the management of resources (human, physical, financial) within a particular function, such as the medical profession or its specialties; the nursing profession; the catering function; or the estates and buildings function. In other words, there is necessarily a strong overlap – in theory – between functions and professions: it might be appropriate to say that all professions have a function or are a function. Alternatively, functions are organized as support services for professionally delivered outputs from the whole system.

Strategic management, as a term, may be used synonymously with general management. However, it is possible for strategic issues to be managed within a functional context: for example, a staff strategy for the medical profession may be considered to be a strategic issue but may be discussed within the remit of the medical function. Strategic management can best be given meaning by distinguishing it from its opposite, *operational* management. The latter concerns the day-to-day working and servicing of patient care services and support services required to provide health care. Strategic management can also be distinguished from *tactical* management. This is another contrast, on another dimension, which distinguishes between rational planning and incrementalism in making management decisions (Lee and Mills, 1982). Generally, tactics are at a lower level of operation within an enterprise or institution – but

not necessarily so. Here, it is important to distinguish between steps that are incremental in nature but in line with a strategic direction and those that are not.

Indeed, it is the job of strategic management to formulate plans to help to achieve strategic objectives, whether management is at the national level or at the level of the enterprise, institution or agency. Strategic management is geared to achieving strategic plans, whether these plans involve the full public provision of facilities or merely the scanning of the environment to seek to identify trends and needs and to seek by one means or another to ensure that these needs are met. The former may be considered to be rational planning, and the latter is often described as a mixed scanning approach to planning (Lee, 1979).

Mixed scanning can use a variety of techniques, such as *network planning*. This sets out a series of variables which influence, and are influenced by, other variables in the environment. The variables may well include *external* environmental factors, but also significant strategic factors affecting the *internal* operation of the organization.

Such an analysis, or approach, helps to scan the environment and is not so much definitive as an aid to decision-making (Gomez and Probst, 1987). The aim is to create strategic plans which rely on significant variables to achieve outcomes, yet seek to minimize unintended outcomes as a result of failing to detect other influences, or counteracting influences. A critical variable, for example, is capable of affecting outcomes (other variables) but is easily affected itself, and therefore plans may have side-effects as a chain-reaction is mobilized if this is not taken into account. Mixed scanning also conforms to the need to be realistic. It is more rational in practice to be selective and systematic about a number of feasible options than rationally to examine all possible choices and variables.

Such a methodology has analogies with a SWOT marketing analysis of strengths, weaknesses, opportunities and threats. Strengths and weaknesses are factors internal to the organization; opportunities and threats are external environmental factors (Argenti, 1980). If one uses the SWOT variables not just to do a static analysis of internal and external variables and their likely effects on the product but also to predict and trace interlocking dynamic trends, one has moved to a network plan. Marketing theory increasingly is embracing this strategic perspective.

Having clarified various aspects of the terminology, what have been the emerging trends? First and foremost, there has been a move away from exclusive reliance upon professional management and functional management towards what is known as general management. This has applied particularly in public sector enterprises, such as health services in the UK, where such an approach had previously either not been considered or had been ruled unsuitable for public services. Why?

Historically, the essence of *professional* management has been that, in a multiprofessional institution such as a hospital, each profession has its own hierarchy, the apex of which could not be readily countermanded by somebody from another profession or from outside the realm of professions altogether. If one moves from career grades known as professions to those known as functions, one can trace a similar logic, though the argument was never as powerful nor frequent.

The logic of *general* management, however, is that at each operational – or indeed strategic – level of the enterprise, all top professional officers are responsible to a general manager. Thus, in the hospital, there is an overall unit general manager or chief executive; below this, there are general managers who are the heads of clinical specialties, normally doctors; and other professions have to accept responsibility to the chiefs of each of these units, who may be known as general managers. (Continuing to resort to terms such as clinical directors and clinical coordinators suggests that the debate between notions of general and of professional management is not entirely resolved.)

In theory, the essence of general management is that professional and functional hierarchies cease to exist altogether. Thus, in the UK, not only is the overall general manager both responsible for, and accountable to, his or her own board (director of finance, director of personnel, and so forth) as well as to the heads of the professions and functions (horizontally), but he or she is also responsible for and accountable to lower-level general managers within the organization (vertically). Thus, the lower tiers of the professional and functional hierarchies, for example the heads of clinical specialties and, below them, individual doctors, may be (and increasingly are) responsible to general mana-

gers for each of the hospital's divisions or specialties. These heads of divisions are then in turn responsible to the general manager.

As a general management-based chain of accountability and responsibility is replacing other chains, what of the top management board itself (of the hospital or institution generally), comprising the director of finance, director of personnel, director of planning and other directorates? Obviously, these are responsible to the general manager or the chief executive of the whole institution. However, it may be asked whether they have responsibilities for their own professional or functional lines or hierarchies. For example, are finance staff, located within clinical specialties or departments, responsible to the director of finance as well as, or instead of, to their local general manager? In a full general management model the answer would be no. The director of finance, director of personnel, director of planning, medical director at the top of the organization are in fact advisory rather than executive *vis-à-vis* their own professional colleagues within the organization. In other words, a director of finance can advise on financial policy for the organization but not be an operational manager, or indeed a strategic manager. Accepting and adjusting to these changed relationships is neither easy nor automatic, or perceived to be acceptable in all cases and for all cohorts of health care workers.

To repeat the message: general management in a hospital may be construed as a vertical chain by which former vertical chains such as professional and functional management have been subsumed or replaced. For example, different medical specialties will be responsible to general management in a hospital. *Within* each specialty or group of specialties, professions and functions generally are responsible to a general manager who is likely to be a clinical director, supported increasingly by a business manager and/or clinical manager.

General management is thus intended to be integrative rather than fragmented into various tiers and chains of both professional and functional management. It is also intended to be both strategic and operational. Obviously, general management needs to be concerned with operational matters concerning the servicing and continuation of functions within its own organization. However, general management does need to be concerned with strategic matters: in other words, the meeting of objectives and the gearing of the organization, or redesign of the organization, to meet objectives. Indeed, the questioning of objectives is also a strategic matter, given that objectives may no longer be consonant with overall aims; indeed, strategic plans may have to be changed as objectives are changed, in line with a need to pursue aims differently. Aims are concerned with the overall mission of the organization – for example, the improvement of the health status of selected groups within the population in health care. The particular objectives by which this may be achieved may change as the environment changes: as causes of ill health change, new diseases come on the horizon, and modalities of care improve.

Yet an essential dilemma still remains: is the shaping of strategy to be promulgated from above or promoted from below? If the former, it always seems a long distance from the articulation of the objectives of the health care system to improvements within a particular specialty, within a particular ward or in a particular community. The emerging orthodoxy in western management circles over the last decade or so has been based on the distinction between the articulation of central objectives (which may be national objectives in the case of the health care system) and local responsibility for achieving these objectives. In other words, one ought to be 'tight' about stated objectives – and certainly about the mission and aims at the broadest level – but one ought to devolve responsibility for achievement to particular agencies, with as much operational and financial devolution as possible.

A number of western countries have seen such trends in their health care systems, often aligned to the introduction of general management. In the UK, the Ibbs Report, *The Next Steps* (Ibbs, 1988), advocated that agencies responsible for delivering services within government or through government-funded programmes ought to be as independent as possible. In New Zealand, the introduction of board-level management within the health care system was accompanied by an attempt to devolve responsibility away from the centre. In the Netherlands, the introduction of greater competition in both the financing and provision of health care has been accompanied by greater autonomy for financiers and providers within the context of national regulation. These are but examples: however, they do represent a discernible trend across national boundaries.

In order to develop managers capable of acting within their own budgets and guidelines received from above as independently as possible, awareness of national policy objectives and awareness of skills required in order to operate at the local level are equally necessary. Hence, a management development programme ought not to make any artificial distinctions between policy and management on the one hand, or strategy and operations on the other. Instead, they ought to be seen as a continuum, different parts of which are relevant for different people at different times.

Both at the national level and at the level of the providing institution (e.g. hospital or community health service), overall aims ought to be set out in what has come to be known as the mission statement. Without it, the correspondence of centre and periphery may be illusory. Equally, however, such statements need to be owned by all those working within the organization to which they apply, and need to be translated into objectives and sets of action – commonly through the production of a strategic direction document (say 3–5 years ahead), and a business plan of action for the next trading (annual) plan.

In short, the business plan links the proposed courses of action within the system to the objectives of the whole system (whether the hospital or the health care system as a whole). For example, objectives may be translated into particular targets of provision for specialties within a hospital. This may be part of a publicly planned system or part of a private sector system which is gearing anticipated demand in the marketplace to supply to be offered through the hospital's specialities. As a result, a business plan will link resources for investment and recurring costs across different specialties and functions in order to render the plan operational, and in order to allow the plan to be compatible with budgetary and other constraints and opportunities. Below the level of the business plan, one is then into the realm of operational management, seeking to 'grease the wheels' of the system and to ensure that it is routinely performing to its specification.

The dimensions of management

There are many differing perspectives on the scientific status of management studies, as Section 9 will clearly show. Some would even deny that management can be studied scientifically at all, and that it is a subjective art. Others would argue that management principles are geared to the achievement of ends, and that quantitative measures can be derived to monitor the success or otherwise of management tasks with given ends in mind.

One may make, for instance, a distinction between *management studies* and *management science*. The term *management studies* embraces a broad area of enquiry including the overall objectives of management; the different schools of management; the political, economic and social environments within which management operates; and perspectives on organizations. *Management science*, on the other hand, focuses on the empirical and quantitative skills, and the analytical methods, which can be used by managers, or commissioned by managers, from professionals, scientists and statisticians, as tools geared to the achievement of ends in an organization. Studying management will, therefore, be a broader engagement than studying management science, which is a component of the task of management.

Management is often contrasted with *administration*. Administration refers to the servicing of an organization's needs given an acceptance of its current direction – an often legalistic 'hand on the tiller' – as opposed to management's concern with determining and reassessing objectives and changing direction (with all that that implies for changed internal practices) when necessary.

British public life is peppered with references to either administration or management which reflect either overt or hidden assumptions as to the style of operation of an organization. The term, the administrative class of the civil service, points to the original ethos of administration as opposed to general or professional management. Until the Griffiths enquiry reported in October 1983 and was accepted by the government, the NHS did not have a system of general management to steer its components, but was serviced by a system of administration reflected in the titles of regional administrator, district administrator, and so forth. An important question then is, what has instituted and formalized a change from the age of administration to the age of management? It would be dangerous to see such (contemporary) historical trends as inevitable or indeed automatically rational. However, there have been compelling forces behind such change

in the UK over the last decade, and it is important to understand them.

The first issue to be considered is that of *policy* and its *implementation*. One can consider the framework of policy at two levels. First, there is government policy which affects the management of the organization; and second, there is the internal policy devised by, and for, the organization. It is important to distinguish policy-making in both those senses from implementation. Policy is – on its own – mere intention; implementation affects results and outcomes.

To explore this matter a little further, in policy and organizational analysis, three central terms are *inputs*, *outputs* and *outcomes*. At the political level of making policy – for example, through passing legislation – inputs refer to the factors which affect the policy-making *process*: for example, the relative strength of political parties in a legislature, the effect of interest groups, the contribution of academics or think tanks with a realm of ideas, are all likely to provide examples of inputs to policy-making. At the political level, the key output is the accomplished legislation or regulation. However, it is only when thinking of outcomes that one addresses the scope for effective implementation. Laws may achieve unintended results, or little result at all. Regulations may not work as expected. The way in which policy is implemented determines what might be called its social outcome.

Using the terms in a different context, one can apply the language of inputs, outputs and outcomes within an organization, for example in a private firm or a service. In a manufacturing process, inputs are the factors of production – capital, labour and so forth. Outputs are the products made, and outcomes can be considered to be either the longer-term results for the company (for example, in terms of the profits and incomes received), or for the public in terms of the availability of goods and their ability to satisfy preferences and live a certain lifestyle.

In the NHS, inputs to the production process are also reducible to labour and capital; in this case, one is talking about doctors, nurses, and other professions and cadres of labour; at the level of money, one is talking not just of capital investment but of revenue budgets, as indeed in private firms. Outputs refer to the services delivered, for example, the number of operations, number of home visits by district nurses in a community setting, number of cervical smears carried out, and so forth. Outputs, however, are not the same as outcomes here either; outcomes refer to the effect upon the health status of the population which the provision of a health service has had (notoriously a difficult thing to measure, when one considers the many effects upon the health of populations, groups and individuals which have to be disentangled).

Just as the implementation of policy affects how outputs are transformed into outcomes at a political level in society, how services are delivered affects outcomes in an 'industry' like the NHS and how products are marketed affects outcomes both for the firm and for society in the private enterprise.

Within a publicly funded and owned organization, such as the NHS, it is no surprise to find that the *political* aspect of strategic management is often direct and visible. That is, in an arena such as the NHS, the influence of the government and politicians upon the delivery of services is more direct than is the case with the private sector. This is not to deny the influence of politics in seeking to set the parameters within which private enterprises operate.

Yet increasingly, public enterprises and public corporations that do operate in the business world have generally copied the management structures of private enterprises, at least at a formal level. The large corporations in the public sector, like their parallels in the private sector, have a corporate board with a chief executive, whatever the exact form of the title is. In some cases, the chief executive will also be the chair of the board or company, though the merits and demerits of separating these two roles in two individuals is actively being discussed in both the public and private sectors of industry, trade and commerce at the present time. This corporate board will have, as its key members, a director of finance, director of corporate affairs/corporate planning, director of personnel, director of operations or their equivalents.

As noted earlier in this chapter, services in the public sector have no tradition of a similar form of strategic management. It is only recently, for example, that the NHS was given first a management board (in 1983–1984) and subsequently a management executive (following the White Paper of 1989; Department of Health, 1989) to direct and oversee the service.

The NHS management board then and the NHS management executive now have to be reviewed alongside the traditional civil service control or administration of the NHS. Prior to

the Griffiths enquiry and its acceptance in 1983, it is not too wide of the mark to state that there was no apex for strategic management of the NHS. There was a Secretary of State responsible to Parliament, with the 'top of the office' of DHSS civil servants (on the Department of Health side of what was then the Department of Health and Social Security) responsible to the minister for the administration of the department first and the NHS second. Strategy was a centralized process, albeit informed by the NHS, at the policy and planning levels, but in the opinion of many, there was a basic lacuna where strategic management was lacking. This situation, of course, went to the heart of the distinction between traditional administration and modern general management.

The advent of the Griffiths Report and the move to management from administration still leaves open, of course, the question of the role of the political process. The splitting within government of responsibility for policy (through the NHS policy board) from management action (through the NHS management executive) is one step along the rubric of 'letting managers manage'. At the same time, politicians are responsible to Parliament: the NHS is a politically very visible and popular service, such that the interaction of policy, planning and management is crucial and will remain so. The slogans 'Keep politics out of health' and 'Keep health out of politics' remain just that – slogans. Likewise, to delineate the issue by saying that policy is about *ends* and management is about *means* is equally simplistic and naive.

But, if politics is an omnipresent force, has the role of the enthusiastic amateur finally been laid to rest? As early as the middle of the nineteenth century, the North–Trevelyan Report (1853) had called for the professionalization of the civil service, and their recruitment by open and meritocratic methods. This led to a reformed civil service in 1870 which Sampson (1983) described as 'the first great British meritocracy'. At that time and until fairly recently, the model was that civil servants would be generalists providing lay advice to ministers and lay administration of their departments, while relying upon technical and specialist advice where necessary.

Yet throughout the twentieth century, and as the economy has become more specialized and the responsibilities of the civil service have increased dramatically, the ethos of lay administration has been seen to be increasingly unsuitable. The

Fulton Committee reported in 1968, and made proposals for the reform of the civil service, confirming a widespread belief that the civil service structure and the education of its senior officers were geared to another age.

The change of culture, however, dates only from the 1980s. Until recently, civil servants at the 'top of the office' dealt in general policy and advice to ministers while, at lower levels, administration was internal and not related specifically to the efficient management of services. With new initiatives by government (e.g. the Rayner Scrutinies) to investigate cost savings achievable in specific programmes within government departments, these soon became identified for their profound implications to the civil service. Subsequently, various initiatives known in the language of acronyms as VFM and FMI (value for money and financial management initiative) reinforced the ethos of efficiency and financial management and were specifically implemented in the NHS, as elsewhere.

More specifically, in terms of health care, the Griffiths Report of 1983 advanced the view that general management should be introduced at the apex of the NHS to provide a management board with corporate direction for the service, as other private and public industries had. The implications were radical and the consequences for the civil service and for the separation of policy matters from management issues is a recurring theme.

To summarize, at the national level, some of the significant changes to date, in managerial terms, can be listed as follows:

1 The growing size and importance of the NHS management executive and its influence on the management of the NHS.
2 The diminution of the centre in proffering traditional lay advice on policy matters.
3 The diminution in the functional provision of services.
4 The infusion of private sector techniques via management efficiency studies within government departments.
5 The opening-up of the service to advice explicitly from think tanks and secondment of individuals (working alongside official civil servants).

Modern approaches to management

Any move towards strengthening the management structure and management performance of an organization is likely to focus upon a limited number of key issues. For example, what should be the organization's approach to shaping its future, i.e. strategic planning? What should be the organization's approach to decentralization of managerial decision-making? What should be the core values of the organization, and how best does it address matters of quality? This section explores trends and their impact upon health care management.

On the first question, the 1980s saw an increasing questioning of the conventional wisdom that centralization of planning and control within large companies makes for effective management or good outcome. In consequence, decentralization into units within companies, with separate responsibilities or separate markets, has been the developing norm. Centralized planning, for example with a divisional structure, with all divisions responsible upwards to a central board, has not been considered flexible enough to meet the needs of markets. Strategic planning, in many western companies and not a few governments, was born in a flurry of optimism and industrial growth in the 1960s and early 1970s. Every business aspired to have a strategic planning staff and every business had a planning curriculum. Health care was similarly characterized, whether the evidence is drawn from the Netherlands, the USA or the UK. But, by the 1980s, the fashion had shifted. The new buzzwords were corporate culture, quality and implementation.

The decline of interest in, and commitment to, strategic planning was not based necessarily on some sort of theoretical inadequacy which it might be considered to have, but on its failure to operate in practice. Similarly, in public services, or public industries meeting populations' needs, it became increasingly evident that strategic planning had failed to deliver or meet the claims and expectations held of it. The reasons are many but included the fact that many such plans were constructed outside of the managerial framework necessary to implement them, as well as the lack of financial realism underpinning the plans as the economy became an increasingly difficult place to conduct business in.

To see planning outside the managerial system was to invite a set of plans and actions drafted by staff members, not managers, and ones that were not necessarily owned by those whose efforts were necessary to carry them out. In consequence, planning became increasingly seen as a function of management, with the production of plans as a necessary but not sufficient condition for their implementation.

Planning, therefore, became increasingly seen as a component activity of management, with parallel moves towards financial decentralization. If units were to be given operational control for their production of services or products within the overall company, financial decentralization had to be given to empower staff locally with the flexibility to invest and finance their revenue budgets as required. If every budget were to be functionally ascribed from the top of the company, then decentralization is a myth and the decentralized unit has responsibility but not power. Therefore, flexibility in decisions over finance, over personnel, over product mix and over particular operational systems of control is necessary in order to meet output goals.

Logically, what follows is that financial decentralization is accompanied by decentralization of decision-making about how much labour to employ, what types of labour to employ, and indeed what reward systems to operate. Most typically, such decisions will not be wholly free but within a spine or system of constraints imposed by the company headquarters. Just as national wage bargaining and centralized wage bargaining within firms have fallen into ideological disrepair, centralized decision-making, including decisions about employment and terms and conditions of service within public industries and public services, is also being questioned increasingly.

The theory, in any organization, is that decentralization downwards is accompanied by accountability upwards. As decentralized units may well have targets for performance (based on performance indicators), overall criteria within which they have to manage their resources (systems of resource management or norms for efficiency), and overall norms for achieving planning goals, the question remaining for any one enterprise is how the mix of devolution downwards and accountability upwards works in practice. Is it closet centralism? Or is it a creative relationship, or creative tension, between centralism and devolution?

Part of the answer rests on the extent to which the overall goals of the organization are shared throughout the organization. Not surprisingly, perhaps, public enterprises and public services have followed private corporations in developing and refining mission statements and statements of core values. The objective here is to unify the different labour groups engaged in the design, production and delivery of products into meeting overall company objectives. At the end of the day, in the commercial world, the aim is to improve market share, improve quality, and – through integration of activity – to improve efficiency also. Thus, in the public sector, organizations are seeking to define their mission in terms appropriate for a public sector organization, and with a set of core values that should characterize their approach to their workforce, their customers and to society itself. The extent to which they are successful hinges not a little on there being a shared vision of the future and how they best shape their organization to the challenge and opportunity ahead.

A key element in such an approach is to have regard to the quality of the product (goods or service) produced, as much as to the cost (resources) to be incurred in its production. In the private sector, albeit rather simplistically stated, the firm or corporation's incentives will generally involve the production of maximum profit within given organizational constraints, and given trade-offs, for example, between the short term and long term. A company may seem to maximize net profits by producing a small output of high quality at high prices or, as in mass production, through maximizing quantity given a minimum definition of quality, yet less than in a high-quality market.

Likewise, in the context of a public service or public corporation operating within organizational and budgetary constraints, there may be expectations of a certain quantity to be produced and, likewise, expectations as to quality. It may be that the stated objectives, as to both quantity and quality, are unrealistic. Efficiency improvements will always, albeit with diminishing marginal returns, make the reconciliation of quantity and quality easier, yet there is obviously a limit as to what can be achieved within given resources.

A health service, for example, may have an implicit or explicit obligation to deliver a quantum of services – acute hospital services, mental health services, community services, general practitioner services, and so forth – to a population or a whole country. If the resources within which those services are provided are limited, then there will be corresponding limits on what quality can be produced. Furthermore, by quality, do we mean something intrinsic to the output or outcome – for example, a higher-quality operation leading to greater quality of life or longer life for a patient – or do we mean quality in support services, for example, a pleasant room and good food when one is in hospital?

Historically, all planning activity has tended to concentrate on the quantifiable and, hence, the measurable. Indeed, centralized planning often has to deal with the provision of norms, whether to be obeyed or merely used for guidance, or aspirational purposes, in the provision of services. Decentralization, by contrast, does in theory permit (and encourage) managers to determine their own product mix and therefore implicitly the trade-off between quantity and quality. Naturally, especially in public services, simply to state this is to gloss over the complexity and political difficulty of managing freely, and begs the capacity of present-day management to seize the opportunity of so doing. Management is necessarily the subject of adaptation, compromise, bargaining and reconciliation of conflicting interests but that is not to say that the reconciliation of goals, values and interests is not possible or desirable, or that it is unattainable.

Public sector management and the purchaser–provider relationship

A fundamental institutional change is running through the public sector in western Europe nations, central and eastern Europe and in the Third World, and is reflected in a movement from centrally controlled functional divisions of corporations and organizations to contractual relationships with autonomous agencies. In part it is a debate about what is public and what should be. It is also a debate about how services are provided and managed in the public service itself (Culyer *et al.*, 1990; Ellencweig, 1990; Paton, 1992; Saltman and von Otter, 1992).

In some cases this has resulted in privatization; in others the creation of an agency relationship whereby public bodies purchase or commission from public services (and/or the private sector) given the task of delivering services of various kinds.

The essential aim of creating *management* agencies (e.g. NHS trusts) to replace functional divisions of large *administrative* departments was that greater cost-effectiveness should be achieved in meeting certain goals. If one starts with large,

centrally planned, functionally organized departments there is a tendency to make the work fit the inputs, rather than hiring inputs to do the job. In other words, if one defines cost-effectiveness as achieving a given output or outcome with minimum cost inputs, it is not sensible to start with already determined, centrally ascribed or functionally ascribed inputs. Instead, the argument runs, the virtues of competitive forces ought to inform the purchasing of inputs and the production of services. On the other hand, competitive forces may lead to biases in the type of work attractive to the provider, and these may have to be carefully reconciled with social objectives.

This assumes, of course, a given set of objectives and that these can be translated into outputs or outcomes. If one has a given quantum of inputs (for example, direct labour employed by a department, fixed financial resources and fixed use of these resources, i.e. with little virement between alternative uses), then a definition of cost-effectiveness incorporating the notion of efficiency would argue that the maximum output ought to be achieved from given inputs. However, it seems to make sense that, given that it is up to the policy-makers to take responsibility for the goals, it is then up to the strategic managers to devise the best strategy for meeting those goals efficiently (recognizing that these same strategic managers may well have helped to determine these strategic goals).

The essence of the reform recently promulgated in the NHS, as a result of the White Paper *Working for Patients* (Department of Health, 1989), and the 1990 NHS Act, has as its rationale a split between purchasing and providing in the NHS. By giving responsibility for the purchasing of health care to district health authorities and to fund-holding general practitioners, providers can, it is argued, use greater financial flexibility in tendering for contracts to provide stipulated services (in price, quantity and quality terms). Again, the other side of the coin is that terms and conditions of employees may have thereby to be protected, to prevent competition undermining conditions.

Strategic management by *purchasers* consists in environmental scanning to assess – and predict – need, and of course to make the necessary value judgements, about priorities (of population groups, of services, of conditions) given that needs are always likely to exceed resources available to address them. Strategic management by *providers* consists in transforming their organizations given *their* new environment (which includes *needs* translated into demands by purchasers) to compete against alternative providers for business and on the basis of the superiority of the product. In this new environment, both purchasers and providers have to think strategically, whether through 5-year strategic plans or through the business planning machinery. In consequence, it would be unhelpful to view one party (the provider) operating in a purely passive manner to the explicit requirement of the other party (the purchaser).

According to the theory underpinning the reforms, closer attention than before will be given to the product, the production process, and the issue of what business the NHS is in. A desire to concentrate on *outcomes* – the health status of individuals, groups, classes and the population as a whole – led to the White Paper, *The Health of the Nation* (Department of Health, 1992), which set targets for achieving reductions in mortality and morbidity from specific diseases. The product, therefore, is seen increasingly as 'health gain', not simply health services. The challenge for the future is to ensure that targets are meaningful and ambitious enough to allow significant changes in health outcome across all classes.

The achievement of quantified outcomes is perhaps the touchstone of scientific management. In health care, effective management therefore requires a similar approach in theory, even if the practice is infinitely more complex than in, say, a one-product industry. One means of bringing about better outcomes is by scanning the environment to identify likely trends, alternative possibilities in production methods, and therefore alternative futures, i.e. future outcomes when trends are mediated by appropriate health care interventions. The Department of Health has recently shown interest in established programmes in the Netherlands' Ministry of Welfare, in this regard. Likewise, purchasers are beginning to address the strategic task of assessing needs, involving the public, evaluating the effectiveness of services, and beginning to use purchasing power to change how services are provided. Priority-setting is one of the key challenges for the future in which health authorities are envisaged less as managers of people and resources and more as champions of the people and guiding where resources should go.

Value judgements, here as elsewhere, are important in deciding priorities even when, or if,

trends are known, as the Oregon state experiment to introduce a form of rationing of health care into its Medicaid programme amply illustrated. The QALY (quality adjusted life year), on which the Oregon formula was based, is rapidly becoming the best-known methodology which senior policy-makers and strategic managers use for 'hard choices'. Essentially, the QALY is a composite expression of the longevity of life and the quality of that life likely to be obtained (i.e. benefit received) by a patient (or patient group) from receiving a particular treatment regime. This expression of benefit is then compared to the cost (resources consumed) in so doing, to derive an overall cost – benefit calculation. As such, it is intended to assist decision-makers in determining which treatments are the most effective and give the most value in terms of quality of life. None the less, it is a *tool* which involves *value judgements*, and therefore contains the essential combination of science and art which defines strategic management.

The territory of management reviewed

This final section of the chapter seeks to draw together some of the threads of the argument advanced so far, and offers some indicators on challenges facing health care management in the future. In the first place, the point has already been made that there has been an irreversible trend away from administration and towards management; indeed, this has been an international one. Titles such as Peters' *Thriving on Chaos* (1988) and Handy's *The Age of Unreason* (1989) imply that challenges facing both private business and public management are to do with managing change in conditions of uncertainty rather than administrating familiar structures in conditions of stability. As with all detected trends, there may be hype as well as insight here. Nevertheless, whether such a prophecy is self-fulfilling or not in all its detail, there is no doubt that public managers are facing ever more demanding jobs.

Perhaps the single most important change has been the move to 'manager as a guarantor of outputs and outcomes' rather than 'administrator as a mediator in inputs and processes'. One unintended consequence, perhaps, is that of manager as scapegoat (Harrison, 1989). In any centralized political system such as that in the UK, and in publicly controlled enterprises, the political imperative drives hoped-for policy outcomes, and it is then up to managers to deliver them.

Secondly, when the achievement of policy is even partly a political imperative (such as allowing the NHS to survive without significant increases in finance), then managers will often find that they are carrying a heavy responsibility for achieving much within finite resources. And, indeed, much of the emphasis on good management today is, in effect, an emphasis upon good husbanding of resources, i.e. 'coming in on the bottom line'. This is not only a British phenomenon: in the USA, managers of both public and private programmes are finding the exigencies of cost control to be their most pressing problem. The conclusion is that the health sector is under the most pressing of economic problems, ever-increasing needs and a lowering in propensity to pay from the public purse.

Thirdly, managers in the public sector are finding that the emphasis on results, specifically interpreted in terms of cost-effectiveness, cost efficiency, and cost minimization, is leading increasingly to a separation of the roles of the provider and the purchaser. Increasingly, the budget holder for a particular government programme is responsible for producing a product and for contracting for the inputs geared to producing that output. That is, a process of competitive tendering in order to maximize efficiency has both nationally and internationally become the characteristic of the age.

Thus, in the USA, budget holders and managers of government programmes such as Medicare and Medicaid, the health programmes for the elderly and poor respectively, find themselves charged with the responsibility of 'shopping around' in the market place of provision to ensure that government money buys the most economical deal for the programme's clients. In the UK, the essence of the NHS and Community Care Act of 1990 is to separate the commissioning for health care and certain community services (carried out by a purchaser, still the state acting on behalf of its people) from the provision of health care, in order to attempt to institute a process of competitive tendering for services to achieve efficiency in provision. In New Zealand, health boards constituted in line with the principles of general management British-style are being charged with a similar responsibility to health authorities in the UK.

Thus, fourthly, although at the risk of over-generalization either across all different policy areas or across all nations, there are significant trends throughout the world towards this approach of a managerial imperative. Even in the former communist countries of central and eastern Europe, the concept of the market place, with a unified purchaser acting on behalf of the public, contracting with competing suppliers, is becoming dominant in the provision of goods such as health care which have traditionally been provided through social administration. Public service has typically presumed that improvements are generated through good will, formal control and clear thinking. Management, almost by definition, was therefore less relevant in the past. The last decade has witnessed, in that sense, the most critical examination of the assumptions underlying public service and the motivation of those who work in it.

Fifthly, could competition between providers and the clear separation of the purchasing function from the provider function provide the answer? The theory (and ideology) underpinning these moves derives from a belief in competitive forces and also a belief in decentralized budgeting to achieve efficiency and to improve incentives to provide. What is the main argument against such moves? A major problem in a number of areas has been the limited existing and potential supply in provider markets. How can hospitals compete to offer care if there is no surplus capacity? How can schools compete if they cannot expand and contract freely; likewise, hospitals? Often, government regulation prohibits fully free markets, or rather markets as free as possible. Market failures often prevent the operation of effective provider markets. Not surprisingly, the term managed competition is used to imply that adjustments will be made to the free flow of market forces. As is well-recognized, the assumptions and conditions of the perfectly competitive model do not hold, and even if they did, the result, though technically elegant, might not be acceptable (Lee, 1991).

The theory of public management, associated with the trend towards strategic management, tends to be one which identifies top-down responsibility for the making of policy and bottom-up responsibility for implementation, or at least decentralized responsibility for implementation – local freedom but within strict limits and along strict lines. It should be pointed out that this type of approach has implications for democratic theory. There has grown up a conventional wisdom that the 1970s in the UK were characterized by what was known as corporatism. At its most general (and often pejorative), corporatism implied the smoke-filled room whereby representatives of the strong institutions, in dealing with controversy, got around a table and hammered out some sort of compromise, yet it at least allowed for pluralist representation.

So, what of the future? Almost irrespective of the country setting and of the ideology of its chosen government of the day, all health care systems will be under the closest scrutiny in respect of their managerial capacity to deliver high-quality services in an efficient and effective manner. At the same time, the very infinity of health needs and the finite resources that can be brought to bear upon those needs suggests strongly that management systems in general and managers in particular will increasingly be expected to deliver the impossible, especially in the public sector – health for all, but with limited and (possibly) shrinking resources.

To prevent this happening, much will depend on how needs are articulated, by whom, and whether or not priorities are expressed in resource terms and, if so, by whom. In the private sector, the invisible hand of the market allocates (and rations) resources according to ability and willingness to pay; in the public sector, the allocation (and rationing) process has been neither so explicit nor automatic.

In the future, the vocabulary is one seemingly of explicitness: in management structure and processes; in management roles and responsibilities; in management information systems and performance measurement. The attempt at separation of policy from management at the central level in the NHS, and that of commissioning from providing services at the local level, will clearly bring new challenges and opportunities. The articulation of government policy through national health policy documents, as has been seen in the Netherlands, Sweden and the UK in recent times, does set the strategic context for the management of the public health industry that has not always been noticeable before. Yet, such initiatives are now required to be matched at the local level; however, as the policy becomes more focused on local communities, the choices do inevitably become more stark and decisions increasingly uncomfortable to take.

Be that as it may, devolution of the delivery of services to local units, e.g. trusts, and the move to try to establish clear lines of accountability

provides both a *challenge* and a *concern* to managers of what are undoubtedly highly complex organizations.

The *challenge* towards the year 2000, for constructive and progressive health service management, is for management to harness an *advocacy* role with its purchasers (government and its nominees); a leadership role with its staff; and, a proactive role with its customers (the population it serves).

The need is also for management to be aware of, and *concerned with*, different ideologies, possibly different forms of political structure in the future, and different interest and pressure groups that will continue to play a part in shaping health policy – as much as does the availability of financial resources, technological developments and wider social and economic factors. In consequence, both shaping the implementation of health policy and questioning it where necessary are constructive responsibilities for management, but not theirs alone.

It might be appropriate then not to look for either politics or management in health care, but for a synthesis of the two. Any conceivable variant of management will not of itself produce health, but any weakness on its part will seriously endanger the capacity of health services to deliver. 'Better management, better health' has become something of a cliché; none the less, one does recognize management when one sees it and one does suffer when it is absent.

References

Argenti J. (1980) *Practical Corporate Planning.* Allen & Unwin, London.

Culyer A.J. *et al.* (1990) *Competition in Health Care.* Macmillan, London.

Department of Health (1989) *Working for Patients.* NHS White Paper. Department of Health, London.

Department of Health (1992) *The Health of the Nation.* Department of Health, London.

Ellencweig A.Y. (1990) *Analysing Health Systems.* Oxford University Press, Oxford.

Gomez P. and Probst G.S.B. (1987) *Thinking in Networks for Management: An Integrated Problem-Solving Methodology.* International Management Institute, Geneva.

Griffiths, R. (1983) *The NHS Management Enquiry.* Department of Health and Social Security, London.

Handy C. (1989) *The Age of Unreason*. Business Books, London.

Harrison S. (1989) *Managing the National Health Service*. Chapman and Hall, London.

Ibbs R. (1988) *The Next Steps*. The Ibbs Report. HMSO, London.

Lee K. (1979) Health care: planning, policies, and incentives. *Futures* **11** 482–490.

Lee K. and Mills A. (1982) *Policy-making and Planning in the Health Sector*. Croom Helm, London.

Lee K. (1991) Competition versus planning in health care: implications for corporate and individual incentives, efficiency and control. *Australian Health Review* **14**, 9–34.

Paton C.R. (1992) *Competition and Planning in the NHS: The Danger of Unplanned Markets*. Chapman and Hall, London.

Peters T. (1988) *Thriving on Chaos. Handbook for a Management Revolution*. Macmillan, London.

Saltman R.B. and von Otter C. (1992) *Planned Markets and Public Competition*. Open University Press, Buckingham.

Sampson A. (1983) *The Changing Anatomy of Britain*. Coronet, London.

Section 3

Management of the NHS

3.1 NHS management structures before Griffiths

3.1(a) Hospital management committees and consensus management, 1948–1984

Brian Edwards

The early years of the NHS

The NHS, created on 1 April 1948, was the product of nearly 50 years of debate and argument about the formation of a unified network of health services in the UK. The voluntary hospitals sectors' financial difficulties in the interwar years created some of the pressure for change, as did the experience of the Unified Emergency Medical Service between 1935 and 1945. But perhaps the most powerful force of all was the mood of the nation at the time as it fought and emerged from the Second World War and began the search for a better, more caring world.

When Nye Bevan became Minister of Health in 1945 he inherited a set of proposals from his predecessors that had been so compromised in the negotiations with all the vested interests that he judged them to be unworkable. He produced his own White Paper in 1946 which committed the government to a free and comprehensive health service and went on to propose the nationalization of all hospitals in order to create a truly national service. Bevan's plan met with furious opposition from the British Medical Association, who were worried about the dangers of state control of medicine and of an enforced salaried service for general practitioners. The voluntary hospitals did need a financial rescue plan but worked to retain their independence. Local government wanted to run the NHS by simply absorbing the voluntary hospitals. As we now know, Bevan won the day and the NHS Act was passed into law in 1946 with an implementation date of 5 July 1948.

The principles upon which it was founded were as follows:

1 A health service financed by general taxation and contributions paid when people are well.
2 A national service in the sense that the same high quality of service, but not a standardized service, should be provided in every part of the country.
3 The service should secure full clinical freedom for the doctors working in it.
4 A service centred on the family doctor team.

The organizational structure was formed in three branches (tripartite) (Fig. 3.1.1).

The regional hospital boards, boards of governors, hospital management committees and executive councils each had lay members appointed for a 3-year term, including representatives from

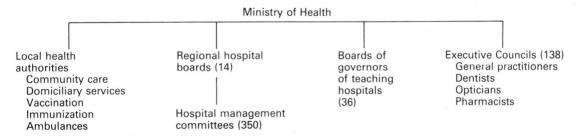

Fig. 3.1.1 Structure of the NHS when it was established in 1948.

the professions. Local health authorities were part of local government. Each board had its own chief officers and worked through a system of subcommittees, which was the principal method of decision-making.

General practitioners retained their independent status and contracted their services to executive councils (who also contracted for the services of chemists, opticians and dentists).

Almost as soon as the new service started, it ran into financial difficulties. By the end of 1948, 40 million people had registered with a general practitioner and doctors were reporting a marked increase in the demand for their services. Many more patients were referred to hospital outpatient departments. Opticians and dentists were almost overwhelmed by patients asking for dentures and spectacles. Perhaps not surprisingly, the first year of operation produced a 35% overspend against target. In the second year, the anticipated budget of £228 million turned out to be £305 million. There was inevitably a major political row, with Winston Churchill (then leader of the opposition) accusing the government of 'wild miscalculation' and 'grave carelessness'.

The government intervened by imposing a ceiling on expenditure (£352 million for 1951–1952) and introducing charges for spectacles, dentures, dental treatment and drugs. The forerunner to the cash limit had arrived with a vengeance.

A committee of inquiry chaired by C. W. Guillebaud was appointed in 1953. When it reported 3 years later, they assessed that the NHS had not been extravagant. Indeed, as a proportion of gross national product, expenditure had actually reduced from 3.75% in 1949 to 3.25% in 1953–1954. The early estimates of the cost of the NHS had clearly been too low.

Underlying the financial debates was a crucial misreading of the economics of health care. It was argued by many at that time that better health services would result in improved overall health in the community, reduce sickness absence from work and, after an initial rise, expenditure would be self-limiting. We now understand that demand for health care has few practical boundaries and the connection between the overall health of the community and day-to-day work of the NHS is often quite tenuous.

The new NHS also included a system of national pay bargaining undertaken through the mechanism of joint management and trade union committees called Whitley. This was of particular value to nursing and ancillary staff from the voluntary hospital sector who had generally had less favourable terms and conditions than their colleagues in local authority hospitals. In practice, the British Medical Association bypassed Whitley and negotiated directly with the Ministry of Health.

Hospital doctors have always had a system of distinction awards. The awards are made at four levels (C, B, A and A+). A top award (A+) can almost double the base salary. Despite criticism over the years, the system has survived. The Royal Commission on doctors' and dentists' pay reported in 1960: 'We consider the awards system is a practical and imaginative way of securing a reasonable differentiation of income and providing relatively high earnings for a significant minority'. About half of all consultants receive some level of award during their careers.

By 1960, expenditure on the NHS was 30% greater in real terms than in 1949, although it represented a slightly lower proportion of gross national product. Hospital activity had however risen sharply: inpatients treated rose from 2.9 million to 4.1 million; over the same 10-year period, outpatients rose from 36.1 million to 41.7 million.

The earlier years of the service also produced significant shifts in the shape of general practice. At the start of the service, about half of all general practitioners worked on their own, but by 1960 the proportion of general practitioners in partnerships of three and more had risen to 35%. The health centre development programme that was designed to bring together under one roof general practitioners and other community-centred health professionals moved ahead much more slowly. There were still enormous geographical imbalances in service and the best-provided regions in the country were still receiving nearly twice as much per head of population as the poorest regions.

The number of doctors working in the NHS had been a controversial matter for some years. The number of hospital doctors more than doubled between 1949 and 1974 but the growth in general practice (36%) was more modest. The profession had consistently taken the view that too many were being trained, and this view was confirmed by a committee appointed by the government in 1955, who recommended a 10% reduction in the number of medical students. With the benefit of hindsight, we now know that they misjudged the levels of emigration and the UK became heavily dependent on immigrant doctors in the late 1960s and 1970s. The Todd Report in 1968 recommended an increase in the number of medical students and during the next 10 years, a series of new medical schools was created. The Royal Commission on the NHS, reporting in 1979, concluded that the level of investment at that time was about right at 4000 new students per annum.

As Britain's economy improved throughout the 1960s, the NHS got a higher rate of development and services began to expand quite quickly. In 1962 Enoch Powell published his *Hospital Plan*, which was designed to improve Britain's ageing and dilapidated stock of hospital buildings, 45% of which were by that time more than 70 years old. Bed provision for the acute sector was set at 4 per 1000 population and capital investment did, for a short time, increase. In 1969 the Bonham Carter Report had expanded the idea of the district general hospital, capable of providing comprehensive care to a defined community. In a related series of ministerial initiatives, local authorities and health authorities were asked to produce 10-year development plans, which they did in a mood of considerable optimism.

Outside the hospital sector, the services provided by local authorities and those provided by general practitioners had been growing steadily together. Many medical officers of health had by this time seen the value of developing a more integrated primary care team, and even where there was no health centre development they began to attach the nursing and health visiting staff to general practices. This would eventually blossom into the concept of the primary health care team, led by the general practitioner.

In 1965, the GPs' charter, as it became known, radically changed the method of remuneration for general practitioners and introduced the General Practice Finance Corporation which made loans to general practitioners who were buying, building or improving their premises. There were also new financial incentives for doctors working in unattractive areas and for those working in group practice. During this period the number of health centres climbed to 523 in 1973, by which time about one doctor in seven worked from a health centre.

Maternity services had changed to the point where, by 1974, 90% of all deliveries took place in hospital (66% in 1960). This led to the closure of many small maternity units, usually after a furious public row.

Mental health services were also changing as new drugs made it easier to control and relieve symptoms. A major piece of legislation in 1959, The Mental Health Act, reduced sharply the number of patients admitted on a legal order. From that date, local magistrates played no part in compulsory admissions. Responsibility for these decisions was now placed firmly on the shoulders of doctors and social workers. The number of inpatient residents in the large mental illness hospitals had by 1974 fallen by nearly a third from the levels that existed in 1948. Lengths of stay had shortened dramatically – over 50% of patients were admitted for less than a month.

The crude death rate had hardly shifted between 1938 (the last full year of peace) and the early 1970s, and was stuck at around 11.6. But there had been a dramatic drop in infant deaths from 53 per 1000 in 1938 to 17 per 1000 in the early 1970s (in contrast, by this time Sweden had got its rate down to 11 per 1000). Tuberculosis had been largely defeated, producing large numbers of empty hospital beds in the old tuberculosis sanatoria (many of which were converted for use by the elderly) and the hospital service was beginning to reap the benefits of new technologies.

The management approach of the first 25 years was public administration in old style, using a network, sometimes a myriad, of standing and *ad hoc* committees of the statutory authorities. Even very small financial commitments required committee approval, as did new staff posts. The bureaucracy and delay were a regular source of irritation and criticism. A leader in the *Lancet* in 1959 captured the picture: 'we are certainly right in preferring the committee system to authoritarian rule, but the health service is only one of many organs whose efficiency is impaired by having too many committees with too many members'.

At the hospital level, a series of reports had developed the notion of tripartite management: a 'blended team' of doctor, nurse and administrator, 'each one supreme in his or her own sphere'. This fitted comfortably with traditional professional territories and was the usual system found in the voluntary hospital sector before the NHS. It worked quite well in practice. The medical superintendent (which had been the model commonly found in the pre-NHS municipal hospital service) had gradually disappeared in England, although it remained in Scotland for longer.

In what was regarded at the time as very radical, a King's Fund Working Party proposed in 1967 a new structure for the *Management of Hospitals in 1980*.

1 A clear administrative chain of command.
2 A reduction in the number of committees.
3 A positive link between the district hospital and community services.
4 The appointment of a general manager who should be a member of the board.
5 The appointment of a medical director.

The King's Fund Report was not welcomed by the professions. In the event, not a great deal changed, despite regular attempts by the Ministry of Health to clamp down on the inexorable growth of the committee structures. Real change had to wait until the 1974 reorganization.

The late 1960s and early part of the 1970s was a ferment of ideas and proposals for structural change in the NHS. Most had one dominating theme – that of integrating and unifying the tripartite structure.

When the government did finally make up its mind to go for integration into all-purpose area health authorities there was little resistance: it felt right, it had a natural and inexorable logic to it and the service was ready for change.

The 1974 reorganization and the Grey Book

As the health service grew in size and complexity, it became increasingly clear that the most sensible way forward lay in trying to integrate its various component parts into a more unified structure. Managing the boundaries between hospital and community care was becoming increasingly important, particularly in specialties like paediatrics, psychiatry and care of the elderly. In the period between 1962 and 1973, a series of proposals emerged for creating unified authorities which would be accountable for the totality of health services within a given geographical locality. These ideas led eventually to legislation and on 1 April 1974, 700 different authorities were swept away and replaced by 90 area health authorities which, within their localities, managed the community health services, the hospitals, the ambulance services, as well as holding the contracts of general practitioners, opticians, dentists and chemists.

The Grey Book

As the implementation date of the 1974 reorganization approached, the Department of Health turned its attention to the internal management arrangements of the new area health authorities. A large multidisciplinary steering group was created, chaired by the then Permanent Secretary, Sir Philip Rogers. Their report which was published in 1972 came to be known as the Grey Book. The Secretary to the Group was Eric Caines, who some years later became the Director of Personnel for the NHS. The report represented an amazingly detailed prescription for the management of the NHS. The role of members, membership of planning teams, the organization of nursing, works, pharmacy, speech therapy, supplies, catering and primary care services all got a mention. It dealt with the allocation of responsibility between levels, problems of overlap and specified roles for everybody involved in the new management teams.

The statutory framework was a network of 90 area health authorities (including some teaching area health authorities) which were all accountable to 14 regional health authorities, which in turn reported to the Department of Health. The area health authorities were geographically coterminous with local government counties, metropolitan districts and London boroughs. Each area health authority was required to set up a family practitioner committee to administer the contracts of practitioners within its boundaries. In most area health authorities provision was made for another tier of management – local district management teams, which were accountable directly to the authority. So, for example, Cheshire area health authority functioned with an area tier (with its own team of officers) and five operational districts in Chester, Crewe, Macclesfield, Warrington and Halton (each with its own team of officers). Leeds area health authority had two districts, Leeds East and Leeds West. Others like Doncaster had no district management teams at all and managed with a single area organization.

Community health councils were established to represent the views of the public to the area health authorities with a member drawn from each of three constituencies of interest: local authorities, voluntary organizations and regional health authorities.

The Grey Book rejected the notion of chief executives as inappropriate to a complex organization like the NHS. Instead they recommended multidisciplinary management teams at regional, area and district levels.

These ideas were certainly in tune with the overall theme of the 1974 reorganization, which was integration. The provision of health care on the ground was often a team activity and the same was said to apply to management.

The precise membership of the teams varied between the organizational levels (Fig. 3.1.2) but the principles were common to all.

1 The national organizational prescription was to apply everywhere in the NHS.
2 The teams were consensus bodies, that is, decisions needed the agreement of all members.
3 Each team had a chairperson who was either appointed by the authority or, more usually, elected by the team and then approved by the authority.

4 If a team could not agree on an important matter, it was referred to the authority for a decision.
5 District management teams, the operational arm of the authority, were accountable directly to the authority and not to the authority's chief officers (the area team).

The statutory health authorities themselves at regional and area levels had lay members appointed either by the Secretary of State or the regional health authority. Their role was described as one of critical policy-making, planning and resource allocation. They were strongly encouraged to delegate operational decisions to their team of officers.

The Grey Book also described a new planning system for the NHS with an annual cycle that was focused primarily on the district.

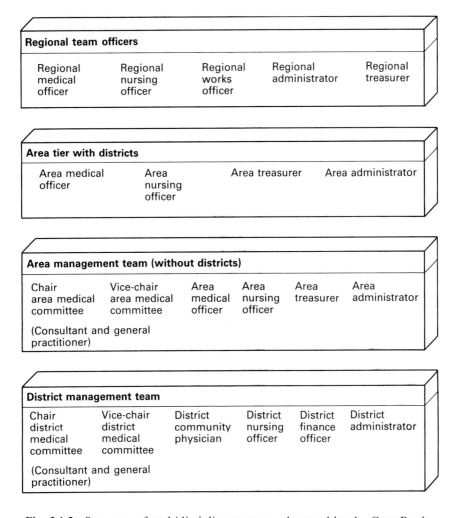

Fig. 3.1.2 Structure of multidisciplinary teams advocated by the Grey Book.

The District is the lowest level at which it will be possible to make a comprehensive assessment of the health needs of the community and to plan and deploy the broad range of health services required to meet their needs and it will be at District level that clinicians will be directly involved in the planning process.

The 'ideal' district had a population of around 250 000. One of the most attractive new ideas was the creation of health care planning teams (for services such as for children or the elderly) which drew managers and professionals together in reviewing existing services and charting a way forward.

The professionals were well-represented all round in the new organization. Doctors and nurses had established seats on management and planning teams, as well as being represented amongst the members of the statutory authorities. There were statutory medical and nursing advisory committees at regional and area levels and, in order to bring primary and secondary care together locally, new district medical committees were established with general practitioners, consultants and doctors in community medicine as members. The chair and vice-chair of the district medical committee automatically became members of the district management team.

Executive councils, which had held the contracts of general practitioners, dentists, opticians and chemists since 1948, had been abolished and each area health authority was required to appoint a family practitioner committee in its place. The chief administrator to the family practitioner committee was accountable to the area administrator. The contractor professions retained their dominant role amongst the membership of the new family practitioner committees.

The White Paper itself was reasonably well-received within the NHS but soon ran into serious difficulties. The prime problems were:

1 The sheer complexity of the new arrangements.
2 The tension between area teams and district teams as they struggled with their complementary roles.
3 The movement of talented staff up the organization to district and area left the units with junior and relatively inexperienced staff. This was at a time of particular pressure on hospital managers, coping with a difficult industrial relations climate. They also had to cope with a growing battery of functional managers operating at tiers above them (district catering managers, works officers, domestic managers, district heads of paramedical services, district pharmacists, etc.).
4 Members of health authorities were often not content with a strategic role and wanted some oversight of often quite important and controversial operational decisions (e.g. closure of beds) which were being made in their name by teams of officers.
5 There were some highly publicized rows amongst management teams where consensus was impossible.

Despite their heavy involvement, the doctors became increasingly dissatisfied with the new arrangements and began to complain vigorously about slow decision-making, bureaucracy and administrative overheads. These pressures, perhaps more than any other, led first to the removal of the area tier of management in 1982 (Patients First), and eventually to the Griffiths Review and the introduction of general management.

But any judgement about this period in the history of the NHS should not be wholly negative. It sensitized the professionals to managerial processes; it brought general practitioner influence to bear on the management of hospitals, it introduced new thinking about comprehensive planning of services for defined communities. The NHS continued to develop – as it did, the managerial challenge grew more demanding. The Prime Minister appointed Roy Griffiths and the NHS waited for him to report.

3.1(b) Introduction to general management

Roy Griffiths

The year 1982 saw the NHS once more subject to intensive attack. There were many questions in Parliament as to its efficiency. NHS staff numbers had increased by 30% over the past decade with higher rises in all departments, with the exception of ancillary staff, whose numbers had been contained by a series of questionable productivity deals. Government spending on the NHS over the same 10 years had risen in real terms by over 28%, despite a substantial reduction in the number of beds and an increase of only 27% in patient cases. The problems had been intensified by two major industrial relations disputes within the previous 3 years.

The background to the questioning was an increasingly hostile attitude towards the whole of the public sector, not simply the nationalized industries – in short a basic questioning as to whether the public sector *per se* was capable of performing at a sufficiently high level. The consequence was that many senior politicians were examining the case for replacing the NHS with a mixed system of public and private insurance.

All this was not surprising. The thrust of the Thatcher government – indeed some of the factors which brought the government to power in the first place – was to question whether there was sufficient motivation in the public sector towards adequate performance. The NHS was increasingly regarded as centred round the professions, with inadequate regard either to the community as a whole, or to the patients as individual consumers and with no overall accountability for performance. The administration, whose numbers had increased by over 50% in the past 10 years, came in for particular censure as being overweight, slow in response and tardy in action, given to the essence of bureaucracy to ensure that everything was done according to the rules and regulations and quite alien to the concept of management in the private sector, the essence of which is to look constantly for improvement in the care of those using the service.

The response of the Secretary of State, Norman Fowler, was to ask Roy Griffiths, Managing Director of the retail chain, Sainsbury's, to head a team of four businessmen, all with experience of large-scale organization, to give advice on the effective use and management of staff and related resources in the NHS. Whilst the remit as originally discussed was to look at staffing levels, since this had been the focus of much of the attacks, it was quickly pointed out that if the use of human resources was ineffective then the problem was one of overall management. There was some initial scepticism as to the appointment, largely because of the election which was in the offing and it might have been thought a move to defuse the problems of the NHS until a later date. The team were not initially asked to provide a report but simply to advise, but it was only when the level of decibels reached a level unusual even for the NHS that the Prime Minister asked for a report to be written. There had been from the outset a constant reiteration by critics that business methods were alien to the NHS and consequently there were considerable reservations as to the whole exercise. Since all the members of the team were still employed full-time in their private sector activities, the methods of working were quite unlike that of a Royal Commission – formal evidence was not taken, management consultants were not used and there were no major background papers called for.

On the other hand there had been almost endless papers written previously on questions of organization and indeed an enormous number of initiatives had been established. Estate management was being examined. Scrutinies under the aegis of Sir Derek Rayner had covered *inter alia* catering and use of nursing accommodation. There had been some attempt to set targets for staffing levels and there had been much activity by the Körner committee to establish statistics and performance indicators. It was almost immediately clear to the members of the team that the great problem was how to translate the fragmented aspects of this work and indeed of overall policy into effective action. The team in its approach was extremely careful not to use the language of business; nor was it fortified by any belief that it was possible to translate wholesale solutions from the private sector to the NHS. Nevertheless, it could and did place across the NHS certain templates giving rise to some simple analyses of effectiveness. First, how well was the NHS looking after its patients, its staff, the community and the taxpayer? Second, what were the strategies and priorities of the NHS and how effectively were these taken through the stages of planning, implementation and monitoring? Third, how did it assess the quality of the work done and the efficiency with which it was carried out, and how well were staff motivated, not only towards quality and efficiency, but also to taking on board any major changes?

The team eventually accepted the more difficult remit of writing a short report and this proved to have its advantages. It meant that the recommendations had to be distilled to those importantly necessary and the report had to be written in a style which would command attention. Essentially the report pinpointed the main faults of the present system. Consensus management meant that there was no one with personal responsibility for ensuring that at each level all the resources of the NHS were being effectively mobilized in support of the professionals immediately providing the care. Decision-taking was slow and, worse, many important areas where improvement might be achieved were being ignored. The absence of any overall general management function was distilled into the subsequently much-quoted comment, 'If Florence Nightingale was carrying her lamp through the corridors of the NHS today she would almost certainly be searching for the people in charge'.

The team felt that much greater efficiency savings could be made and could be sustained, with the result of providing more resources for the direct care of patients. Many problems could be resolved by involving professionals more closely in management, particularly the medical profession, whose decisions about individual treatment actually dictated the use of resources. The main recommendations for action involved the centre, the setting up of an NHS supervisory board and a management board. The role of the supervisory board was to strengthen existing arrangements for determining policy for the NHS; strategic decisions; approval of overall budget and resource allocation; and receiving reports on performance. The recommendation was that, in addition to the Secretary of State

and the ministers and senior permanent officials, it should include a chairperson of the NHS management board and two or three non-executive members with general management skills and experience.

The role of the management board would be to plan implementation of the policies approved by the supervisory board; to give leadership to the management of the NHS and to control performance. It was felt that in order to provide the necessary catalyst to effective action, some members of the management executive should come from outside the NHS and the civil service, so that the necessary expertise in introducing effective change might be achieved. At regional and district level the accountability was to be strengthened, particularly by the identification of a general manager charged with overall responsibility for management performance. At unit level the same approach was recommended, and particularly the involvement of clinicians in decisions about priorities in the use of resources. The essence of these recommendations at unit level, in particular hospital level, was to ensure that there were clear responsibilities, strengthened accountability and structures and budgets which would enable improvements in quality and efficiency. There were separate recommendations on the importance of the personnel function, long neglected in the NHS, and also for a major reorientation in the handling of the NHS estate to ensure that procedures for handling major capital schemes were streamlined and speeded up and the whole function given a more purposeful approach. There was a key recommendation that the chairperson of the NHS management board should undertake a general review of levels of decision-taking in the NHS.

Much of the background for the recommendations is probably best illustrated by extracts from the report, as follows (Griffiths, 1983):

> One important prelude to the recommendations: we believe that a small, strong general management body is necessary at the centre (and that is almost all that is necessary at the centre for the management of the NHS) to ensure that responsibility is pushed as far down the line as possible, i.e. to the point where action can be taken effectively. At present devolution of responsibility is far too slow because the necessary direction and dynamic to achieve this is currently lacking.
>
> The Management Board and Chairmen should ensure that it is central to the approach of

management in planning and delivering services for the population as a whole, to:-

- ascertain how well the service is being delivered at local level by obtaining the experience and perceptions of patients and the community: these can be derived from CHCs and by other methods, including market research and from the experience of general practice and the community health services.
- Promote realistic public and professional perceptions of what the NHS can and should provide as the best possible service within the resources available.

The clear similarities between NHS management and business management are much more important. In many organisations in the private sector, profit does not immediately impinge on large numbers of managers below Board level. They are concerned with levels of service, quality of product, meeting budgets, cost improvement, productivity, motivating and rewarding staff, research and development, and the long term viability of the undertaking. All things that Parliament is urging on the NHS.

The NHS does not have the profit motive, but it is, of course, enormously concerned with control of expenditure. Surprisingly, however, it still lacks any real continuous evaluation of its performance against criteria such as those set out above. Rarely are precise management objectives set; there is little measurement of health output; clinical evaluation of particular practices is by no means common and economic evaluation of those practices extremely rare. Nor can the NHS display a ready assessment of the effectiveness with which it is meeting the needs and expectations of the people it serves.

Above all, of course, lack of a general management process means that it is extremely difficult to achieve change. To the outsider it appears that when change of any kind is required, the NHS is so structured as to resemble a 'mobile': designed to move with any breath of air, but which in fact never changes its position and gives no clear indication of direction.

A general management process would be enormously important in:

(i) providing the necessary leadership to capialize on the existing high levels of dedication and expertise among NHS staff of all disciplines, and to stimulate initiative, urgency and vitality.

(ii) Securing proper motivation of staff. those charged with the general management re-

sponsibility would regard it as vital to review incentives, rewards and sanctions.

It is not for the centre to engage in the day-to-day management of the NHS. It must make sure that the statutorily appointed Authorities do so effectively in accordance with the requirements of Government and Parliament. Sufficient management impression must be created at all levels that the centre is passionately concerned with the quality of care and delivery of services at local level. As a coherent management process is developed, of planning, implementation and control, the DHSS should rigorously prune many of its existing activities.

To effect change some outside catalysts will be required; but there are enough people at all levels within the NHS enthusiastically committed to wanting change and capable of making a contribution to ensure that it can largely be effected from within.

The team's objectives in making the recommendations were against their background in the private sector, geared so as to be in their opinion capable of implementation.

The government accepted the report in principle immediately, subject to appropriate consultation and gave the formal approval for implementation in June 1984. Inevitably the report did not find immediate favour with the professions. The doctors for the most part uneasily felt that linking the question of clinical care and management struck at the basic concordat between government and the professions, i.e. that if the government provided reasonable funding then the doctors would be free to set priorities and take clinical decisions within the confines of the money so provided. The nurses in particular were hostile, feeling that to mention care and money in the same breath was in fact wrong. Substantively they realized that the strengthening of the management function and some of the specific recommendations would militate against the career ladders which had been established, particularly by the earlier Salmon report. Some nurses took advantage however of the exciting career opportunities which were provided within general management and saw that the report gave them a much greater opportunity than previously to contribute to the overall running of the NHS.

Acceptance by the government of the report was one thing but to implement it was quite another. The first problem was how to effect the necessary changes. The report contained a fundamentally different philosophy of running the NHS and this needed to be explained throughout the service with the appropriate reassurances both to the public and to the staff. General managers were appointed at regional, district and unit levels, accountable for the total performance. Work on management and budgetary systems was set in train. There was a limited introduction of performance-related pay and individual performance review, all geared towards higher achievement and the search for improvement. The authorities took advantage of the recommendation that they be given greater freedom to organize as they wished, by, e.g., appointing senior managers to take specific responsibility for quality assurance and quality control. A heavy emphasis was given to training as part of the overall drive to manage people more effectively within the NHS. The report's recommendation was followed that the Whitley council system for establishing pay and conditions of service at a national level should be reviewed to ensure greater devolution. Implementation was making progress in the right direction, but was a hazardous exercise. Managers were having to learn how to effect change at the same time as implementing the proposals. The need for, above all, effective communication and motivation of staff was appreciated in concept but not in the enormity of the task to be undertaken. The professional bodies showed themselves in the early stages to be much more effective in putting across their own message to staff than did the NHS itself.

In the absence of such communication the managers were in danger of becoming a separate estate of the NHS realm. This was quite contrary to the intention of the business team, whose main objective was to suffuse the whole of the NHS with an effective management process. One of the other outstanding problems was that the recommendations for change at the centre had been accepted intellectually but without real commitment. In particular, the orderly process of determining priorities and bringing policy documents and effective indicators of overall NHS performance to a supervisory board was not fully understood, or at least not carried out. Importantly, the substantive work of organization and job analysis to enable effective devolution from the centre to appropriate levels within the NHS was not implemented. Substantive progress, however, was made. There were enough catalysts within the NHS itself to understand and to move the NHS in the new directions. There were enough initiatives and interest in quality and performance to evidence a whole new approach and, with the greater clarity of responsibilities, certainly many of the managers felt newly liberated.

The great problem with the process of change was to get an understanding that it is a long process and could not be confined within the electoral cycle. At the same time the changes were being introduced when the pressures on funding were considerable, not least because of the advances in medicine. Arguments as to funding reached new heights and resulted in the Presidents of the Royal Colleges presenting a strongly worded protest to Downing Street. The Prime Minister's response was to announce that she was setting up her own review of the NHS.

3.2 The role of doctors in policy-making

Cyril Chantler

Introduction

Overall policy for the NHS is determined by government. This is bound to be the case because the health care of the nation is an important responsibility of government. Benjamin Disraeli stated in 1872 in a speech in Manchester that the first responsibility of a minister was for the health of the people.

As long as health care is provided by an NHS substantially funded by general taxation, so the funding of the service remains the responsibility of government under the political process. We may wish to separate the NHS from politics but this is unrealistic, for ministers have to reflect on political debate and then make decisions, often difficult, concerning the allocation of resources to different national priorities for which they are accountable to parliament, not to doctors. None the less, doctors and indeed other professionals have a contribution to make in providing professional advice at all levels in the NHS and it is important that this advice is effective.

The relationship between politicians and managers on the one hand and the profession on the other has become strained over the last decade. In spite of ever-increasing resources devoted to the NHS and a steady increase in the proportion of gross domestic product allocated to it, the gap between what professionals wish to spend and what government is prepared to provide has widened as medical technology has developed and the number of people requiring health care has increased with an ageing population. Previously it was as though the politicians and managers provided resources and the professionals spent them with only muted criticism of each other. As professionals have become increasingly strident in their criticism of politicians, so politicians have begun to question whether the professional's right to determine expenditure should go unchallenged. These arguments culminated in a review by Mrs Thatcher and her government which did not involve formal consultation with the profession and the implementation of the proposals led to further conflict.

Society no longer accords total respect for a professional opinion; Schon (1991) has noted that this phenomenon applies to other professional groups, not just doctors, and has suggested that the old contract whereby infinite respect was accorded in return for infinite wisdom has been broken, not least because the infinite wisdom has been shown to be flawed. Doctors too often have been thought to be arguing from a narrow professional interest, or even self-interest, rather than from a disinterested position. Discussions about the organization of the NHS have concentrated on the adequacy of funding rather than confronting the real dilemma, experienced all over the world, of demand for the services exceeding the funding available, and the need for choices to be made with a clear identification of priorities and even the necessity of rationing. Terms and conditions of service of professionals which are, of course, an entirely legitimate discussion, have been allowed to intrude or at least have been thought to be influencing views on the organization of patient care.

It is not in the interests of patients, health authorities or governments for professional advice not to be sought and heeded. None the less, if doctors are to influence policy at all levels they will need to be aware of how the NHS has changed and is changing and how best to exert their influence. As long as the advice is given responsibly, they will find NHS policy-makers at all levels anxious to listen because, in spite of the conflicts, it is recognized that doctors have a knowledge and influence over patient care which is unique. I have no doubt, personally, that politicians of all persuasions are anxious to work with and not against the profession.

The structure of the NHS

Knowledge of the structure, function and responsibilities of different parts of the NHS is imperative. There is no other single organization in the world which is so large and decentralization with clear responsibility and accountability at all levels is essential if it is to work effectively.

The political strategy for the NHS is determined by government, and the civil servants at the Department of Health have the responsibility for designing policies to ensure that the strategy is implemented. The actual implementation of the policies is the responsibility of the NHS management executive. Both the permanent secretary at the department and the chief executive of the NHS management executive report to the Secretary of State who delegates political oversight for different parts of the service to fellow ministers.

Whilst there is a potential for confusion of roles and conflicts between the civil service and the management executive, this has been minimized in recent years (Griffiths, 1983). An NHS policy board meets monthly, chaired by the Secretary of State, to consider general issues of policy within the confines of the overall government strategy. The policy board's membership includes all ministers, the permanent secretary, the chief executive, the chief medical officer, the chief nurse and a number of other members. Recently these have comprised two chairs of regional health authorities, three members from industry and the commercial world, all with considerable experience of management of large organizations, and a doctor.

Well over 100 doctors are employed by the Department of Health under the overall supervision of the chief medical officer. They assist both in the formulation of policy options for presentation to ministers and in the implementation of policy through the NHS management executive. The deputy chief medical officer has a seat, as medical director, on the management executive, as does the director of research and development, who is also a doctor.

The chief medical officer and colleagues have a number of specific roles within the department. Historically and importantly, the primary function is to monitor the health of the nation, evaluate factors that may influence it and encompass this within an annual report. In carrying out this task, the medical function in the department contributes to government policies designed to promote health, both through the Department of Health and by offering advice to other government ministries and agencies.

Doctors also provide expert medical advice on the development and evaluation of health care policy and some of this work may be highly specialized, for instance in relation to the pharmaceutical industry or in relation to scientific or statutory bodies. The chief medical officer and staff have certain statutory functions for which they are accountable to Parliament and he or she is called on from time to time to provide evidence to parliamentary committees. There is no clear separation of powers within the British parliamentary system between the legislature and the executive, but in recent years parliamentarians have requested and been provided with much more information concerning the background to government policy through parliamentary questions and standing committees. Where these questions concern medical matters, it is often the responsibility of the doctors in the department to provide the answers. Doctors from the department also contribute on behalf of the government to many international discussions and this aspect of their work is perhaps becoming more important in relation to the European Community and concern about the environment.

Doctors in the Department of Health have to operate within the rules of the civil service which require, at least in public, loyalty to the government of the day and the utmost discretion in public discussion of government policy. It seems likely that some feel uncomfortable at times with these restrictions and one reads with interest the views they contribute to the general discussion on health care policy after their retirement! Whilst in office they have to act as the interface between the profession and the government, attempting to explain government policy to professional bodies and represent the views of professionals to ministers. In spite of these restrictions there is no doubt that many doctors do find their responsibilities within the department rewarding because of the wide spread of responsibilities and the opportunities to influence health policy. In my view, it is important for the nation's health, for the proper workings of the NHS and for the profession that the chief medical officer and staff should continue to have a strong influence on government policy and in collaboration with the director of research and development to influence health care and medical research.

The intermediate tier

England and Wales are divided into 14 regional health authorities (RHAs). The chairs report directly to the Secretary of State or other ministers, and the general managers to the NHS chief executive as well as to the regional chair. Usually doctors will serve on the RHA in a personal capacity rather than representing a special interest, though experience in academic medicine will usually be sought in filling one place, bearing in mind that all regions have at least one teaching hospital within their authority. The regional director of public health will of course be an executive director on the RHA. Similarly, doctors will be involved in non-executive as well as executive roles on the boards of district health authorities, trust hospitals, community health services and family health service authorities. Where their appointment is as a non-executive member, it is important for them to remember constantly that they have been chosen for their special experience or knowledge, not as the representative of a special interest, nor should they attempt to interfere with, undermine or assume the responsibilities of those with executive roles.

The new NHS (HMSO, 1989)

The main theme of the NHS changes which were instituted in 1991 concerned decentralization with clear responsibility, authority and accountability at different levels of the service. The NHS is mainly funded through a revenue and capital allocation to each of the 180 or so district health authorities according to the population concerned, weighted for age and health status (weighted capitation). This system, which is being introduced over the next 3 years, will lead to major shifts of funding away from some inner cities and some shifts from the Thames regions to other parts of the country. The requirement to account for the funding as well as maintenance of capital is a new feature for the NHS, though normal practice in commercial life.

The district health authorities are responsible for commissioning health care from provider hospitals and services in their locality or outside and their role is now separated from the management of hospitals in their district, whether or not they are trust hospitals. Given the problems of providing community care for the handi-capped, aged and infirm, and the high cost of maintaining people in beds in acute hospitals, it is likely that there will be a progressive change in expenditure into small community facilities and away from large district general or teaching hospitals.

Other changes which have been introduced include the emphasis on clinical audit in hospital and in primary care and resource management, underpinned by a massive investment in information technology. The purpose is to improve the efficiency of the use of resources and to determine more clearly which health care interventions are effective. These initiatives have been supported by the appointment of a director of research and development to the NHS with a seat on the NHS management executive, whose task is to coordinate research into health care interventions throughout the service. The appointment of regional directors of research and development links into local initiatives in clinical audit and resource management. A national clinical standards board has been created to ensure the drive for efficiency is not at the expense of quality of care and this board may also be useful in assisting RHAs adjudicating in disputes which could potentially arise between commissioners and providers regarding the adequacy of resource to support a required clinical service.

Finally, the concept of general management introduced in 1983 (Griffiths, 1983) now operates throughout the service. In this respect it is vital to note that when Sir Roy Griffiths recommended general management he did not intend a new profession of managers to be created: rather that doctors, nurses, administrators and other professionals would take on general management responsibilities (Griffiths, 1992). Moreover, he intended that doctors should influence and be involved in decisions at all levels of the NHS.

Choices, priorities and money

If society contributes through taxation for the funding of the NHS, it seems inevitable that they will wish to exert influence over choices, priorities and funding. This they do at national level through the political debate and through the access that their professional organizations, such as the British Medical Association and the Royal Colleges, have to senior levels of both government and of the management of the health service. This access is both formal, through bodies such as the joint consultants committee, as well as through informal contacts. These organizations as well as individual doctors also have access to members of health authorities and officers at region and district level, to those who control local community services, to community health councils as well as to the media. Whilst the concept of choices, priorities and even rationing is appreciated by all of us when well, few acknowledge it when ill. We all expect our doctors to do everything humanly possible to care for us under these circumstances. There is no doubt in my mind that the increased expectation of modern medicine by the population, coupled with the constraint in spending, has increased enormously the stress on doctors over the last 15 years and I believe that politicians, the media and the profession should do more to explain these issues to the public rather than arguing that the problems of the NHS relate solely to inadequate funding. We need the support and understanding of society to do our job properly and to reduce the pressure which we all now feel in our day-to-day work.

It is always tempting to influence the allocation of resources by uncritical promotion of research or technological advance but this can be dangerous in that it serves to increase the expectations of the population, making day-to-day practice more difficult, and destroys public confidence if the raised expectations are not fulfilled. Some peer review of such claims before public discussion is usually advisable.

Decentralization of management and funding of the NHS offers a way of managing this conflict. Broad decisions of priorities and funding can be made at district health authority level, whilst leaving clinical teams the freedom to choose appropriate therapies for individual patients within a global budget allocated to that clinical service.

For most doctors it is their influence on local funding and policy decisions which matter most because these influence the clinical care of their patients. Assumption of responsibility with others for a clinical budget brings with it the authority to determine usage of the resource as well as accountability for the efficiency and effectiveness of the service provided.

The natural basic unit of management of a hospital is a clinical service which is often, though not always, based on one ward. The acceptance of a managerial role at this level by

a clinician should also bring with it the opportunity to influence the policy of the hospital as a whole and all clinical directors at Guy's Hospital sit on the hospital management board, which is chaired by a clinician and meets monthly. Clinicians in my view should resist models of hospital management which give them responsibility as a clinical director or chair of service but which do not provide authority over the use of resources and the right to influence overall hospital authority (Chantler, 1990; Disken et al., 1990). A medical advisory committee, though a useful forum for consultants to seek to influence policy, is not an adequate substitute for involvement in management. It is the acceptance of accountability which comes with the role of clinical director which determines the authority and confers the right with other clinicians to advise central hospital management. Likewise the medical director of a hospital has a crucial role on the executive board in determining policy, because again the acceptance of responsibility and accountability increases the authority of the advice.

General advice

There are certain general points to be noted if advice is to be sought and welcomed.

1 *Always seek professional consensus.* One of the banes of life for a general manager of a hospital is the differing advice and conflicts that arise from consultation with professionals. Doctors in the same specialty frequently disagree, at times vehemently, and make little attempt to make policies with other professionals such as nurses, therapists, finance staff, administrators, etc. Policies which have been discussed and, if possible, agreed with colleagues and arrived at with equal participation from other staff will not only be more likely to be accepted; they will usually work better, if only because by spending time formulating them, it is more likely they will be widely understood. Apart from anything else, a united professional voice carries great authority.

2 *Try to avoid self-interest.* Obviously few doctors argue for policy directly beneficial for themselves personally but the responsibility to one's own patients can sometimes blind one to the needs of patients of colleagues. Again, policies formulated for a single interest tend to cause conflict and lead to inefficiency or failure. It is usually possible at ward, outpatient or hospital level to arrive at policies which are mutually acceptable if time is

taken to discuss the problems with all who are affected. If self-interest is involved, at least declare it, if only to acknowledge it to oneself.

3 *Accept that responsibility, authority and accountability always go together.* Where resources are limited, as they always will be in the NHS, it becomes an ethical responsibility to strive for efficiency and effectiveness in clinical practice. Advice which is given without responsibility for the outcome in terms of cost as well as clinical benefit, whilst it may be appropriate and even heeded, is much less powerful than when responsibility for the outcome is shared.

4 *Do your homework.* Flashes of inspiration as one reads papers during a meeting are often unreliable. Time spent considering the issues, seeking advice and marshalling facts is usually well-spent. As more information becomes available in the hospital service, so arguments will be developed more effectively for a given course of action. Disraeli once said that the man with the most power is the man with the best information. This is important at all levels of the service and for the Secretary of State it is essential if he or she is to convince the Treasury that a larger proportion of the country's wealth should be devoted to the NHS (Chantler, 1992).

5 *The higher up the service, the more general the responsibility.* In any decentralized management there is a role of operational management to deliver the service and a strategic role to advise about general policy. The roles are often mixed but should not be confused. It is dangerous to argue from a narrow operational concern for a change in general policy and, whilst individuals may be chosen to advise about general issues because of a particular professional experience or knowledge, they should be careful to maintain perspective.

6 *Maintain lines of communication.* The responsibility to advise on behalf of others confers an obligation to inform and consult with the various groups who will be affected by the decisions that are made. The aim is to reach the best decision for the whole organization and it will rarely be possible, or even at times desirable, for the individual who carries the responsibility simply to propose a course of action which will cause the least dissatisfaction. Leadership, as has been written, requires courage, imagination and sensitivity. But even if the final decision is contrary to the wishes of those who have been consulted, the fact that they have been consulted and the reasons for the decision explained will often ensure their cooperation with the action required (Harvey Jones, 1988).

7 *Try to keep an open mind.* Obviously there are points of great principle where compromise is neither possible nor desirable, but frequently a discussion can reveal alternatives which were not apparent to anyone beforehand. The determination to achieve one's own solution, reached privately beforehand, is rarely helpful and can be destructive (Heirs, 1989).

8 *Loyalty to group decisions.* Any management group will at times have to take difficult decisions which are not universally welcomed. The management process is impossible if those party to the decision do not accept the responsibility to explain and defend the decision. Some decisions will be wrong and will need to be changed but this should be argued within the management group rather than undermining the group by mobilizing dissension.

Conclusion

Doctors have an important responsibility to assist in the formulation of policy at all levels of the health service. They should seek to persuade by argument and by marshalling facts rather than opinions. They should strive for consensus with colleagues and, most importantly, with other professional groups. Conflict between professionals means that their influence is minimized and their views may be ignored. Recognition and understanding of the responsibilities of those who are accountable for the management of the health service at all levels are essential if advice is to be sought and acted upon.

References

Chantler, C. (1990) Management reform in a London hospital. In: Carle, N. (ed) *Managing for Health Result.* King's Fund, London.

Chantler, C. (1992) Management and information. *British Medical Journal* **304**, 632–635.

Disken, S., Dixon, M., Halpern, S. and Shockett, G. (1990) *Models of Clinical Management.* Institute of Health Services Management, London.

Griffiths, R. (1983) *NHS Management Enquiry. (The Griffiths Report).* Department of Health and Social Security, London.

Griffiths, R. (1992) Seven years of progress – general management in the NHS. *Health Economics* **1**, 61–70.

Harvey Jones, J. (1988) *Making it Happen (Reflections on Leadership).* William Collins, Glasgow.

Heirs, B. (1989) *The Professional Decision Thinker and the Art of Team Thinking Leadership.* Grafton, London.

Schon, D.A. (1991) *The Reflective Practitioner.* Avebury, Aldershot.

HMSO (1989) *Working for Patients: The NHS Reforms.* HMSO, London.

3.3 The role of medical directors in trusts

Mark R. Baker

Introduction

Hospitals have existed for many centuries, doctors for almost as long, nurses – as we know them – rather less so and effective treatments for a shorter period still. One may be excused, therefore, for disregarding history in analysing the relationship between doctors and the management of hospitals in the modern idiom.

By the end of the decade, 60% of consultants will have been appointed since the reforms of the NHS were implemented. Although philosophical opposition to the reforms remains commonplace, necessity will ensure that doctors play an active role in forging the future shape of NHS facilities and services and an accelerating pace of change can, as ever, be anticipated.

One of the structural nuances of the reforms is to advance the managerial status and responsibility of selected doctors through their appointment as directors of a trust, usually as medical director and less often as non-executive directors.

Rationale

The organization of health services in the modern era has mainly been driven by the need to bring into apposition the skills of the clinical professions and the patients' needs for those skills. It is not surprising, given the age of the different clinical professions, that doctors were pre-eminent in identifying the need for organization and playing a leading role in promoting and implementing the solutions. Although health politics is a relatively recent phenomenon, even that was initially led by a doctor.

The zenith of medical leadership was reached during the period 1926–1948 when the large majority of health services were managed by medical officers of health and medical superintendents.

The creation of the NHS, anticipating moves towards a planned service, and occurring in an age when societal power balances were shifting, signalled the end of medical dominance in health structures, though the intangible power of the practitioner has continued to be the single most powerful influence on health development.

The first two decades of the NHS saw revolutionary changes in health services led by pharmacological and surgical advances, accompanied by plant renewal and technological development. The relative prosperity of much of the period meant that management was conducted through queueing rather than choices. The end of national economic prosperity in 1968 led to changing attitudes to managing public services, including health.

In order to render feasible the tougher decisions to be made during the 1970s and later, deliberate efforts were made to engage hospital doctors in the management processes through 'cogwheel' machinery and later through membership of management and authority boards.

Professional behaviour, however, changes only slowly and the severe and direct management pressures of the 1980s often ran ahead of the sensitivities of clinical practitioners.

Modern medical managerial history

The last decade has witnessed a number of parallel but interrelated themes in the development of medical managers, especially the processes which culminated in resource management, the introduction of general management and the reforms.

Resource management

Recognizable budgetary management systems are a recent innovation in the NHS. The first attempts to manage resources at clinical department level were conducted around 1980 and were finance-led. The clinical commitment was at the level of permissiveness rather than leadership. However, the next generation, known as clinical budgeting, saw professional leaders much more engaged in the process and resulted in the rather unexpected spectacle of clinicians passionately selling clinical information systems to their peers.

Although not primarily intended to reduce gross expenditure, this initiative was explicitly adopted at Guy's Hospital to help reduce costs and eliminate the hospital's deficit. Cause and effect have not been demonstrated but there was little doubt that clinical and resource information could be used together to improve cost-effectiveness of services and the key to delivering this ideal was clinician leadership.

The roll-out of these principles under the resource management banner shifted the focus from information leading to change towards a less tangible clinical leadership issue. Resource management may be regarded as a management system led by clinicians and driven by information rather than a transposition of these roles as envisaged earlier.

The structural sequel to this analysis was the creation of a hierarchy amongst clinicians based on clinical and managerial accountability rather than seniority on grounds of age, excellence or achievement.

General management

The introduction of chief executive-style general management at district and unit level in 1985 gave doctors the opportunity to seize the managerial reins after years of publicly proclaimed disfranchisement.

The appointment of consultants to these posts was actively favoured by the government and several instances of positive action were evident. Doctors, it was considered, would sweep away bureaucracy and bring a touch of clinical realism to hospital management. However, the most powerful motive was to empower medicine's leaders to exert influence on their peers to change practice.

The initiative met with some success but the frustrations of managing the unmanageable took their toll and the 1987 financial crisis persuaded many to return to clinical medicine. By 1990,

medical managers at the top of the NHS were once again becoming anachronistic.

The NHS reforms

Conceived during a financial crisis, implanted following perceived unprofessional shroud-waving and delivered after a long and leaky confinement, the reforms fell upon the professions like a nuclear storm. The replacement of collectivism by explicit competition was anathema to professions which prided their false image of equality. For medicine, the firestorm was fanned by many features: the rising power of lay managers, threats to national pay bargaining and the sacred monopoly of the DDRB, medical audit, the premature judgement on the success of resource management, the *primus inter pares* of fundholding and, most of all, the competitiveness created by the internal market and promoted by NHS trusts.

Sources in government expressed surprise that the expected knee-jerk opposition from the British Medical Association took 3 weeks to emerge. In reality, the profession was, from the outset, split between a small visionary and/or predatory minority and the slower-changing majority who preferred the unsustainable status quo. The unparalleled political opposition led staff to believe forlornly that the reforms were not real. It was, as ever, the medical leaders that created the reality.

Markets are created by choice and marketing is described by price, focus and differentiation. The first and last of these are largely in the control of clinicians. It is obvious that the cost of hospital services is determined mainly by the cost of what doctors do or influence. Still more important is differentiation. Prices can always be undercut but service style, innovation and quality are harder to beat. Not only are doctors the principal source of innovation and differentiation, but they are also the sales force for a trust.

Doctors have always been competitive; from entering medical school through training to consultancy, private practice and distinction awards, positioning and competitiveness are at the heart of success. In the past, it has been the success of clinical promotion of innovation which has been blamed for failure of cost control. Thus, doctors emerged as the natural leaders of service marketing in the emerging NHS market and, of course, some are better than others.

Whether much of this was recognized at the outset is questionable. None the less, the historical precedents and the opportunities created by resource management and the reforms have served to create medical director posts of profound importance to trust organization. Although seen in their early days as sinecures, doctors on the trust board now stand alongside the finance director and chief executive as architects of the organization's culture and success.

Doctors on the trust board

In most trusts, the executive medical director will be the only doctor on the board. In exceptional circumstances, another executive position will be filled by a doctor. More often, a non-executive directorship will be given to a clinical academic. In such cases, some minority responsibilities fall naturally to the non-executive (e.g. research coordination) but in general the activities and relationships outlined here are those vested in the medical director.

Internal

The closed nature of executive groupings tends to create an *apparatchik* mentality which must be avoided. To retain credibility, medical directors must remain members of the medical staff and cognizant of the community they represent. There is a natural expectation that medical staff will look to the director to represent their views in management and the converse is also true. It is this dichotomy which makes the role so challenging.

Increasing political and economic pressures place inevitable demands on an organization. The incompatibility of rapid technological and therapeutic advances with the 40-year career of medical staff creates interesting tensions which are not easily resolved in a commercial environment. Rightly or not, the medical director has a role to play in easing the pressures due to commercial and technological change for staff who do not wish to participate. It is not a matter of taking sides but of easing the effects of inevitable change.

External

The board as a whole must determine the overall direction of the trust, including issues of investment and service focus. These decisions are informed by two principal factors – the market's demands and the hospital's internal strengths and capacity. While the latter depends on the medical staff, the former is also influenced to a large extent by the relationships forged between consultants and general practitioners and the wider community.

The medical director has a particular role in harnessing clinical strengths and potential to meet wider organizational goals. In some instances, the director has a singular role to play in developing, and sometimes repairing, intraprofessional relationships which are a key component of the marketing strategy. The capture and retention of general practitioners' 'business' is one of the tasks at the heart of the reforms. It has already been exercised explicitly with fundholders but, as volume-related contracts with district health authorities become commonplace, will soon affect dealings with all general practitioners. Indeed, medical directors may well become embroiled with the detail of service specifications and contracts, especially qualitative and outcome aspects.

A key component of this approach is the selection of new medical staff, especially consultants. Most directors will be familiar with the interview process of the AAC but less so with the more active and important elements of the process, including competitive 'head-hunting', which is usually necessary if the organization is really positioning itself in the market.

Partnerships and transition

There are a number of important functions of great importance to trusts but whose control is independent of providers. The most important examples are medical audit, research and development and postgraduate medical education. In all cases, the regional health authority is the responsible organization and the repository of funds, but the manner in which the funds are dispersed is of critical importance to trusts. Furthermore, trusts have relatively little power in controlling the investment and disinvestment strategies for these functions.

Medical audit is still in its early stages. Few audit cycles begin with defensible standards and audit is practised actively by a small minority. The whole process is costing £40m annually in direct costs and probably 10 times as much in opportunity costs. Yet the whole exercise is ill-conceivedly considered as an educational endeavour. The only legitimized purpose of audit is to change practice in ways that improve clinical outcome and/or reduce costs. Eventually management will recognize the catalogue of wasted opportunity and expect the medical director to do something about it.

Research and development is not recognized as a universal NHS trait, although many doctors think they do research. Amongst the NHS's less laudable characteristics are the subjectivity of most managerial and many clinical decisions and the absence of a framework for applying new technologies in a managed and coherent fashion. The NHS research initiative is intended to correct this; operating in a harsh economic climate, it will seek disinvestment from unproductive areas to enable reinvestment in more promising areas. This agenda is by no means specific to medicine but the impact of change will be particularly felt in medicine due to refocusing of existing – mainly medical – research funds and the greater direction to service development which the programme will produce.

The greatest difficulty, however, comes from the postgraduate dean's office. With shorter junior doctors' hours and greater training expectations, the traditional fabric of cover is under severe threat. How hospital services adapt to stricter control of junior staff is perhaps the single most important determinant of their capacity. This factor alone can be used to justify what is now referred to as 'rightsizing' – reducing the bed complement of hospitals to that required by the marketing position.

The problem here is that the number and quality of junior medical staff has a profound impact on service quality, not only through their direct contribution but also by making a hospital attractive to consultants and stimulating changes in practice.

In all these areas, the medical director represents the best way of influencing the complex machinery which makes decisions for one set of reasons but which are vital to the trust for another.

Relations with clinical directors

The near universal presence of clinical directorates or equivalent groups can both help and hinder the medical director. On the one hand, they provide a recruiting field for the post; conversely, all clinical directors think they can do the board job better, even if they don't want it.

In some of the more hierarchical structures, the medical director emerges from the clinical board, often as its chairperson. This is not always the best model. As indicated above, their external and troubleshooting roles are big enough without having their extensive line management responsibility too.

None the less, clinical directorates offer a genuinely alternative powerbase for the profession, and the medical director, and other doctors on the board, must square their position with their peers.

Career issues

As if the job were not big enough, the appointment creates two real paradoxes – the hours and the future.

In large acute hospital trusts, the medical director role can easily be made into a full-time post, yet the logic of the post relies on the continuation of practice. Similarly, the innovative nature of many tasks attracts consultants in mid-career, leaving them with unattractive prospects during the latter part of their career. These problems have not been resolved and individuals will be left to make their own solutions. However, if the NHS takes medical directorships seriously, it will have to learn to manage career transitions better.

Whence medical directors?

Some trusts are now advertising externally for medical directors. Appointees from outside a hospital have a steep hill to climb in building the relationships with clinical staff which would enable them to fulfil some sometimes unpleasant duties. I can think of no ideal circumstance which would make it preferable not to appoint someone from the staff. Even if an external appointment is made initially, the goal must be to develop internal candidates for the future.

In fast-changing times, the duties of doctors on trust boards are bound to change in future years, rendering succession planning even more difficult. There is a tendency to regard possession of an MBA degree as a passport to success. I can only point out that the British and Americans have many more such graduates than the Germans and Japanese.

Section 4

Hospital funding

4.1 Financing the NHS – from Bevan to Thatcher

Malcolm J. Prowle

Introduction

During the 45 years of the existence of the NHS, one of the most politically and managerially demanding tasks has been financial resource allocation. It must be appreciated that the financial resources available to the NHS in any one year are strictly limited and indeed the NHS, historically, has a first-class record of containing its spending within the resources available. Throughout the life of the NHS it has always been the case (and still is the case) that the vast bulk of its funds come from the national exchequer but it is beyond the scope of this section to discuss, in any detail, the processes whereby central government decides the overall levels of public expenditure in any one year and the distribution of that expenditure between different programmes (e.g. education, health, defence). What can be said, however, is that such decisions are predominantly based on a combination of political and economic judgements about the country as a whole and thus the expenditure needs of the NHS have to compete against the needs of other government programmes.

Given that the NHS has finite resources available to it, NHS finance has been largely concerned with deciding the most appropriate way of allocating a fixed sum of money between different parts of the country and between different types of service.

The history of resource allocation in the NHS can be considered in three distinct eras:

1 Pre-Resource Allocation Working Party (RAWP) – 1948–1977.
2 The RAWP period – 1977–1991.
3 The post-RAWP period – 1991 onwards.

The period from 1991 onwards concerns the approach known as weighted capitation (see Section 4.2). This chapter concerns itself with the earlier periods. However, before doing this a brief description of the different types of resource allocation in the NHS is in order.

NHS resource allocation

Resource allocation in the NHS can be considered in two parts:

1 the Family Practitioner Service (FPS).
2 the Hospital and Community Health Service (HCHS).

The FPS will be dealt with briefly. FPS expenditure levels were determined by the various professional groups concerned (doctors, dentists, opticians and pharmacists) who were reimbursed for the activities they had undertaken according to a detailed schedule of payments. Until 1991 the FPS was one of the few areas of public expenditure (together with welfare benefits) that were not cash-limited. FPS expenditure was described as demand-related in that the expenditure incurred by practitioners would always be met without any limit being imposed. Since the introduction of the 1991 NHS reforms, FPS spending has become much more tightly controlled.

With regard to the HCHS, there are three different types of allocation:

1 Revenue allocations – funds required to finance day-to-day spending on such items as pay costs, consumable costs, etc.
2 Capital allocations – funds required to finance new buildings, equipment etc.
3 Earmarked allocations – allocations made for specific purposes such as joint financing of projects with local authorities.

The bulk of this chapter will be concerned with revenue allocations, with some comment on capital allocations.

HCHS: pre-RAWP 1948–1977

The formation of the NHS in 1948 involved bringing together different types of hospital (e.g. voluntary hospitals, local authority hospitals etc.) under a structure of Regional Hospital Boards (RHBs) and Hospital Management Committees (HMCs). Not surprisingly, in the early years, resource allocation in the HCHS involved the allocation to the then RHBs and HMCs of funds necessary to meet the estimated running costs of those existing hospitals for which they had taken responsibility. The lack of precision involved was illustrated by the fact that, unfortunately, in the first year of its existence the running costs of those hospitals were more than twice the original estimate (Rigden, 1983). Where new hospitals were constructed additional funds were allocated to meet the additional running costs according to a formula approach known as the Revenue Consequences of Capital Schemes (RCCS).

The major weakness of the above approach is, of course, that funds were being allocated to RHBs mainly according to the expenditure needs of their existing hospitals rather than the needs of their population. Similarly, the approach took no account of the impact of major population shifts (such as the large-scale movement of the population out of London) on the health needs of a particular area. Thus there was an increasing mismatch between the resource needs of an area based on its population and the resources being devoted to an area according to the expenditure of its existing hospitals. This mismatch is essentially one which still exists in central London, due to the high preponderance of teaching hospitals, and which has been addressed by the Tomlinson report.

The Crossman formula

This combination of policy inertia and demographic drag engendered a situation of considerable inequality, between different parts of the country, in the distribution of health resources. Such a situation was seen as unacceptable in the NHS with its concept of equal access to health care for all. Indeed, in 1945 Aneurin Bevan had said: 'We have got to achieve as nearly as possible a uniform standard of service for all' (Memorandum, 1945). Ironically, it was even said that there were greater inequalities in the so-called *National* Health Service than there were in the education service administered by quasiautonomous local authorities working under central guidance (Research Paper, 1978).

The first attempt to remedy this situation was made, in the early 1970s, by the then Health Secretary, Richard Crossman. He introduced an approach based on allocating funds to an area on the basis of a formula comprising factors such as population served, beds provided and cases handled. In spite of its good intentions, the Crossman formula was not really a success in terms of reducing inequalities. This was because most of the additional funding that could have been used to reduce such inequalities was pre-empted for two main purposes:

1 to finance the RCCS of new hospital developments;
2 as a guarantee that each RHB would receive at least 0.25% growth in revenue funding, each year, in addition to RCCS.

Thus the Crossman approach was essentially a failure and the next few years saw the introduction of the topic which subsequently dominated the issue of NHS resource allocation, namely the RAWP.

HCHS: the RAWP Period: 1977–1991

In 1975 the then Health Secretary, Barbara Castle, set up the RAWP to look into resource allocation in the HCHS. It is important to note that in its terms of reference the RAWP was not asked to comment on the adequacy of the total funding available to the HCHS, nor was it to concern itself with how funds allocated to health authorities were to be deployed. Its main task was to consider how best a fixed amount of resources might be distributed between health authorities.

The RAWP report, published in 1976, recommended the use of a formula approach to NHS resource allocation in England. Similar approaches, entitled SHARE and RAWG, were ultimately adopted in the health services in Scotland and Wales respectively. The various elements of the RAWP formula were designed to reflect the *relative* (as opposed to absolute) need for health resources of different geographic areas in the country. The formula recommended by the RAWP comprised the following five elements:

1 Population size.
2 Population structure.
3 Morbidity/mortality.
4 Cost weighting.
5 Cross-boundary patient flows.

Population size

As health services are supplied for people then clearly the population size of an area must be the primary consideration. Thus the starting point for the RAWP formula was the mid-year population estimate of an area.

Population structure

It can easily be demonstrated that different segments of the population have different needs and place different demands on the NHS. Elderly people have greater needs and place more demands on the NHS than younger people, while men have differing needs to women. Thus the age/sex structure of the population is an important element in the measurement of relative need and this is recognized by the RAWP formula.

Morbidity/mortality

It is self-evident that the greater the degree of morbidity in an area, the greater the need for health care. This factor was recognized by the original RAWP report but unfortunately the working party, having looked at many possible indicators of morbidity, found it difficult to agree on what would be suitable comprehensive and objective measures of morbidity for an area. Thus the RAWP approach adopted the use of mortality data (standardized mortality ratios or SMRs) as a surrogate for suitable morbidity data. Throughout the RAWP period much of the debate about the formula has concerned the appropriateness of using mortality data as a surrogate for morbidity measures but unfortunately no universally acceptable alternative could be identified.

Cost weighting

Different clinical conditions cost different amounts to treat. Thus, area A, although having the same overall level of morbidity/mortality as area B, might have a greater relative need for health resources because the prevalent clinical conditions in A are more expensive to treat than those conditions prevalent in B. Although this point was recognized by the original working party, the problem at the time was the paucity of financial information in the NHS about the relative cost of treating clinical conditions. However, over the years it has proved possible to incorporate such relative cost measures into the RAWP formula by means of cost data produced through the statistical analysis of hospital cost statements.

Cross-boundary patient flows

For a number of very good reasons the boundaries of a health authority cannot be regarded as sacrosanct and it is common for patients resident in one health authority area to obtain treatment in another area. For example, a patient may need to attend a teaching hospital in another district health authority (DHA) for treatment not available in his or her authority of residence. Hence, in looking at the relative need for health resources of an area, adjustment must be made for the numbers of patients who have migrated in or out of the area for treatment purposes. Although the working party recognized this point, the problems were again practical. Although data about cross-boundary flows of inpatients were readily available, data on outpatient and day-patient cross-boundary flows were not. Thus, the RAWP formula could not fully take account of such flows.

Applying the RAWP formula

Taking the population of an area as the starting point, various weightings could be applied to take account of the factors of health need, referred to above. This process would produce, for each area, a weighted population which could be regarded as a measure of the relative need, of an area, for health resources. These weighted populations could then be used to calculate what was referred to as the RAWP target of an area.

Let us use regional health authorities to illustrate this process. What RAWP did was to take the total funds available to the HCHS in 1976–1977 and notionally share those funds between regional health authorities (RHAs) in proportion to their weighted RAWP populations. This calculation produced what were referred to as notional RAWP targets, being essentially the funds each RHA should receive if the total HCHS funds were shared out according to the RAWP measure of relative need. In 1976–1977, what was then done was to compare those target allocations with the actual allocations being received by RHAs. The overall picture produced was that:

1 The four Thames RHAs were receiving allocations of funds well in excess of what they should have been receiving according to their RAWP target allocations. Oxford RHA had an allocation marginally in excess of its RAWP target allocation.
2 All of the other nine RHAs in the country were receiving allocations which to a lesser or greater degree were below their RAWP target allocation.

This then was confirmation of the picture referred to earlier of an NHS containing considerable inequalities in the distribution of health resource across the country. It is important to recap on what was being said here. Nobody was suggesting that the above-target RHAs had too much money. However, what was being said was that, using the RAWP approach to measuring relative need, those RHAs were getting more than their fair share of the resources available and, conversely, below-target RHAs were getting less than their fair share.

The existence of these inequalities dominated health service resource allocation for the next 15 years and it became the policy of all governments to allocate resources in a manner that made progress towards the eradication of those inequalities.

The RAWP approach: targets and allocations

Much academic research gives the false impression that the detailed intricacies of the RAWP formula are the only important issue in HCHS resource allocation. This is not the case and what is of more importance is how funds were actually allocated each year in order to try and meet the RAWP objective of eradicating inequalities over a 10-year period. This is a very complex process and the interested reader is referred elsewhere for further details (Jones and Prowle, 1987). However, a brief summary of what is involved is given below.

Basically, the approach to eradicating RAWP inequalities between RHAs was *not* to be achieved by taking existing funds away from above-target RHAs and giving them to below-target RHAs. Such an approach – robbing Peter to pay Paul was impractical in a health service where patient needs and demands are increasing every year in all parts of the country. The policy adopted could best be described as one of directed differential growth. What this means is that whereas, each year, all RHAs would receive some element of growth monies, those RHAs below RAWP target would receive a much higher rate of growth than those RHAs above their RAWP target. Thus, over a long enough period of time, this policy of differential growth in resources would ultimately achieve RAWP equalization. Clearly, the higher the total rate of growth monies available, then the faster equalization could be achieved. However, even when relatively high rates of resource growth were available, political pressures often meant that part of this growth money might be siphoned off to finance specific items with sensitive and short-term political considerations. It is worth keeping in mind that most in-year announcements by politicians about additional funds to meet the latest headline problem do not usually imply additional funding for the NHS as a whole. What is more likely to have happened is that funds have been transferred from elsewhere within the health programme, possibly from the funds earmarked for RAWP equalization.

These last comments show the basic weakness of the RAWP approach. RAWP equalization policies require resource growth to work and the limited growth available in the 1980s inhibited the speed with which equalization could be achieved. There is also the tendency for funds originally planned to be available for RAWP equalization to be spirited off for other purposes.

Interregional RAWP and subregional RAWP

Up until now, our discussion of RAWP has been concerned with its use in allocating revenue funds to RHAs. This is usually referred to as interregional RAWP. However, it was also possible to compute RAWP targets for each DHA within an RHA and to compare actual DHA allocations with their target allocations. What this showed was that, in addition to inequalities in resource distribution between RHAs, there also existed large inequalities between DHAs within a particular region. Thus, within some of the Thames RHAs (which were themselves well above RAWP target), it was possible to find pockets of relative deprivation in terms of DHAs whose actual revenue allocations were well below their RAWP target. Thus, in addition to interregional RAWP, there was also the process of subregional RAWP concerned with promoting equality of resource distribution within regions.

How did subregional RAWP differ from interregional RAWP other than in scale? In broad terms, the two approaches were very similar but at the detailed level the following changes should be noted:

1 Quite often RHAs, in making subregional allocations, would make modifications to the national RAWP formula to reflect particular local circumstances. For example, an RHA might modify some of the weighting used in the formula or might add additional factors such as a measure of social deprivation.
2 Whereas with interregional RAWP the formula was used to allocate revenue funds to all health services, sometimes with subregional RAWP the formula approach was only applied to acute services. Funds for psychiatric services or services for the mentally handicapped might be allocated by a service planning mechanism.
3 Quite often, RHAs may still have retained RCCS allocations within a framework of revenue equalization through RAWP. The use of RCCS inhibited the speed with which revenue equalization could be achieved.

RAWP and capital allocations

Until now our discussion of RAWP has concerned its use in the allocation of revenue funds. However, a few words are required about the RAWP report's recommendations with regard to capital allocations within the NHS. The RAWP report recommended an approach to capital allocations which was broadly similar to that for revenue allocations. This involved using a formula to calculate the share of the total value of NHS capital stock (buildings, equipment, vehicles) that a particular region should possess and comparing that with the actual capital stock in the region. As with revenue RAWP, this approach showed considerable inequalities between the various regions in England. However, clearly it is not possible to eradicate such inequalities by moving buildings and equipment from one part of England to another. What can be done, however, is progressively to steer new capital funds into those RHAs below target and away from those above target. In broad terms, this was the approach adopted. In this way, over a long enough period of time, inequalities in capital stock distribution would be eliminated.

RAWP developments

The original report of the RAWP was only the start of the RAWP process and subsequently a number of amendments to the formula have been proposed and or implemented. Two specific initiatives should be mentioned:

1 Following the RAWP report, the Health Secretary set up the Advisory Group on Resource Allocation (AGRA) to advise on possible changes to the RAWP methodology. Over the years the AGRA has recommended a number of changes which have subsequently been implemented. An example is the inclusion of a factor to reflect differences in labour costs between regions.
2 In 1987 the Department of Health initiated a major national review of the RAWP approach to resource allocation. This report identified a number of technical changes to the RAWP formula, the most significant of which concerned the issue of social deprivation. For many years it had been argued from several quarters that if the RAWP formula was genuinely to measure the relative need for health resources, then it needed to incorporate a factor concerned with the relative social deprivation in the various populations. The RAWP review suggested that this be done by the use of what were termed Jarman indices which were, in effect, composite measures of social deprivation. Clearly the outcome of this national RAWP review was overtaken by events, through the publication of the government's reform proposals as set out in *Working for Patients*.

Conclusion

The implementation of the NHS reforms and the move towards resource allocation based on weighted capitation principles formally ended the RAWP period. Looking back, one can take two differing views about the success or otherwise of the RAWP approach. On the one hand, the inequalities between RHAs, referred to above, were substantially less at the end of the RAWP period than at the beginning and this could be regarded as a success. However, the RAWP approach failed to achieve its initial objective of eradicating inequalities over a 10-year period and at the end of the period the basic pattern of inequality was the same, with the four Thames RHAs being above target, while the rest of England was below RAWP target.

Overall, this author was a supporter of the RAWP approach in that it tried to bring some degree of equity and objectivity to NHS resource allocation, in preference to an approach sometimes referred to as resource allocation by deci-

bel. Whether future approaches to resource allocation are any more or less successful than RAWP remains to be seen.

References

Department of Health (1989) *Working for Patients*. HMSO, London.

Jones T.W. and Prowle M.J. (1987) *Health Service Finance: An Introduction*, Chapters 3 and 6, 3rd edn. Certified Accountants Educational Trust.

Memorandum by the Minister of Health to the Cabinet, 5 October 1945. Public Records Office, CAB 129/3.

Research paper no 3 of the Royal Commission on the NHS (1978) p 3. HMSO, London.

Rigden, M.S. (1983) *Health Service Finance and Accounting*, Chapter 2. Heinemann, London.

4.2 Hospital finance since the 1990 reforms

Elizabeth Hunter Johnson

Ownership of assets

A fundamental difference between NHS trusts and directly managed units (DMUs) is that the NHS trust owns its own assets – that is, land and buildings, equipment, furniture, etc. When it is established, an order is made (under Section 8 of the NHS and Community Care Act 1990) transferring to the trust from the Secretary of State 'such of the property, rights and liabilities of a health authority or of the Secretary of State as, in his opinion, need to be transferred to the trust for the purpose of enabling it to carry out its functions'. These are then the property of the trust board.

Deciding what the trust owns is not always simple. The main buildings and equipment used may be obvious but the appropriate ownership of peripheral buildings where, perhaps, a few clinics are held may be unclear and can give rise, if everyone is not sensible, to heated territorial disputes, even if common sense in the end prevails. Common sense is also needed to sort out whether it is more appropriate to own or to lease certain buildings. Either way the trust will have to earn and hence charge a return on capital for the building concerned, and it is likely that the lease payment or the interest paid on the building if owned will be similar. The decision therefore tends to be made around the question of what will happen when the building is sold. The trust has to weigh up the advantages of being sole beneficiary of any land sale against the disadvantages of the management time that may be involved in the sale (obtaining planning consent can be an administrative nightmare); the effect on its financial performance of making a loss if the sale of the building realizes less than its notional value (see below); and the complications if other units have an interest in the services provided in that building. Moreover, although it might appear that raising capital from a land sale is a way round the process of bidding to the centre for capital, the position is not that simple. The process of bidding to the centre for capital is described more fully below, but provided the trust can make a good business case for capital, whether or not the source of funding is a land sale may be a minor consideration. If the NHS management executive does not approve the capital expenditure, the trust may find the proceeds of the land sale locked in by means of an adjustment to its external financing limit or even, under Paragraph 6 of Schedule 3 to the NHS and Community Care Act, extracted from it.

Having established what the trust should own, the trust should arrange with solicitors for land and buildings to be conveyed to it: other assets are transferred by order, which will be arranged by the NHS management executive.

The value of the trust's assets is then determined according to the rules for capital charging. The district valuer values land and buildings: the values of other assets are taken from the capital charges register. Once audited accounts for the district from which the trust has come are ready, two further items are known – inherited creditors (to whom money is owed, hence a liability to be deducted from the total value of assets) and debtors (from whom money is owed, hence an asset to be added to the total value of assets). Many of the problems in sorting out opening assets of trusts have arisen because of disputes about these two items.

Originating debt

The trust is not given these assets for nothing. In return it is considered to owe to the government an amount equal to the value of its assets. This is called the *originating debt*. The trust has to pay interest on an interest-bearing part of this debt at current long-term government lending rates (the rate will be a fixed one for the whole period of the loan) and has to pay off the loan over 25 years. This latter provision need not cause too much concern: if the trust cannot afford to pay off 1/25th of the loan in any particular year, it will simply borrow to raise that amount, thus rolling forward the debt at *current* long-term interest rates.

Assets donated since 1948 and works of art do not form part of the originating debt as the trust does not have to earn a return on them.

Interest-bearing debt/public dividend capital

Part of the originating debt will be given not as interest-bearing debt (IBD) but as public dividend capital (PDC). This is the government equivalent of share capital, and on this portion of its debt the trust will thus pay a variable dividend rather than an annual fixed amount. Some years it may not pay anything at all – but the Treasury presumption is that *in the long term* the trust will pay just as much in dividends as it would have done in interest had that part of the debt been interest-bearing.

The split between IBD and PDC is usually 50–50. This has the virtue of simplicity, but actually results from the interest rates that were current when the trust financial regime was designed. These were then about 12% and trusts are only allowed to earn from the NHS a return on capital of 6%. This 6% is, essentially, the amount they have out of which to pay interest and therefore to have had to pay 12% on *all* their originating debt would have taken about twice what they had available. Consequently only half the debt was made interest-bearing, thus using up the return on capital in this interest payment, and it was presumed, for year 1, that trusts would not pay a dividend. By the time subsequent waves of trusts came along, interest rates had fallen but it was decided to keep the 50–50 split and balance the figures – i.e. plan to extract approximately the 6% rate of return – by requiring the trust to pay a dividend. This is the crucial part to note: it is the government that tells the trust what dividend to pay; not, as is usual with shares, the trust's decision as to what it chooses to pay.

Exceptionally, a trust may be given a split other than 50–50. This would usually be because it had a major building programme and was therefore having to pay interest on assets in the course of construction (which form part of the originating debt) but was not earning a rate of return on them out of which to pay interest (assets in the course of construction do not attract a capital charge or have to earn a rate of return). A scheme would probably have to be very large indeed to push a trust into deficit in this way and the NHS management executive would discuss the necessity for a different IBD-PDC split with the trust concerned.

Financial duties

The first financial duty on a trust is to achieve value for money in its activities. It also has three specific statutory financial duties to meet. These are:

1 to break even;
2 to earn a predetermined return on its assets (currently 6%);
3 to live within its external financing limit.

It is on the performance of these three financial duties that the whole accountability system for trusts rests, and provided the trust delivers these three duties *and* meets its contractual obligations to the satisfaction of its purchasers, its managerial freedoms are, if not total (certain national priorities, procedures and guidance will continue to be imposed on trust management), at least very considerable. It is against this background that the financial regime needs to be understood. The trust financial regime is frankly not to be regarded as a major 'freedom' for a trust: rather it is a tightly controlled system which ensures that the managerial freedoms offered to trusts do not lead them into expenditure which could make the NHS as a whole breach revenue or capital funding limits that have been voted by Parliament. The combination of having to make a fixed return on capital, of having to break even and of having to live within an external financing limit is more of a financial straitjacket than a financial freedom – and is meant to be such. The real freedom left in the finance field is the freedom to plan expenditure – on both capital and revenue – within these constraints, to the best effect; i.e. the freedom to be efficient. This is not as paltry a freedom as it sounds: the absence of bureaucratic constraints or requirements to go along with certain procedures imposed from above which have been found to be unhelpful or irrelevant can make trusts much more flexible and responsive in their financial control.

Break even

The first requirement on a trust board is to break even. The wording of the Act is:

> Every NHS trust shall ensure that its revenue is not less than sufficient, taking one financial year with another, to meet outgoings properly chargeable to revenue account (NHS and Community Care Act 1990 Part I Section 10(1)).

This means that, after paying all the costs of providing its services, allowing for depreciation (which counts as expenditure in the accounts although *cash* may not actually have been spent), and after paying interest and dividends, the trust must either show a surplus or at least *not* show a deficit. The accounts might look like this:

Category A income (contracts)	40	
Category B income (extracontractual referrals)	3	
Category C income (service increment for teaching and research, etc.)	7	
Total income		50
Pay expenditure	35	
Non-pay expenditure	5	
Depreciation	5	
Total expenditure		(45)
Surplus before interest		5
Interest receivable	1	
Interest payable	(3)	
		(2)
Surplus/[deficit] before extraordinary items		3
Extraordinary items (e.g. a loss on disposal of a piece of land)		Nil
Dividends on PDC		(2)
Surplus/[deficit] for period		1

This trust has thus met its first financial duty: it has broken even.

Rate of return

The second financial duty is to earn a specified rate of return on capital. Both this and the duty to live within the external financing limit are covered by the general provision in the NHS Act that:

> It shall be the duty of every NHS trust to achieve such financial objectives as may from time to time be set by the Secretary of State with the consent of the Treasury and as are applicable to it; and any such objectives may be made applicable to NHS trusts generally, or to a particular NHS trust or to NHS trusts of a particular description (NHS and Community Care Act 1990 Part I Section 10(2)).

One financial objective that is required under this provision is to earn 6% on an average of opening and closing net assets.

$$\frac{\begin{array}{c}\text{Value of what trust} \\ \text{owns} \\ \text{at beginning of year}\end{array} + \begin{array}{c}\text{Value of what trust} \\ \text{owns} \\ \text{at end of year}\end{array}}{2}$$

Of course, this means that it is not possible until after the end of the year, and after audited accounts are available, to know whether the trust met this particular duty. The point is that the trust needs to *plan* to do so, setting its prices to include a 6% return on capital and then (and this is the crucial part so far as the monitoring of financial performance is concerned) ensuring that this 6% is not 'leaked' into subsidizing the trust's ordinary revenue expenditure but remains available to meet interest payments, dividends or to form part of the trust's surplus for that year.

The importance of this is that the 6% return on capital that trusts have to charge is, unlike the capital charge for DMUs, not just a paper flow of money round a closed system. It is *real* money, charged by the trust to health authorities, which therefore has to be put into the hands of those health authorities by the Exchequer. However, except for any part of the 6% rate of return which the NHS management executive chooses to fund from its capital allocation, this 6% is *not* part of the money voted for health care – whether revenue or capital. It is simply, so far as the Treasury is concerned, a neutral flow of funds whose purpose is to inject economic realism about the costs of using capital. The Treasury expects the 6% rate of return that it funds to be matched (apart from the transfer from the NHS capital allocation mentioned above) by the payments to it of interest and dividends, plus the surplus kept by trusts which must remain in approved investments (see below). Provided all the 6% can be accounted for in this way there is no problem, but if a trust applies some of the 6% to bailing out its revenue expenditure, there will be a shortfall in the money returning to the Exchequer or remaining invested, and action will have to be taken to recover this. It may seem strange that the trust's investments are not regarded as money lost to the Exchequer but the point is that the money held by trusts in approved investments has not left the public sector.

The 6% rate of return is, inevitably, somewhat of a moving target. No one expects it to be hit spot-on. It may be a little above or a little below; it may even be significantly different without that being the responsibility of the trust. That can arise where asset values change after prices are set so that what was planned to be a 6% return becomes a higher or lower percentage. This can best be illustrated by the following example.

A trust sets its prices to recover:

$$6\% \times £\ \frac{30 + 32m}{2} = 6\% \times £31m = £1.86m$$

but land values fall and in fact average of opening and closing net assets is:

$$£\ \frac{26 + 28m}{2} = £27m$$

£1.86m is nearly 7% of £27m but since the purchasers were funded for the full £1.86m, that must be returned to the Treasury or invested and *not* spent as a windfall. In practice the likelihood is that the money will be returned to the Treasury by means of a dividend payment. It should however be noted that this does not reflect any discredit on the trust, which will not be considered to have breached a financial duty.

The 6% is meant to be an upper as well as a lower limit for NHS work, but the trust is free to charge whatever the market will bear for private work and either use this, in effect, to cross-subsidize for non-NHS work (one of the few cases where cross-subsidy is allowed), or to make a higher overall return than 6%.

External financing limit

This is the most important of the three financial duties since the NHS as a whole is accountable to Parliament for delivering the global external financing limit for the NHS. This global financing limit is made up of pluses and minuses so that any failure to meet an individual EFL affects the total.

An external financing limit is set each year for each trust by the NHS management executive. Put simply, it is a form of cash control which limits the extent to which a trust can borrow to supplement funds it generates by its own trading operations. It is probably best explained by an example:

Trust *X* sets its prices so as to obtain £40m income. This is to cover costs of £35m, depreciation of £3m and a return on assets of £2m. Out of this return, it has to meet interest payments of £1.5m and a dividend of £0.25m.

Very simplified, its accounts will show:

	£m	
Income		40
Expenditure		
Cost	35	
Depreciation	3	
Interest	1.5	
Dividend	0.25	
		(39.75)
		0.25

£0.25m is the *surplus* earned by the hospital. (In a commercial organization it would be called the *profit*.) However, depreciation is shown as expenditure in the income and expenditure account, but is not actually a cash item: its appearance in the accounts does not relate to any actual expenditure of money. The cash position of the trust is therefore different.

	£m	
Income		40
Expenditure		
Costs	35	
Interest	1.5	
Dividend	0.25	
		(36.75)
		3.25

Leaving aside working capital changes (which are dealt with below), this trust has £3.25m either to spend or invest. If it has to invest it all, it will be given a *negative* external financing unit of £3.25m (£ – 3.25m), indicating *not* that it has to return money to the centre, but that it has to invest that amount in approved securities. The list of approved securities includes government securities, local authorities, nationalized industries, building society deposits and shares, and banks. It is for trusts themselves to decide where to invest, bearing in mind the need to avoid risking public money.

If a trust wishes to spend more capital than it has generated itself, it will need a positive external financing limit so that it can borrow the difference. To take the example above, if the trust wished to fund a £10m capital development, it would need to borrow £10m *less* £3.25m, i.e. £6.75m, and would therefore have to be given a positive external financing limit of £6.75m.

If a trust sells assets it will be generating resources internally and thus lower its borrowing requirement. The sale of any asset will affect the trust's external financing limit. Those over £1m have to be approved by the Secretary of State. If the NHS management executive does not consider further capital expenditure appropriate, the proceeds of the sale can be 'locked in' to the trust by giving it a more negative external financing limit and hence requiring it to invest the proceeds.

Changes in working capital also affect the external financing limit. Working capital broadly means the capital that is tied up in stock or in the increase in debtors (from whom money is owed, hence an asset) over creditors (to whom money is owed, hence a liability). If a trust requires more working capital (e.g. because its stock levels increase or debtors rise) it will need to increase its external financing limit. The effect of this working capital position on the external financing limit is not just of mathematical interest. One of the performance indicators for financial management in the public sector is keeping creditor levels down so that the public sector is not driving small private businesses into bankruptcy by not paying bills. However, a trust that is having difficulty living within its external financing limit may want to take the easy option of stopping paying bills and letting creditor levels (normally measured in terms of weeks) rise. Members of trust boards would therefore do well to look carefully at creditor levels – bearing in mind that the public sector aims to keep them below 8 weeks.

Negative external financing levels can be used to repay debt or to build up reserves by investing money. There are special provisions that mean that paying back debt early will rarely benefit the trust, but it should be considered. All trusts have to pay back their debt, both originating and subsequent, eventually, however, and this will be reflected in their external financing limit. If they have to borrow to pay back the debt, this will have a neutral effect on their external financing limit since the payback has a negative effect and the borrowing a positive one.

If a trust finds it is in danger of breaching its external financing limit it has three real options. The first is to curtail expenditure – capital or revenue. The second is to use a permitted flexibility to overshoot its external financing limit with NHS management executive approval by up to 1% of its total turnover plus fixed asset expenditure. This additional cover will automatically be deducted from the next year's external financing limit so can only be regarded as a short-term measure. The third option is to ask the NHS management executive to arrange brokerage so that a trust that is likely to undershoot its external financing limit, in effect 're-turns' this to the centre to be handed out to an overshooting trust. The sums will simply be reversed the following year so that the over-shooting trust pays back the undershooting one. Again, therefore this is only a short-term solution. It does, however, offer a real benefit to the *under*shooting trust since undershoots of external financing levels are not otherwise carried forward. If, therefore, a capital scheme is slipping, a trust may well want to offer brokerage so that it is guaranteed the funding for the following year, and does not lose it for ever.

Borrowing

Where a trust has a positive external financing limit, it is allowed to borrow from wherever it chooses. However, trusts have an overriding duty to obtain value for money and in practice the government usually lends more cheaply than any other source. There is a loans section in the NHS management executive which arranges the loan when it is required and finance departments have full details of how to apply. An alternative is to borrow from the private sector with a government guarantee, which lowers the interest rate asked. Private finance will usually be necessary for very short-term borrowing (a night or two), when the trust may simply need to use a bank overdraft facility. They should, however, ensure that they have a guarantee to keep this as cheap as possible. If a guarantee is sought, the trust has to demonstrate that the loan offers value for money. The most important point to remember is that *all borrowing, from whatever source, is covered by the external financing limit.*

Trusts are not allowed to borrow in advance of need. They cannot, for example, borrow money from the government at one rate and then earn interest on it by investing it at a higher rate. They must therefore use their invested funds before borrowing any further items. They are also not allowed to borrow in any currency other than sterling without the consent of the Secretary of State and the Treasury. Such consent would normally only be given if there was a flow of income in that currency into the trust (e.g. from overseas patients) to remunerate the debt.

Further PDC

All borrowing subsequent to the trust's establishment is usually in the form of interest-bearing loans. Exceptionally, further borrowing may be given as PDC. This is most likely to happen where there is a major capital development being undertaken on which no rate of return will be earned while it is still in construction. The NHS management executive will consider all such cases individually in the light of that trust's financial position.

Temporary borrowing limit

Sometimes trusts need to borrow to cover temporary cash fluctuations, and these may even exceed the external financing limit cover, which is an end-of-year figure. Trusts therefore need to apply for a *temporary borrowing limit* which allows them to borrow in-year to cover these temporary cash shortages. Again, they should ensure that they apply for a guarantee where this will give them a lower rate of interest.

Capital allocations

The external financing limit is the mechanism whereby a trust's access to capital is controlled. As has been explained above, it is affected by several things, including the amount of depreciation charged by the trust, any invested surplus held by the trust, movements in working capital, repayment of debt and land disposals, and all these will be taken into consideration by the NHS management executive when it is set each year. Many of these points are quite technical and may be of little interest to most hospital staff and patients but the one issue that will interest them as external financing limits are set is the amount of capital that the trust is allowed to spend (whether borrowed or generated internally).

Again, this is set annually by the NHS management executive for each trust individually. The NHS is allocated a global amount of capital each year, which is determined as an outcome of the Public Expenditure Survey and announced in the Chancellor's autumn statement in early to mid November. During the latter part of November and early December the NHS management executive decides how to divide this capital amount between regional health authorities and trusts and then how much to give to individual trusts. Decisions about the amount given to individual trusts and to the trust sector as a whole are made on the basis of the business cases submitted to the NHS management executive. These business cases will usually be the end-product of a period of discussion with the NHS management executive, including agreeing with them the *Strategic Direction* for the trust (a formal published document produced every 3 years) and subsequently producing option appraisals of the best way of meeting the need for investment that has been identified. The record of the NHS in capital investment is not a good one: for too long the tendency has been to regard large capital expenditure as an indication of a successful hospital. The introduction of capital charges and the equivalent for trusts was intended to introduce the NHS to the discipline of regarding public sector assets as a resource that has to be paid for and accounted for and should therefore be used as efficiently as possible. If a trust has to charge 6% on the value of every asset to its purchaser, some difficult decisions have to be made, in consultation with purchasers, about whether they can afford a smart new building or whether they would prefer an existing building to be upgraded and use their purchasing power for something else. Whatever a business case provides therefore – and professional help will probably be needed in analysing options and preparing a business case for more complex and costly capital developments – it should provide evidence that purchasers are signed up to both the capital and revenue consequences of the development. The business case will also need to demonstrate that the trust can afford any borrowing required or can generate the funds internally, but this is secondary to the question of affordability to purchasers.

This is not to say that all capital decisions are taken on purely financial grounds. It is true that it may be easier to make a good business case for a scheme which has a quick pay-back (where spending capital quickly produces revenue savings that outweigh the capital expenditure). However, purchasers will also consider the non-financial value of quality improvements and may be willing to pay for this 'added value'. They will also be considering NHS management executive priorities which may, for example, encourage the provision of a new facility or more of a kind of facility quite apart from purely financial considerations.

Schemes under £1m are known as minor capital and into this category will fall most of the routine backlog maintenance and minor upgrading, of which so much of the NHS has been in such need for so long. The new capital regime is designed to encourage units to spend a higher proportion of capital in this way, which quickly produces quality improvements for patients and properly maintains public sector assets, rather than tying up limited capital resources in a few major schemes.

Once the external financing limit is set, the trust is theoretically free to manage within it, for example by shifting around sums for capital schemes. However, in practice capital expenditure is monitored quite closely, at least for schemes over £1m, since resources are tight and if money that has been allocated to one scheme on the basis of a business case is not used for that scheme, the funding for the scheme will not be supplied in a subsequent year.

Funding a major scheme frequently has implications for several years and this is understood by the NHS management executive who will, so far as the Public Expenditure Survey system allows, guarantee to continue funding for a scheme once committed.

In all areas of capital funding, trusts should work closely with both the NHS management executive outposts and their purchasers from the inception of a scheme to its delivery.

Accounts and audit

Trusts have to produce commercial-style accounts in a format laid down in the *Trust Accounts Manual* which largely follows the disclosure requirements of the Companies Act and relevant Statements of Standard Accounting Practice, and Financial Reporting Standards. These accounts are audited by auditors appointed by the Audit Commission (usually a professional firm of auditors). The National Audit Office is responsible for auditing the consolidated accounts of NHS trusts and laying them before Parliament. Both the Audit Commission and the National Audit Office may conduct value-for-money studies in trusts.

The audited accounts together with the annual report have to be presented at an annual public meeting, as well as submitted to the Secretary of State. Accounts are the corporate responsibility of the trust board, although they will be prepared by the director of finance and are the direct responsibility of the trust chief executive.

Contracts and pricing

The rules for trusts are exactly the same as for non-trusts. The prices charged to purchasers must cover the trust's costs of providing the service plus depreciation of its assets plus a 6% return on capital. DMUs charge costs plus a capital charge which covers depreciation and a 6% return on capital. This leaves only the question of whether there are certain costs associated with being a trust which could put it at a disadvantage. Non-executive members of trust boards are paid small remunerations which have to be earned from purchasers.

Functioning as an autonomous unit may well increase the management costs of a trust that was formerly run by a district health authority. Trusts are also permitted to insure against risks other than medical negligence (claims related to which have to be met by borrowing, with a consequent increase in the external financing limit) and business interruption and therefore have to meet insurance costs. In discussion with their purchasers, trusts must ensure that all these costs are recognized and funded. Where it is simply a question of a block of management moving from district to trust level, this should cause no problem. However, trusts are likely to have robust negotiations with their purchasers, who will expect to see the benefits of trust status in increased efficiency which may at least in part outweigh these extra costs.

Business plans

A basic planning tool for every trust is its annual business plan, in which it sets out its management agenda for the year ahead. Business planning is a continuous process and one to which any lively trust will need to devote considerable management time to ensure that it is responding to its purchasers' requirements as efficiently as possible.

Each trust needs to take stock periodically of where it is going and its strategy for getting there. In discussion with its purchasers it needs to be clear about any major changes that are required or major developments in terms of the services it provides and how and where it provides them. Trusts are required to produce these *Strategic Directions* every 3 years and submit them to the NHS management executive for agreement that they are sensible and tie in with the NHS management executive's broader understanding of the NHS market and national and local priorities. The *Strategic Direction* should cover the next 5 years in some detail and the following 5 in outline. Once the NHS management executive has given its approval to publish, the *Strategic Direction* then becomes a public document.

It will be updated each year in an annual business plan which the trust has to submit to the NHS management executive by the end of 31 October of the financial year before that to which the plan relates. The plan has to be finalized by the end of the following February, by which time contracts should virtually be finalized and the external financing limit will have been set. Given the *Strategic Direction*, the contracts and the external financing limit, the annual business plan will almost write itself: it will be a brief management agenda of its priorities for the year and how it will achieve these. A summary of the plan is published once the NHS management executive has agreed that it is a sensible business plan for the year.

Monitoring and accountability

Performance of the trust's financial duties is carefully monitored by the NHS management executive. The considerable management freedoms enjoyed by trusts are predicated on their observing their three statutory financial duties:

1 to break even;
2 to earn 6% on capital;
3 to live within their external financing limit.

At least every quarter, and for some trusts every month, a trust has to submit to the NHS management executive a set of financial tables reporting on its financial performance in that quarter or month and its projected outcome for the year. Returns have to be submitted no later than 15 working days after the end of the period to which they relate.

The returns are analysed by the NHS management executive and any queries on them raised at an appropriate level with trust management. Returns which show that the trust is in danger of not meeting its financial duties are taken extremely seriously and taken up with the chair and chief executive of the board by an appropriate level in the NHS management executive. There are sanctions available to the NHS management executive – board members can be replaced or even a trust dissolved – but in practice the NHS management executive will normally offer advice and support as the trust takes the necessary management action to rectify the problem. In some cases there may be an issue for the NHS management executive to explore with the purchaser – not to bail the trust out but to ensure that the market is working as effectively as possible.

When trusts were first established their line of accountability was direct to the NHS management executive in Whitehall. With the growing number of trusts, this proved impractical and six outposts of the NHS management executive were established around the country, each covering two or three regions, to undertake the NHS management executive's role in monitoring trusts and dealing with business plans and capital allocations. Trusts can expect a good deal of routine contact with the outposts as part of the monitoring process but are still free to manage themselves in the most appropriate way to deliver their agreed objectives.

4.3 Capital charging

Rob Peters

Background

In common with all organizations, the NHS needs to acquire and use a mixture of consumable and durable (or capital) items. Within the NHS the range, volume and value of capital assets are vast. However, the accounting methodology for capital expenditure within the NHS before 1991 was wholly inappropriate to deal with this. The methodology failed to record the volume and value of capital assets held; it failed to recognize the consumption of capital assets and, most importantly, provided no incentives for good management of those assets. Indeed, it was possible to recognize perverse incentives which appeared to encourage poor management decisions. The most significant of these perverse incentives was that the majority of capital expenditure was funded from resources outside the direct control of local managers. Thus it was possible to develop plans to spend large sums of capital (the responsibility of someone else) in order to save minor sums within revenue budgets controlled locally.

These failings in the system led to an environment in which capital, both existing and proposed additions, was widely regarded as a free good.

During the 1980s numerous reports had highlighted the inadequacies in the system and the related poor performance in management of assets. These reports exhorted managers to take more responsibility for capital assets and suggested various changes to accounting arrangements which might be introduced to encourage progress. Whilst some health authorities took an initiative in reviewing their use of capital assets, it was apparent that the situation would not significantly alter without action by the Department of Health to implement fundamental revisions to accounting and funding procedures.

The wide-ranging reforms to health service management introduced in April 1991 were partly designed to make health authorities more business-like in their approach to the provision of health care. This package of reforms offered an ideal opportunity for a thorough revision of all NHS accounting arrangements, including those for capital expenditure. Thus, as part of these reforms, a system of capital charging was implemented to introduce a normal commercial discipline of charging for the use of capital assets.

Objectives

The primary objective of the capital charging scheme was to ensure that managers recognized that the possession of capital assets has a cost and that action on acquisitions, disposals and usage has a direct impact on that cost. This objective would be achieved by requiring managers to pay a direct charge based on the volume and value of assets under their control. There were two subsidiary objectives. First, the scheme would provide a comprehensive record of all fixed assets held within the NHS. This will be of considerable benefit both locally and centrally for a variety of purposes. At a local level the availability of a comprehensive asset record should bring benefits in assigning responsibility for assets, security, ensuring safe and optimum usage of the assets and preparing plans for replacements at appropriate times. The availability of a comprehensive database of NHS capital assets at a central level for the first time should enable the Department of Health to assess far more accurately the needs for and timing of additional resources for capital expenditure. More rational assessment of needs at both local and central level will of course not automatically bring forth additional resources. However the availability of the information does enable a reasoned case to be presented.

The second subsidiary objective was to ensure that all statements of the costs of health services within the NHS were comprehensive, in that they reflected the costs of using capital; this had previously been omitted from all cost information.

The market for health services being introduced as part of the wide-ranging reforms, of course envisaged the purchase (by health authorities and general practitioner fundholders (GPFHs)) of services from NHS trusts, directly managed units (DMUs) and the private sector. For this market to operate it was essential that the cost base of all providers was consistent. The private sector already reflected the cost of capital within overall costs and thus, to be comparable, cost constructions for the NHS needed to be altered. The capital charging scheme introduced provided a cost basis comparable with the private sector, although it must be said that alternative systems could have achieved this objective.

The capital charging scheme

Asset registers

The first requirement for the introduction and operation of the scheme was for the construction of comprehensive asset registers for each hospital and other health care facility. In the interests of consistency and comparability, instructions were issued to health authorities explaining which assets should be regarded as durable goods and recorded as fixed assets for this purpose. As additional assets are acquired after introduction of the scheme, the existence of those assets and their recording in an asset register will be an automatic process. However, at the time of introduction of the scheme, the NHS had vast numbers of assets which had been acquired over many years but had never been properly recorded. Asset registers are required to include all land and buildings and all durable equipment. For administrative simplicity it is appropriate to exclude from the scheme those assets which, whilst technically of a durable nature, have a value too low to justify the effort involved in maintaining records in this way. Initially this minimum figure was set at £1000; this is a purely arbitrary figure which can be easily altered and was raised to £5000 in 1993. Construction of the initial asset registers was completed by mid 1990 and this revealed that across the NHS in England alone, almost 2 million separate assets had been recorded.

NHS authorities are required to maintain these asset registers to reflect acquisition disposals and other changes and the asset registers will be subject to verification by auditors.

Valuation

The capital charges payable under the scheme relate directly to the valuation of assets and it is thus essential that consistent methods of valuation are operated across the NHS. The capital charging scheme is based on current valuations of assets. These current valuations are based on the original acquisition price of assets uplifted, by an index, to reflect changes in monetary values over time. The current gross value of assets is then reduced (depreciated) to reflect the reduction in worth of the assets caused by passage of time or usage and the resultant net value forms the basis on which the capital charges are calculated. At the introduction of the scheme the NHS of course had vast numbers of assets, the values of which had not been recorded at all. In the interests of consistency, instructions were issued to health authorities concerning the method of valuation for those assets. The valuation of land and buildings is a complex task which requires the input of specialists. The initial valuation of all NHS land and buildings was therefore undertaken by district valuers working under the guidance of the chief valuer's office of the Inland Revenue. To ensure that the recorded values of land and buildings remain in line with movements in property markets, it is intended that the NHS estate will be subject to revaluation by district valuers every 3 or 5 years. When the initial asset registers for the NHS were completed in mid 1990, it was revealed that the current net value of all assets recorded in England alone exceeded £25b (at 1990 values). The gross replacement value of these assets would clearly have been considerably in excess of this figure.

Capital charges

The capital charge (i.e. the new cost item) has two separate components: depreciation and interest. Each of these figures is calculated by reference to the current value of assets held by a hospital. Depreciation is an accounting concept which is designed to reflect the consumption or wearing-out of the value of an asset. This consumption may be due to the passage of time or usage or a combination of both. Within the NHS capital charging scheme, depreciation is measured by reference to the passage of time and is based on standard asset lives for equipment and remaining lives, as assessed by district valuers for buildings. The use of standard asset lives was intended to produce some consistency across the NHS in rates of depreciation. As local managers develop knowledge about the actual rates of depreciation (based on the maintenance of asset registers), it is likely that discretion will be allowed to vary these standard lives at local level. There is no depreciation charge on land as this is deemed to have an infinite life.

The interest component of capital charges is designed to represent a rate of return on capital used. An alternative view of the interest charge is as an 'opportunity cost'; resources within the NHS (as elsewhere) are limited and capital used in one place cannot be used elsewhere. The interest rate for the capital charging scheme was initially set at 6% per annum. A common misunderstanding concerning the scheme relates to the size of this interest charge. It has been claimed that this is an unrealistically low figure when compared with typical commercial interest rates. However, typical interest rates include an element reflecting the effects of inflation as well as a rate of return. The interest charge within the capital charging scheme is based on asset values which have already been increased (by indexation) to reflect the effects of inflation and the required rate of return is therefore not a direct comparator with typical rates of commercial interest.

The depreciation and interest charges are calculated each quarter by reference to the current value of assets held at the end of the accounting quarter. The sum calculated is payable to the host regional health authority and appears as a cost of a department in exactly the same way as all other costs.

Payments and funding arrangements

To enable hospitals to meet this additional cost (capital charge), funds available to district health authorities for the purchase of health care services have been increased initially by an amount similar in total to the sum of the capital charges estimated to be payable. In the first years of the scheme these additional funds have been allocated to district health authorities broadly to match the additional costs which it is expected they will incur from their local providers. This cycle of payment and funding has been widely misunderstood but is easily illustrated diagrammatically (Fig. 4.3.1).

The primary aim in the early years of the system is to introduce and perfect the mechanics of the system. It was intended that the first year would have a broadly neutral effect, i.e. individual health authorities and hospitals would neither gain nor lose as a consequence of the system.

A key principle of the system is that the allocation of resources from regional to district health authorities (2 in Fig. 4.3.1) is one sum which can be used at the discretion of the district health authority. This allocation should not distinguish between resources available to meet the capital charges element of provider costs and other costs.

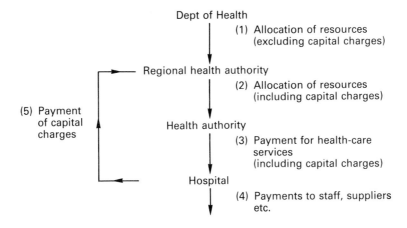

Fig. 4.3.1 Cycle of payment and funding.

This basic mechanism does allow for redistributive effects between regions, districts and hospitals to be introduced. It also allows scope for the Department of Health to alter the balance of costs within the NHS between those relating to retention and usage of capital assets and all others. Redistributive effects between health authorities and hospitals will inevitably occur very quickly after the first year of the system as a consequence of operation of the market. However it remains unclear when the Department of Health might begin to alter the balance between capital and other costs.

NHS trusts

The capital charging scheme was designed to operate for DMUs. However, there is a clear intention that the number of hospitals and other units moving to NHS trust status will accelerate over a few years. The financial arrangements for NHS trusts have therefore been designed to produce the same cost effects and incentives as the capital charging scheme for DMUs. The essential difference is that the depreciation and interest (referred to in NHS trusts as the rate of return) charges are not paid over to the regional health authority, as is the case with DMUs. These funds are instead retained within the NHS trust as a means of sourcing future capital expenditure and meeting charges on loans to the NHS trust. The methods of calculating depreciation and interest charges as they affect individual managers are identical for NHS trusts and DMUs. The effects on costing and pricing of services are equally identical. Managers within all units, whether NHS trusts or DMUs, thus have the same incentives within the system. The funding system makes provision for the fact that capital charges are not paid to regional health authorities by NHS trusts but will be reflected in prices charged to health authorities.

Incentives

All service managers will incur a cost for the capital assets which they use. If additional assets are acquired, the cost will increase. If the quantity (and value) of assets is reduced or if assets are used more extensively (i.e. the cost is spread over more activity) the cost to managers will reduce. Savings which arise from this reduction will be available to utilize in other ways. The way in which savings or additional costs consequent upon changes in volume or usage of capital assets are managed within individual hospitals (and other units) will be a matter for local determination, as with other items of cost.

In time it is intended that allocation of funds to district health authorities (including the new provision for costs of capital) will be by reference to the weighted capitation funding formula. This formula will distribute the total resources available for health care nationally (including costs of capital) proportionate to resident populations weighted for factors such as age and assessed health needs. It is intended that the formula will afford protection to those areas which unavoidably incur higher costs of capital, due to factors such as high land values in central London. However, the basic intention is to ensure that managers have equitable access to capital assets as well as to all other resources.

Summary

The objectives and basic accounting mechanisms for the capital charging scheme are relatively simple. However, the scheme was a fundamental change in accounting arrangements for the NHS and its introduction was not without some initial problems. It was inevitable that initially the efforts of most managers were focused on implementing the mechanics of the scheme. It is appropriate and inevitable that over time some of the technicalities of the scheme will be refined in order to improve the administration of the scheme. However the capital charging scheme is only of value if it encourages different managerial attitudes to capital assets. Whilst there have been examples of the scheme having the desired impact, much more attention is required to this aspect of the subject. The capital charging scheme has ensured that use of assets is at least on the agenda for management. It is important that development and operation of the scheme do not concentrate on administration of the scheme to the detriment of achieving real progress in asset management.

4.4 Mission statements and business plans

Frank Burns

The case for business planning

The terms mission statements and business plans have not captured the imagination of most clinical colleagues. To many doctors such terms are part of the language of the new breed of manager employed by the government of the day to inflict the latest managerial fad on the NHS's hard-pressed professionals.

Although many senior clinicians are now actively embracing management responsibilities, others feel that managers and management processes are intruding detrimentally and unnecessarily into the day-to-day world of hospital medicine. Such doctors may argue that managerial concepts are all right in their proper place but should not be allowed to interfere in the real business of the hospital – the treatment of patients. After all, they might argue, hasn't the effective separation of clinical and managerial processes maintained some sort of uneasy peace in the NHS throughout its recent history?

Such a view, of course, ignores the painful reality of a cash-limited public health service in which health authorities, on behalf of the government, the tax-payer and the wider public, are exercising an increasingly sophisticated control over the delivery of health care. This influence of 'management' over the work of health care practitioners will continue to strengthen and develop irrespective of which particular political philosophy is the dominant influence on policy. Whether through some kind of internal market or through detailed central planning, the aggressive pursuit of value for money in health care is firmly on the agenda.

The business planning process is the mechanism which most private and public sector organizations use to determine and pursue their medium-term service or business goals and is not, of course, the intimidating and vaguely threatening instrument of management control that some may believe it to be. Business planning is in fact a vitally important mechanism through which practising clinicians can exercise their considerable influence over the particular part of the health service in which they work.

Life in a hospital, or in a department of a hospital, is constantly and inevitably subject to internal and external influences which produce a constantly changing working environment. No hospital, department or individual practitioner is immune from these influences.

In summary, therefore, the business planning process embodies a recognition that hospitals and the professional staff who work in them need a mechanism for articulating and developing their ambitions and for responding to the changes in their external environment which are promoting or inhibiting these aspirations.

For a hospital, or a part of a hospital, to have any hope of succeeding in the achievement of its goals requires the active and enthusiastic commitment of senior clinical staff to the business planning process. This commitment to embrace change becomes the difference between making things happen or being surprised (and often disappointed) by unpredicted and unexpected events.

Inevitably – as is the case with most professions – health service managers and the burgeoning corporate management consultancies have infected simple planning concepts with an impenetrable cloak of jargon and 'management speak'. The following paragraphs represent an earnest attempt to demystify business planning processes through the use of language and examples which may be recognizable to clinicians.

Prerequisites for successful business planning processes

Clinicians will, of course, be familiar with the various approaches to, and benefits arising from, the medical audit process. A recurring theme in much of the recent debates about medical audit has been the need to avoid 'cook book' medicine through the use of rigidly applied standard treatment regimes. The conventional wisdom around medical audit requires commitment to, and involvement in, the process by individual practitioners and a willingness to change practice in the light of audit findings. In other words, audit should become an essential and integral part of the clinical process and not some form of 'bolt-on extra'.

The same can equally be said of business planning processes. In a hospital situation there simply cannot be an effective business planning process without the continuous commitment and involvement of the leading health care professionals – the doctors.

Clearly, if medical staff are to have any significant input to planning processes then their input needs to be channelled into areas of service in which they have an influence and an interest. This requirement can be more readily facilitated if the business planning process is applied to individual specialties and departments. Such an approach allows in turn the involvement in business planning discussions of all the different professions and services that contribute to the services provided by the department or specialty concerned.

By making business planning a specialty-based activity, not only can more people be involved but the process is much more relevant to them. The involvement of a wide spectrum of people in discussing the future of services in which they have a direct and personal interest is an absolute prerequisite to the success of the business planning process. Given that these processes succeed more readily when they utilize established managerial and organizational structures, it can be seen how readily the clinical directorate model of management lends itself to the principles of business planning for clinical services.

A fundamental advantage of using the clinical directorate as the main vehicle for business planning is the availability in a mature directorate of a strong managerial infrastructure led by an influential clinical director and including business or information managers as well as clinical managers and specialist accountants. Successful business planning at the specialty or directorate level requires this marriage of clinical ambition with managerial pragmatism. The collaborative working at directorate level of doctors, mana-

gers, accountants, nurses and other professional staff is much more likely to produce a realistic plan for the future than would be the case if one group was planning in isolation.

The stages of business planning

Again, business planning involves a cycle of activity, not entirely dissimilar to that used in medical audit. The standard audit cycle involves an initial observation of current practice, followed by agreement amongst the relevant professionals of an appropriate treatment standard. The audit itself involves the comparison of actual practice against the agreed standard and the introduction of changes to practice, where necessary, to conform with the standard. Medical audit is, of course, a continuous process requiring frequent adjustment to agreed standards as knowledge and practice change within the medical profession.

So too business planning is a continuous cycle in which service goals and objectives are constantly reviewed and adjusted in the light of knowledge, circumstances and experience. This use of the audit cycle to illustrate the cyclical nature of business planning is perhaps particularly appropriate as not infrequently it is changes in clinical practice that fuel changes in service delivery. As a simple example of this, the impact of minimally invasive surgery on the organization of hospital surgical services over the next few years is likely to be profound.

The planning cycle, therefore, has much the same stages as the audit cycle and these are set out in full in Figure 4.4.1 below, in which formal business planning terminology is given, together with simple explanations of the process involved. The framework is described in a way that would be applicable equally to a whole hospital, to a particular clinical directorate or even to a department within a directorate. For the remainder of this chapter business planning will be discussed in the context of a clinical directorate.

As will be seen, the business planning cycle has seven distinct phases, each of which offers a major opportunity to involve key directorate staff in making a personal and positive contribution to shaping the future direction of the service. Essentially the process is a sequential refinement of a broad service ambition to a sharply honed set of personal objectives for key

Formal stages	Explanation
1 Define the *mission* and core purpose of the service concerned	Define in precise terms the extent and nature of the service to be provided in terms of the ultimate and overall service goal
2 Undertake a *SWOT* analysis (strengths, weaknesses, opportunities and threats)	Examine actual and potential capability to achieve the ultimate service goal. This process may result in some modification of the mission
3 Set *major service goals*	Identify specific major service goals necessary for the achievement of the mission (normally covering 3 years)
4 Devise *service strategies*	These will be clinical, managerial and organizational policies designed to effect movement towards major service goals
5 Agree operational and personal *objectives*	These will be specific short-term objectives (normally within 1 year) which are directly related to achievement of major service goals
6 *Monitor* performance	Assess achievement of long-term goals and short-term objectives against the business plan
7 *Review* the plan	This would be done annually with a reassessment of 3-year goals and renewal of 1-year objectives

Fig. 4.4.1 The business planning cycle.

directorate staff. Each of the business planning stages can now be dealt with in turn.

The mission statement

First and foremost, it has to be acknowledged that managers as well as clinicians have some difficulty with the notion of mission and core purpose. Like clinicians, managers spend the greater part of their professional life trying to cope with an ever more demanding set of problems in an ever more difficult environment.

Clinicians, however, as well as managers, must recognize that their failure in the past to find time to look ahead will have helped to create the difficult circumstances in which they find themselves today.

It is simply not good enough to thrash around in the water with the sole objective of keeping afloat. Both managers and clinicians must occasionally raise their heads and establish the quickest way to dry land. Many doctors and many managers think that the core purpose or the mission of a clinical directorate (or even of a hospital) is patently self-evident. The experience of groups of professionals who have sat down to agree a succinct statement of the purpose of their service or department suggests this is not in fact the case. In fact there are any number of variations on the theme.

Whilst of course the mission of everybody in the hospital service is to provide the very best service for their particular patient, we immediately find that the very best is constrained by available resources which cannot be ignored. So we see that immediately the mission must be framed in the context of what is ultimately achievable. Mission is of course fundamentally shaped by the nature of the service to be provided. For example, a paediatric department will have a very different mission from an adult surgical department, given the importance of heavy emphasis on family involvement. Equally, a university hospital will recognize its teaching and research responsibilities in its mission statement compared with that, say, of a district hospital.

The fact of the matter is that the only worthwhile statement of core purpose or mission is one that has been specifically thought through by the people who are daily involved in the particular service to which it relates. The sacrifice, for this purpose, of half a day by the key professional staff in a directorate or department is more than repaid by the energy and clarity of purpose achieved through an open and honest debate designed to achieve a statement of core purpose or mission which encapsulates both a sense of direction and an ultimate goal for the people concerned.

It may all appear theoretical but it's undoubtedly better to make an attempt to define a mission than to continue or embark on a journey with little conscious thought of ultimate destination.

To demonstrate the potential power of a mission statement let us consider the following example.

> The Blankshire Hospital exists to provide a comprehensive range of efficient, high-quality health care services to the people of Blankshire and adjacent communities in a patient-centred environment which respects and rewards the skills of the staff.

If that particular hospital believes its mission statement then it has set for itself a number of significant and demanding goals as follows:

1 A comprehensive range of services.
2 Efficient and cost-effective services.
3 A patient-centred approach.
4 A highly valued and well-motivated workforce.

It will be no accident that this particular hospital makes reference in its mission statement to a comprehensive range of services and excludes reference to centres of excellence. This is clearly because the hospital concerned regards itself as the local district general hospital and values access by local residents to a comprehensive range of hospital services more highly than the development of particular expertise.

For completeness and to illustrate the relevance of mission statements at directorate level, the full version of the paediatric directorate mission statement referred to earlier is as follows:

> The paediatric directorate exists to serve the health needs of the children of the locality in relation to the acutely sick child under the age of 16 years. It aims to produce a personalized, accessible and high-quality service in the most appropriate way, maintaining the family unity at all times.

Neither of the mission statements referred to is offered as a perfect working model. They merely serve to illustrate the application of the concept.

The SWOT analysis

The concept is simple and involves no more than an honest analysis of the strengths, weaknesses, opportunities and threats facing a particular service or department and which must be taken into account in the business planning/objective setting process.

A clinical directorate engaged in any serious attempt to agree and influence the future pattern of service must at the outset recognize those internal and external factors which will have an influence on its plans. Given that the production of the mission statement has produced a broad indication of where the directorate is trying to get to, the SWOT analysis will identify those factors in the internal and external environment which have a bearing on the development of realistic service objectives.

A detailed analysis of this type takes considerable time, effort and openness on the part of those concerned. None the less, the involvement of key professionals in the department or directorate concerned in this kind of appraisal can be of enormous benefit. The process of mapping in detail the service development objectives and opportunities in the context of the external threats and internal deficiencies provides an ideal vehicle for interprofessional team building.

A brief and somewhat incomplete list of the issues that would need to be addressed in a SWOT analysis is given in Figure 4.4.2

External factors

Size of population served

Age and sex structure of the population served

Mobility and socioeconomic circumstances of surrounding centres of population

Morbidity in the population

Potential demand for service (e.g. comparison of actual and expected hospitalization rates)

Existence of other providers

Comparative efficiency against other providers

National service priorities

Regional service priorities

District service priorities

General practitioner attitudes

New medical technologies

Internal factors

Current range of professional skills and clinical interests

Age profile of professional staff

Current levels of efficiency

Utilization of facilities

Management capacity

Staff commitment

Staff morale

Current financial situation

Staff attitudes to patients

Staff attitudes to each other

Fig. 4.4.2 Issues for SWOT analysis.

In the end, the SWOT analysis will assist a department or directorate in taking realistic decisions about service development intentions whilst at the same time identifying those factors in the external and internal environment which need to be tackled to facilitate the achievement of the planned service goals.

Setting major service goals

So far in this business planning cycle we have identified our ultimate service goal (mission or core purpose) and we have also taken a long hard look at our own capabilities and at the external environment in which we have to operate. Inevitably, the mission or long-term service goal will generate a number of specific and major goals which must now be articulated distinctly and clearly as we begin to build up a more specific agenda for action. This particular section is best illustrated by example, so let us take the example of a general surgical directorate in a hospital whose mission statement might well read as follows:

> This directorate exists to provide a comprehensive range of efficient, high-quality general surgical services to the population of Blankshire through a highly motivated and caring workforce.

Obviously the above mission statement, although very broad, does encapsulate some major challenges, especially if the SWOT analysis revealed for example the following:

1 Staff morale is currently low.
2 Other providers appear more efficient.
3 The special interests of the existing general surgeons exclude vascular surgery and paediatric surgery.
4 The department has no accredited urologist.
5 Other providers are actively courting local general practitioners on the basis of higher quality and lower costs.

In these circumstances this directorate might well agree the following as its *major service goals* to be achieved over a 3-year period.

1 To become the sole provider of non-tertiary general surgery to the local (defined) population.
2 To become a major provider of non-tertiary general surgery to a particular neighbouring population.
3 To develop a centre of excellence in the management of breast disease (to reflect high levels of existing cross-boundary referrals).
4 To raise the level of staff satisfaction within the directorate to above 75% on key survey measures.
5 To raise the level of patient satisfaction with the service provided to above 90% on key survey measures.

At first glance it might appear that whilst this directorate has set major goals which align exactly with its mission statement, it then seems to have disregarded the adverse factors identified in the SWOT analysis. In fact this is not the case as it is both inevitable and essential that major goals will incorporate action to overcome the deficiencies identified in the SWOT analysis where this is a realistic possibility. Equally, major services goals should not be pursued if they are manifestly unattainable in the prevailing circumstances. In this particular case it is possible to speculate about major service goals which may have been excluded, viz:

1 No reference has been made to the development of private facilities, presumably on the basis that the local private hospital is too strongly established.
2 No reference is made to the development of new surgical facilities, presumably on the grounds that present facilities are adequate and that the capital charges of major new investment may exacerbate already adverse cost differentials.
3 The development of a supradistrict service is confined to one narrow area of surgery where there is an existing strength.

In summary, therefore, major service goals should be fully aligned with the mission statement and must be within the compass of the directorate to achieve, given a collective determination to overcome the factors which might otherwise prevent their achievement. This in fact is the essence of business planning in that service goals are set and pursued only where they are consistent with the agreed core purpose of the service concerned and where their achievement is a practical possibility which has been properly assessed through a full examination of all the relevant factors.

Even so, we need to refine the process beyond the mere setting of major medium-term goals.

Agreeing strategies and setting operational objectives

Continuing with our example of the general surgical directorate, we now need to take individual major service goals and determine strategies and operational (or short-term) objectives which will result in their achievement.

If we take as our example the first major goal of our mythical surgical directorate, viz: 'To become the sole provider of non-tertiary general surgery to the local population', a number of different *strategies* will be required to bring this about, e.g.:

1 Extend the range of general surgical interests.
2 Improve outpatient and inpatient waiting times.
3 Reduce unit costs per case.
4 Consolidate and improve relationships with general practitioners.
5 Consolidate and improve relationships with the local community.
6 Improve service delivery quality.

In relation to each of these strategies we need to agree specific operational objectives achieveable normally within the time frame of a single year and for which key individuals within the directorate might be held personally accountable. Again, taking a number of the broad strategy areas in turn, we may set the following operational objectives (Fig. 4.4.3).

Similarly, strategies and operational objectives should be established in respect of each of the major service objectives. By way of a further brief example we can look at the service objective which targets significant improvement in levels of staff satisfaction.

The strategies we may employ in this particular case would be:

1 Improve internal communications.
2 Facilitate the empowerment and involvement of the workforce in directorate decisions.
3 Give a higher priority to training and postgraduate education.
4 Provide better staff facilities.
5 Improve terms and conditions of service.
6 Give prompt recognition for achievements.

Again, for each of those broad strategies it would be necessary to agree detailed operational objectives, for instance, in the area of improving communications one objective could be to introduce a directorate newsletter. In the area of training and education a specific target may be set in relation to the numbers of enrolled nurses allowed to do the registered general nurse conversion course.

When this process of converting major service goals to strategies and strategies to operational objectives is completed, all the individual operational objectives must be allocated as the personal responsibility of a senior manager or professional within the directorate. Only at this

Strategy

Improve outpatient and inpatient waiting times to a maximum of 13 weeks and 1 year respectively

Reduce unit costs per case to within 5% of the lowest for the region

Operational objectives

Increase numbers of new patients seen in surgical outpatient clinics by 10%

Set up pooled referrals for simple common conditions

Increase throughput in the surgical day unit to the level of the regional average

Negotiate and carry out waiting list initiatives to deal with 750 routine cases at the back of inpatient lists

Absorb additional throughput without additional staff

Audit lengths of stay for the top five conditions by volume

Reorganize elective inpatient beds to create a 5-day ward

Review nursing skill mix

Fig. 4.4.3 Operational objectives in relation to specific strategies.

stage have we fully established a clear and effective link between the personal objectives of key directorate staff and the long-term goals of the directorate. This linking of action to aspirations is at the heart of the business planning process. Figure 4.4.3 shows the whole process diagramatically.

Performance monitoring

We must now make certain that these operational objectives are pursued and achieved by the individuals concerned, which brings us to the next stage in the process.

When the clinical director has agreed detailed operational objectives with senior professional and managerial colleagues (including all the consultant staff), these then become that directorate's business agenda for the year in question. It now

becomes vital to allocate individual responsibility for the achievement of particular objectives.

It will have been necessary for the clinical director and team to have acquired approval through negotiation from the hospital chief executive and the management board for the major service goals and the annual operational objectives. Just as the chief executive of the hospital will review the progress of the clinical director and colleagues in achieving these objectives, so must the clinical director review the progress within the directorate.

For this process to be effective it requires the clinical director (or head of department) to agree with individual managers and other senior colleagues a set of operational objectives for which they will be held accountable. This agreement should be explicit, quantifiable and encapsulated within a formal written statement of personal objectives for the person concerned. If ultimately the accountability for the delivery of a directorate's or department's medium-or short-term objectives cannot be pinned down on individuals, then the business planning process will end up as an enormous paper exercise.

Equally, if individuals are not held to account for the achievement of these personal objectives by some form of individual performance review, then the business planning process will fail at the very point of implementation.

Reviewing and agreeing the business plan

Clearly, the process of producing a directorate business plan must be fully integrated into the business planning mechanism for the hospital as a whole. In previous years this process in the NHS has been top-down and has been typified by the production of detailed planning documents at district and hospital level with no real, if any, actual involvement of practising clinicians and professionals. Such plans have inevitably failed to materialize in any significant way, as will be the fate of any business plan which has not been written and is not owned by the people who have to deliver it.

In almost all circumstances, if individual directorates do the job properly then hospital business planning will become a genuine bottom-up process and plans will be produced which properly reflect the aspirations and capabilities of the hospital's professional staff. In such an environment it should be neither necessary nor possible for central hospital management to impose their own view of the world on the different clinical departments. The NHS must shake off the legacy of past planning processes which have seen managers and planning bureaucrats fill the vacuum created by the persistent refusal of clinical and professional staff to take an active and realistic interest in their own futures.

The chief executive of the hospital, together with the management board, has a responsibility to pull together all of the different directorate business plans into a single hospital business plan. The chief executive and the hospital board will be a major influence on directorate business plans in two particular respects.

Firstly it is inevitable that the directorate's view of the world, however carefully they ad-

dress the stages of the business planning process, will be tested in negotiation with the chief executive officer and team. The chief executive will want to subject directorate business plans to a searching examination, especially in relation to current resource utilization, against the case for directorate service objectives which require investment of additional resources. This process of challenging, testing and advising on the directorate's business plan is essentially positive and ties the chief executive and the hospital board personally to the objectives which are ultimately agreed.

The second major area in which the hospital chief executive and the hospital board would be influential is in the area of prioritizing new investments. However strong individual directorate business plans may be, there will never be sufficient new resources available to finance all of those aspirations which require additional finance and as a consequence the hospital will have to make investment choices. This crucial process of weaving together individual directorate business plans into a corporate hospital business plan will be greatly assisted by the use of the business planning framework described in this chapter.

In order to ensure that the corporate hospital business plan is not regarded as a centrally imposed alternative to the aggregation of individual directorate plans, it is vital that the chief executive of the hospital involves the clinical directors collectively in fleshing out a corporate business plan.

A new and ultimately powerful planning cycle is thus created. The hospital's business plan draws very substantially on the aspirations expressed in directorate business plans and in turn directorate business plans must take account of the hospital-wide service objectives that have been collectively agreed with clinical directors.

The planning timetable

From a standing start it would take a clinical directorate or hospital department months to move comprehensively and in sufficient detail through all the seven stages of business planning. At the end of this period the directorate should have agreed with central hospital management a mission statement, a set of major service objectives and a detailed set of operational objectives to be achieved in the first year of the 3-year cycle.

In the NHS the planning period equates to the financial year and commences on 1 April. During year 1 of a 3-year plan, the directorate will be actively involved in implementing the current year's operational objectives and developing a modified 3-year plan to begin on the following 1 April. Towards the end of the current year, operational objectives for the first year of the new 3-year plan will also need to be agreed in detail.

Business planning is a continuous cycle of rolling plans. Adjustment of 3-year plans on an annual basis allows the flexibility and adaptability which is essential in the constantly changing environment of the NHS. The renewal and active pursuit of short-term objectives on an annual basis ensure, however, that forward momentum towards service goals and the service mission is maintained at all times.

4.5 Service contracts (including case mix analysis)

Karin Lowson

Introduction

Separating the responsibility for purchasing and providing health care is an important plank of the White Paper *Caring for People*. The purchasing role is to ensure that, within available resources, services are identified and secured for the health needs of the resident population. The provider role is to deliver the health care so identified within health care units.

In the specification of services for the resident population, purchasers will distinguish between:

1 *Core services* – services to which patients will have guaranteed local access, and for which there are not necessarily local alternatives, such as accident and emergency services, or maternity services.
2 *Non-core services* – for which purchasers can exercise choice, such as elective orthopaedic surgery.

By and large, purchaser units will identify the parameters within which providers are to deliver the services, for example the quality and quantity specifications. Purchasers and providers enter into service contracts, which will set out these specifications. The contracting process is shown in Figure 4.5.1.

External service contracts

External service contracts will therefore be the norm between all service provider organizations and all purchaser organizations.

Providers can be directly managed units (DMUs) or trusts and can be organizations providing solely acute care, solely community and longer-term care, or the totality of care, as in trusts which cover whole district services.

Purchasers can be a district health authority (DHA) a consortium of DHAs, general practi-

tioner fundholders (GPFHs), or even private hospitals.

Figure 4.5.2 outlines the areas that are specified in a typical contract:

There are three types of contracts:

1 *Block contracts*, in which the purchaser's residents have access to services from the provider, within a defined range of services and limited volume specifications.
2 *Cost and volume contracts*, in which a specified number of cases will be treated for a specified price.
3 *Cost per case contracts*, in which treatment is paid for as each case presents.

Those patients not covered by contracts are known as extracontractual referrals, and will be paid for on a cost per case basis. For any purchaser and provider, the quantity and case mix of these patients are unpredictable.

Costing issues

The setting of contracts, together with the increasing attempts to define more clearly the products of the NHS, hinge very much around the issues of costing and pricing.

Contracts are based on prices agreed between the purchaser and the provider; these prices are calculated in accordance with Department of Health guidance:

1 Prices should be based on costs.
2 Prices should be calculated, as far as possible, on a full cost basis; marginal costing is only allowed where there is spare capacity for a short term.
3 There should be no planned cross-subsidization.

Costing and budgeting

It is important to distinguish between costing and budgeting:

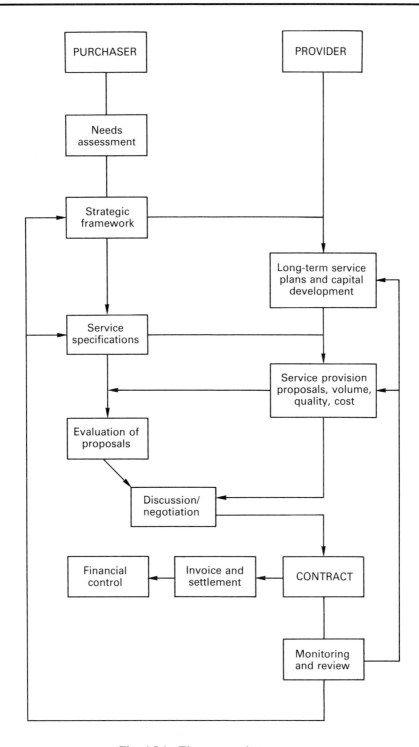

Fig. 4.5.1 The contracting process.

1 *Costs* relate to the loss in value when a resource is used.

2 *Budgets* are quantifications of future costs of planned courses of action over specified time limits.

Typical Contract
Contract for Services to elderly people
provided by
Very General Hospital Trust

Contents

Memorandum of contract
- With signatures on behalf of all parties

Conditions of contract
Containing 18 conditions, each summarized within the contract
- Purpose of contract
- Services to be provided
- Contract period
- Modifications
- Confidentiality
- Statutory requirements
- Indemnity
- Payment
- Fluctuations
- Assignment and subcontracting
- Control and monitoring
- Default and termination
- Arbitration
- Activity monitoring
- Quality monitoring
- Medical audit
- Health promotion
- Patient discharge procedures

Profile of services
Such as:
- Service specifications
  Services to be provided
  Quality of service
  Review process
- Service activity levels
  Services/product
  Measure of activity
  Total contracted activity level
- Information requirements
- Quality standards and monitoring
  Access to service
  Assessment
  Care programme
  Discharge
- Standards for purchaser's reward/retention scheme

Pricing schedule
- Total price of contract, within floors and ceilings

Fig. 4.5.2 Typical contract.

Budgets relate to the responsibility of individual managers and are linked to accountability and performance of agreed objectives.

Costs are recorded at a disaggregated level.

Costs and budgets are used in:

1 Monitoring and controlling the overall resources of the organization.

2 Providing historical data on which to base future costs and planning decisions.

Classification of costs

Two classifications are discussed below:

1 Direct, indirect and overheads.

2 Fixed, variable, marginal and standard.

Direct costs are those which can be directly attributed to a particular activity or product, for example, drugs or operations.

Indirect costs are those which cannot be directly attributed to a particular event or product, but are shared across a number, for example, catering or laundry.

Overhead costs are those of the support service which contribute to the general running of the organization but cannot be directly related to volume of activity, such as portering or estate management.

Fixed costs are those which are constant over a period of time, for example maintenance and heating.

Variable costs are those which vary in direct proportion to changes in volume, for example provisions and central sterile services department packs.

Marginal costs are the variable costs of an additional unit of activity.

Standard costs are a predetermined estimate of how much costs should be under specified conditions.

Standard costing

Most standards are based on efficient, but not perfect, operating conditions. The objective is to provide realistic targets.

Having set standards, the associated standard costing systems will provide for continual comparison of actual costs against standards and thus provide variance analysis. This analysis will be reported to managers who should take corrective action.

For case mix costing, standard costs are calculated for each type of activity or event, which in total add up to a patient's stay in hospital. A standard cost calculation is shown in Figure 4.5.3, which includes costs of labour, consumables and capital. In this way, all the costs of a hospital can be attributed to some standard cost. This is known as absorption costing, and is in accordance with the first principle of pricing, described earlier.

Clinicians and the contracting process

Two questions are pertinent for clinical directors.

Direct labour	
Radiologist – 3 minutes	0.87
Senior II radiographer – 13 minutes	2.51
Direct materials	
Films – size 35 × 13	0.95
Developing costs	0.20
Indirect costs	
Clerical staff support	0.77
Departmental overheads	1.29
Capital costs	1.14
Total costs	7.73

Fig. 4.5.3 Calculation of standard cost for an abdominal X-ray.

1 *Involvement in process*: Were the clinical directors involved in the setting of the external contracts? In other words, was the contract setting bottom-up or top-down?

A totally bottom-up approach would not be appropriate since negotiations with purchasers include:

(a) purchasers setting the agenda for priorities in respect of developments, internal movement of funding, etc.;
(b) purchasers driving down the price, volume or method of delivering a service.

On the other hand, providers attempt to set the agenda based on:

(a) their experience of developing services via new technology or clinical advancement;
(b) marketing different services, or building up market intelligence on competitors or purchasers;
(c) quality improvements which can only be achieved at a cost.

The bottom-up process has therefore to be tempered by the top-down. The contract negotiation process does not involve the provider taking a 'wish list' to the purchaser and looking for a blank cheque. The shopping-list method of planning services has long gone.

2 *Delivery of contract*: Clinical directors are responsible for delivery of the contracts in terms of all the elements shown in Figure 4.5.2. Therefore there needs to be a form of internal service contract, which can be known as service level agreements etc.

How these agreements are internally delivered depends very much on the local organization, but where clinicians play an active management role, for example as clinical directors, they would be very much involved in the specification and delivery of these service agreements.

The assumption for the rest of this chapter is that indeed clinicians are involved in the management process, and therefore are involved in both negotiating and agreeing service contracts, plus agreeing, delivering and monitoring internal service contracts.

Internal service level agreements

For simplicity's sake, and also because this broadly reflects reality, it is assumed that there exist two categories of directorate:

1 Service directorates, e.g. medicine or surgery.
2 Support directorates, e.g. pathology, radiology and theatres.

Figure 4.5.4 indicates the probable flow of goods and services between these directorates.

There are areas where a service directorate becomes a support directorate and vice versa; and the degree and detail of this depend on the internal organization. Two common scenarios are given below.

1 *Pathology as support and service*: The directorates of pathology and radiology are primarily support directorates because they provide tests and X-rays to the service directors, and external purchasers such as general practitioners.

They may also have beds and outpatient clinics, for example, within the subspecialty of clinical

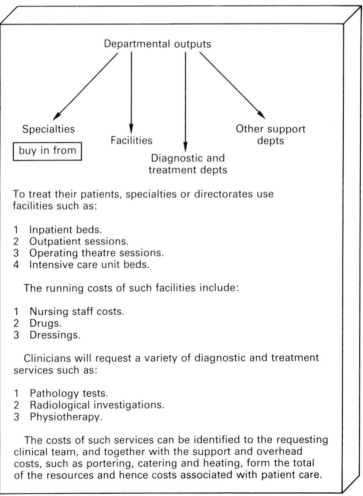

Fig. 4.5.4 Probable flow of goods and services between service and support directorates.

haematology. In the management of this part of their service they have the same management responsibility and obtain the same services as do other service directorates.

2 *Medicine as support to itself*: The service directorates obtain inputs such as X-rays from the support directorates, but they internally provide inputs to themselves. Nursing is one example, in that the medical directorate in this case manage their own nursing staff in terms of skill mix, number of nurses on the ward at any time, the amount of nursing care offered to an individual patient, and so on.

Therefore, there can be internal service level agreements between directorates to deliver internal contracts, and between the service directorates and the provider organization in order to deliver the external contracts.

The role of support directorates

Support directorates will have internal service contracts with other service directorates, and external contracts with GPFHs or with other trusts or DMUs to provide, for example, an X-ray service. These contracts can be block, probably with floors and ceilings, cost and volume, or cost per case/test/procedure.

Internal service contracts may also include different structures and pricing arrangements, according to whether the service directorates are purchasing a 'nine-to-five' service, or out of hours. Two examples of agreements between a pathology laboratory and a service directorate are shown below.

1 A simple agreement under a block contract may specify: provide the service that was provided the previous year, at a price of £50 000. There will be a ceiling on costs of 5%: in other words if the costs of providing this service rise above £52 000, there will need to be negotiations as to the basis for providing the extra workload. This could be cost per test, cost and volume, or, if no additional funding is available, the work may not be performed.

2 A more complex agreement may hinge around marginal and fixed activity and costs. The fixed costs of the pathology laboratory, i.e. the capital associated with the equipment, the fabric and the overheads, the costs associated with the quality assurance functions, and those associated with infrastructure staff, are pro-rated across the customers on the basis of historical usage. This is the equivalent of 'buying into the service'. The pathology laboratory therefore has an assured income for the year. The rest of the costs, associated with junior staff and consum-

ables, are charged out on a cost per test basis. Out-of-hours costs are charged as incurred.

The costs of internal service level agreements need to be reflected in the budgets of the service departments, so that they have the funds available to purchase the tests, X-rays, etc.

The pathology department will have a notional budget which reflects the income derived from the internal service level agreements, whether that be in the form of (1) or (2) above, or indeed any other form of agreement.

Under agreement (1), if the service directorate wishes to reduce the usage of the support department, it will need to give, say, 6 months notice, so that the support directorate can shed staff, or gain additional work.

Under agreement (2), the support directorate can manage the changes more easily within the year, since the fixed costs are already covered.

Section 4.6 discusses in more detail the budget-setting process. The discussion above has merely indicated issues that arise in setting internal service level agreements.

An agreement between a pathology laboratory and a GPFH is likely to be more explicit, as to cost and volume, given the small numbers involved. Also, GPFH's prefer to be more explicit in their contracts.

Support directors may also have contracts to provide direct services, for example beds, outpatient clinics. However, it is often the case that these direct services are provided by a service directorate for example medicine, whilst the medical staff are from a support directorate, for example the clinical haematologists from the pathology directorate. In this case, the service contract for the provision of clinical haematology services will be with the medicine directorate.

The role of service directorates

Their internal service agreements will be the delivery of externally agreed contracts for their service, in terms of agreed volume and case mix. Figure 4.5.5 gives examples of the three contracts discussed earlier.

Block contracts tend to be the preferred option for the first year of contracting; thereafter, when those involved become more sophisticated, the move is towards cost and volume contracts.

Block contracts are still more likely to be the method of contracting for core services such as accident and emergency, maternity, and those services where a large proportion of the admissions are unplanned, such as medicine. Cost and volume contracts are more likely to be in respect of waiting lists, elective surgery and high-cost, low-volume cases.

Clinical directorates are unlikely to accept block contracts where the trend has been towards an increase in expensive and complex cases. The provider's contract is more likely to exclude these complex cases which will be contracted under cost and volume, whilst the greater proportion of the lower-cost and less complex cases will be under block contract. This approach works to the detriment of the purchaser, but to the advantage of the provider.

Example of *cost and volume* contract:
  50 hip replacements for £55 000

Example of *cost per case* contract:
  Each hip replacement costs £1600

Examples of *block* contract:
  £2.1m for inpatient trauma and orthopaedics services within a 10% floor and 5% ceiling on 5000 inpatient cases

---

Fig. 4.5.5 Examples of the three contracts discussed earlier.

Extracontractual referrals (ECRs)

ECRs are more common in provider organizations which historically have had large cross-boundary flows, such as seasonal fluctuations.

ECRs provide a source of extra unplanned income: prices are at average cost, but cost is marginal. However, it is not good business acumen to contract for less than 95–97% of planned activity. ECRs are by their nature unpredictable, and should not be relied on as a stable source of income. A further problem with ECR income is the feeding of it into directorate budgets. ECR income may be seen as a bonus, and directorates, particularly service directorates, often absorb the extra workload and costs without receiving extra income.

Management of contracts

Figure 4.5.6 shows the management of the 'products' of the provider organization. The internal contracts are very much about managing cost and volume in service directorates and cost and efficiency in support directorates, whilst the external contracts are about managing volume and case mix.

Role of support directorates

The support directorate's role within the hospital production function is the responsibility for economy and technical efficiency.

1 *Economy*: This is defined as minimizing the costs of inputs, for example of X-ray films, chemicals, and increasingly the costs of staff.
  A clinical directorate could therefore negotiate improved contracts with outside suppliers in respect of, for example, X-ray films.
2 *Technical efficiency*: This is defined as the mix of inputs to produce a given output. That output could be a pathology test, or a theatre session.
  A clinical directorate could therefore change the skill mix of its staff, and now that capital charges figure more significantly in the equation, the mix of capital, staffing and consumables.
  It is worth reiterating here that service directorates may also have to manage technical efficiency, for example in managing the skill mix on wards.

The support directorates are not responsible for the volume of activity that passes through their departments. This is the responsibility of the service directorate who, for example, send requests for pathology tests, X-rays, or who use their theatres. Additional volume over and above contracted levels, for example, tests, theatre sessions or hours of theatre time, as well as the mix and complexity of tests, are also entirely the resonsibility of the service directorates, or other purchasers such as GPFHs.

The support directorates are only responsible for volume where a clinician or Medical Laboratory Scientific Officer (MLSO) within the directorate takes the decision to extend or repeat tests, X-rays etc. without reference to the originating clinician.

Service directorates

Under most directorate structures, although there are exceptions, service directorates have a support arm.

As explained earlier, the medical directorate, for example, manages wards and outpatient cli-

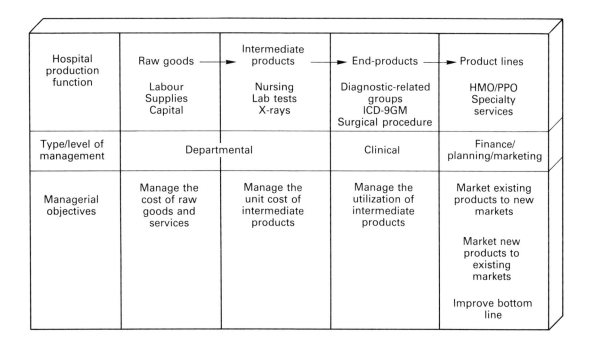

Fig. 4.5.6 The management of the products of the provider organizaton.

nics. This includes provision of nursing staff and purchase of consumables for wards. This is akin to the economy and technical efficiency aspects of the support directorates.

Service directorates are also responsible for:

1 *Volume*: number of patients.
2 *Case mix*: complexity and diagnostic category of patients.
3 *Treatment method*: what combination of events are used to treat a patient.

Clinicians as managers

What information do clinicians need to manage? The clinical director needs information which will help in the operational and strategic management of the services. An analysis of the range of functions encompassed within this management role includes:

1 Financial management.
2 Staff management.
3 Activity management.
4 Planning and development of service, etc.

Financial management

This will include:

1 Controlling a budget which will be fixed according to the contract income gained.
2 Maximizing patient care within the income allocated to the directorate.
3 Improving efficiency.
4 Effective use of resources.

In order to achieve the above, information is required on standard costs, actual expenditure, budgets, trends, etc.

Staff management

This will include:

1 Coordinating the availability and deployment of staff.
2 Agreeing staff structures and grade and skill mix.
3 Managing staff resources within financial resources.
4 Staff recruitment, motivation and leadership.

In order to achieve the above, information is required on numbers, grades and types of staff, turnover, training and education requirements, and professional issues.

Activity management

This will include:

1 Number of patients.
2 Type of patients treated.
3 What happened to the patients.

In order to achieve the above, information is required on individual patients, aggregate patients such as grouped, specialty and directorate totals, trends, and 'what if' models.

Quality management

This will include:

1 Process audit.
2 Patient satisfaction.
3 Outcome measures.

Information is required on individual patients, grouped patients, samples, research and procedures.

Case mix systems

The availability of a case mix system is critical to managing the contract process, particularly in relation to activity, standard costs and variance analysis. It is this core system that enables an organization to pull together in a management information system data from other systems, to monitor *overall* performance on actual activity across a range of indicators against *expected* performance, which is reflected in contracts. It is therefore critical that an organization can understand the integral parts of the contracts, and performance against those contracts.

A case mix system will hold details of:

1 Each patient, e.g. name, address, date of birth.
2 Hospital stay, e.g. date of admission.
3 Relevant diagnostic and operative procedures.
4 Individual events occurring during the patient episode, e.g. date and nature of pathology test.
5 Care profiles, against which actual treatment patterns can be monitored.
6 Standard costs which are applied to actual and expected treatments.

7 Reporting, which can be:
  (a) Patient to aggregate.
  (b) Actual against expected.
  (c) Trends.

Where does the information come from?

Broadly, three elements can be extracted:

1 Personnel.
2 Finance.
3 Activity, including case mix.

Personnel and finance information is, in part, provided via the budgetary monitoring process, and personnel information is also available from workforce information systems. Clinical directors *must* hold budgets for the *whole* of their service.

The allocation of budgets is discussed in more detail elsewhere. Several aspects are relevant to the discussion on service contracts and the management thereof.

1 Budgets must reflect the expected income as well as expected expenditure.
2 Total budget allocation for a directorate will not reflect total income for that directorate via the contracting process. The cost of, for example, a hip replacement will include overheads, the costs of which are incurred by departments other than the service directorate. The income received in respect of the overheads should go into the budget of, for example, the directorate of estates, to cover costs of items such as heating, lighting, laundry, etc.
  It may also include elements that will be recharged to other service directorates.
3 The budget monitoring document should also include income received for the month, as well as budgeted expenditure, against which is compared actual expenditure.
  The reason why actual expenditure differs from expected expenditure is due to variance across five headings:
  (a) Economy.
  (b) Technical efficiency.
  (c) Volume.
  (d) Case mix.
  (e) Treatment patterns.

Variance under heading (a) can be explored via budget statements which show whether what the clinical directorates paid for their inputs was the same as the prices that they expected to pay. For example, were the chemicals more expensive because discount was not obtained from the supplier on the order, or were the costs of the bank nurses that were used to fill vacancies higher than those replaced?

Variances under heading (b) can also be explored via budget statements, together with additional information from departmental management systems, such as the theatre or pathology management systems:

- Budget statements will give cost and mix of inputs, for example expenditure, quantity and mix of inputs.
- Departmental management systems will provide data on quantity and type of output, for example, number of theatre sessions, whether and by how much the sessions overran, number and type of pathology tests, and how many were ordered out of hours.

Variances under headings (c–e) can only be explored by data obtained from a case mix management system, whilst variances under (c) and (d) alone can be explored via a working patient administration system.

Section 7 in this book, which covers computing and information technology, gives more detail on the above systems; this chapter discusses the analysis of volume, case mix and treatment that can be achieved from using these systems.

Describing patients

Volume

The simplest way to describe patients, and quantify them, is as follows:

> Very General Hospital admitted 25 000 inpatients during 1992–1993 and the cost was £30m.

It is unlikely that the most basic external block contract is as simple as the above. It is also inappropriate to set internal contracts such as the above, without floors and ceilings.

The above statement also gives no indication as to complexity of cases; the 25 000 inpatients could be very simple cases, or very complex.

The costs of the 25 000 inpatients and the activity could be subdivided across specialties, or directorates, for example:

> The medical directorate admitted 8000 inpatients and the cost was £12m. Of the £12m, £3m is in respect of overheads such as estates and

central services, leaving £9m for the medical directorate budget.

Case mix

What sort of patients are these 8000 inpatients admitted by the medical directorate? They are certainly not all the same; some will be simple cases, for example they may have only been admitted for an endoscopy, whilst some may have been admitted for major cardiological investigations.

If the contract for the medical directorate expects 8500 inpatients to be admitted, it is important to analyse whether the extra 500 anticipated cases are, for example, simple endoscopies, or complex cardiological cases.

A further way of subdividing patients is via the diagnoses given to them on discharge. The diagnosis could be via the International Coding of Diseases (ICD) schema, or the Read categorization. Alternatively, surgical patients can be described using coding in respect of their procedures. In fact, GPFH contracts for elective surgical cases are described in terms of procedures.

Section 7.2 discusses in more detail the coding of patients.

However, no matter what method of coding or categorization is adopted, it is difficult to describe what is termed the *case mix* of the 8500 patients, which does not involve many hundreds of codes or procedures, each of which only describes a small number of cases. It is therefore equally difficult to aggregate patients for planning or management purposes.

One method of grouping patients, used extensively in the USA is diagnostic-related groups (DRGs). This approach is based on statistical methodology, which combines data items such as primary and secondary diagnoses, together with procedures, method of discharge and, in some circumstances, age and sex, to place patients into larger groupings.

The principles behind the grouping of patients into DRG's are:

1 The groups are medically meaningful.
2 Groups are based on readily available and, preferably, computerized data.
3 There is a manageable number of groups which is both mutually exclusive and exhaustive.
4 Each group, as far as possible, has a statistically stable distribution of length of stay and cost.

Variance analysis within a contract; a case study

This section describes a simple scenario. The effect of changing volume, case mix and treatment regimes is explored. The scenario describes the implications within an orthopaedic directorate.

The orthopaedic directorate admits patients within the following case mix groups:

Closed lower limb fracture and dislocation
Closed upper limb fracture and dislocation
Neck of femur fracture
Primary replacement of major joints
Soft tissue and other bone procedures

The directorate's contracts for 1992–1993 are:

Group	Purchaser	Number	Cost per case (£)	Total cost (£000)
1 Cost and volume contract				
Primary replacement major joints (elective)	Local DHA	112	1884	211.1
2 Block contracts				
Trauma and orthopaedics	Local DHA	715	591	422.6
	Consortium	354	767	271.5
Totals		1181	3242	905.2

The expected case mix for 1992–1993 is:

Case mix group	Number of cases		Cost per case (£)	Total cost (£000)
	Local DHA	Consortium		
Closed lower limb fracture and dislocation	84	36	295	35.4
Closed upper limb fracture and dislocation	291	124	513	212.9
Neck of femur fracture	126	54	1573	283.0
Primary replacement of major joints	112	48	1884	301.4
Soft tissue and other bone procedures	214	92	237	72.5
Totals	827	354	4502	905.2

Actual treatment profile

Inputs	Type	Quantity	Cost per input (£)	Total cost (£)
Length of stay	days	23.0	5.00	115.00
Theatres – major	hours	1.7	226.00	384.20
Radiology – simple	films	9.0	10.80	97.20
Radiology – complex	films	1.0	54.00	54.00
Pharmacy	doses	354.0	1.20	424.80
Biochemistry – simple	tests	7.0	3.80	26.80
Haematology – simple	tests	7.0	3.50	24.50
Histology – simple	tests	1.0	3.20	3.20
Microbiology – simple	tests	7.0	4.20	29.40
Nursing – qualified	hours	32.0	10.00	320.00
Nursing – unqualified	hours	28.0	5.00	140.00
Other services	hours	52.0	4.00	208.00
Total – direct care				1826.90
Add on 10% for overheads				182.63
Total				2009.59

Changing volume
The total number of cases has decreased from 1181 to 1179
but

Changing case mix
The number of cases within each case mix group has also changed.
The total effect is shown below:

Case mix group	Expected volume, case mix and treatments			Actual volume, case mix and treatments		
	Total no. of cases DHA/consortium	Cost per case (£)	Total cost (£000)	Total no. of cases (DHA/consortium)	Cost per case (£)	Total cost (£000)
Closed lower limb fracture and dislocation	120	295	35.4	102	295	30.1
Closed upper limb fracture and dislocation	415	513	212.9	406	513	208.3
Neck of femur fracture	180	1573	283.1	185	1573	291.0
Primary replacement of major joints	160	1884	301.4	188	2010	377.9
Soft tissue and other home procedures	306	237	72.5	298	237	70.6
Total	1181		905.4	1179	4628	977.9

If the following are changed:

1 *Volumes*
2 *Case mix*
3 *Treatment regimes*

then the implications for the costs and contracts can be explored.

Changing treatment regimes

The expected and actual treatment regimes for primary replacement of major joints are:

Expected treatment profile

Inputs	Type	Quantity	Cost per input (£)	Total cost (£)
Length of stay	days	19.0	5.00	95.00
Theatres – major	hours	1.5	226.00	339.20
Radiology – simple	films	9.0	10.80	97.20
Radiology – complex	films	1.0	54.00	54.00
Pharmacy	doses	345.0	1.20	414.00
Biochemistry – simple	tests	7.0	3.80	26.60
Haematology – simple	tests	7.0	3.50	24.50
Histology – simple	tests	1.0	3.20	3.20
Microbiology – simple	tests	7.0	4.20	29.40
Nursing – qualified	hours	29.0	10.00	290.00
Nursing – unqualified	hours	28.0	5.00	140.00
Other services	hours	50.0	4.00	200.00
Total – direct care				1712.90
Add on 10% for overheads				171.29
Total				1884.19

Fig. 4.5.7 Case study based on Very General Hospital, taken from the HERMES reference training manual.

A further development of DRGs in the UK has been the healthcare resource group (HRG). The work in this field has been lead by the National Casemix Office, which is part of the NHS management executive's information management group. The development of the groupings has been done in conjunction with the Royal Colleges, and groups of clinicians working within specialties. The objective is to develop a set of groupings which hold to the same principles as DRGs, described above, yet are more appropriate to UK medical practice, and hence are more acceptable to UK clinicians.

The design criteria for HRGs were that they should:

1 be clinically acceptable;
2 be more homogeneous in resource use than DRGs;
3 reduce the chance of misclassification;
4 be nationally applicable (based on Körner data);
5 produce benefits that outweigh the costs;
6 be preferable to maintaining international compatibility.

They were also designed for use with patient data which is routinely available within hospitals' information systems; in practice, the provider's minimum data set.

Experience of the pilot versions of HRG grouping suggest that:

1 Some 85% of hospital records can be assigned to a predefined HRG.

2 HRGs will be most productively used to aggregate past activity and to analyse that activity by length of stay.

Treatment profiles

A profile of care represents the expected treatment profile for a particular case mix group, or ICD, Office of Population Censuses and Surveys or Read patient category. An example of a profile of care for primary replacement of major joints is given in the case study below.

Treatment profiles and contracts

A contract to deliver a given quantity of service within a cost and quality envelope depends as much on the expected treatment profile as it does on the actual quantity of cases, and the degree of complexity of the patients. This is because the cost per case is based on the expected treatment profile. If the length of stay was increased, or the type of prosthesis used was more expensive in treating the patient then it is unlikely that the contract will be delivered within the cost framework, because the actual cost per case of the patients treated will be much higher than that expected when agreeing the contracts.

4.6 Allocating clinical/service budgets

G. C. McGarrity

Introduction

Budgets are plans describing the activities of a department in financial terms and can only be prepared by evaluation of that department's activities for the coming year. Budgets in the health service have been largely calculated on an incremental basis and not adequately related to clinical workload. The emergence of the purchaser/provider roles will eventually make identification of accurate costs an important factor in relation to the negotiation of contracts. With the advent of serious clinical involvement in budget management and the closer scrutiny of budget calculation, it is vital that the individual budgets realistically reflect workloads that are planned and will change if the planned workload changes. They need to be agreed and understood by the budget-holder. The amounts to be devolved to clinical directors' budgets should be as much as possible within the ability of information systems to provide appropriate supporting data.

The holding of a budget identifies responsibility and accountability in one place. The delegation of budgets can motivate the holder by either the element of competition with colleagues, i.e. a budget-holder does not wish to be seen as unable to control costs, or by incentives – more efficiency allows money to be directed to other sections within the budget-holder's department. In addition, ownership and control of a budget allow greater flexibility in managing. Often a department's expectation in its business plan may not be able to be met by the income available, and choices will need to be made, depending on priorities and the use of efficiency savings. Further, the effect of one department's plans on another needs to be taken into account. The health service is a demand-led organization, so many service departments such as laboratories, radiology departments, theatres will need to review their budgets if inpatient activity increases, e.g. by greater bed utilization. The type of contract negotiated could affect opportunities to obtain more funds from purchasers. A block contract could reduce such an opportunity unless adequate thresholds were included to trigger increases in the block sums to provide additions to the base budget.

In a large directorate, there are many complicated professional and personnel issues to deal with, not least with other consultants. Whilst they support the clinical director in general, it needs to be recognized that the clinical director is a managerial appointment and is responsible to the chief executive for managerial functions. But the clinical director is a clinician among clinicians and part of his or her role in the directorate is to examine, with colleagues, the impact of clinical practice on the directorate. They should achieve agreement as to what will normally be the best approach in dealing with specific issues. The directorate will need to pay regard to hospital policy, current clinical practice, local outcomes, purchaser requirements and the balance of resources involved.

Consideration must be given to the type and level of support that are required to enable the directors to manage a budget that can be between £0.5 and £5m – the equivalent of many small businesses. By definition, the clinical director is clearly part-time in his or her management role. The directorate needs full-time management and administrative staff who will be of sufficient ability to respond to major managerial challenges. Directorates may be managed through a single-role senior manager who is accountable to the clinical director or by a business manager and clinical manager working together for the clinical director. Either system can achieve the desired result, but if the clinical directorate scheme of things is to be more than a token arrangement, the managers involved should be of sufficient calibre to run a major undertaking. It is common for hospitals to have between nine and 16 directorates and it is neither economical nor practical to support each director with his or her own accountant.

Currently it is good practice to have an identified accountant who will support a group of directorates – the number depending on their size and complexity.

To survive effectively, the directorate needs to have regular, timely and correct financial information via a general ledger system. Directorates should have on-line access to the general ledger, for perhaps read-only enquiries, to speed the process and increase the understanding and trust between directorates and the finance department.

In allocating budgets, the health service has historically used the incremental approach. The starting point has been the previous year's budget. Changes for the current year would be made based on identified pressures, e.g. increased activity or inflation increasing beyond expectation. While each of these and others would be challenged and required to be substantiated, an increase (or decrease) may be agreed over the previous year. This approach ignores the effect of such borderline issues as changes in practice in other departments unless the effects are quite sizeable. It encourages budget-holders to conceal underspending, but, more importantly, it is not measuring outputs and their effect on unit costs. These are key interests to the corporate organization in achieving its contract income.

The primary alternative to incremental budgeting is zero-based budgets, which is a procedure whereby no budget is automatically carried forwards without explanation and investigation. Outputs and costs are related to the activities of the department. The benefits of the outputs are assessed by the larger corporate organization and the most beneficial succeed. However, it is difficult to assess some benefits in a 1-year or even longer budget time scale because fixed costs are, of course, not flexible and such a procedure can be expensive and time-consuming. This may be overcome in practice when certain elements of a budget are zero-based each year, depending upon the impact on the budget and activity levels. Normally the nursing budget would be included because of its size, as would drugs and medical and surgical supplies and equipment, because of their complexity and the impact of small changes in practice.

The clinical budget is now an instrument for monitoring these areas of activity, together with the support of case mix systems which identify the complexity of patients' illnesses.

The directorate, i.e. the clinical director and senior managers, is therefore fully involved in the budget-setting process. Each year in November/December they begin the process which culminates in a meeting with the chief executive. By this time objectives will have been set and incorporated in a written agreement forming an internal contract with the directorate. This agreement will be an integral part of the hospital's business plan and become part of the external contract with purchasers.

Within the hospital, some service departments may agree to recharge the cost of services to users against agreed workload, thus leaving the service department totally recharged. It is recognized however, that if savings can be achieved in a user department, service department savings can only be claimed at the margin because, although reduced demand affects costs, infrastructure costs cannot be reduced instantly.

Finally, clinical directors need to become involved in the corporate process and have their actions monitored by a corporate forum of peers. This is necessary because in the budget process the actions of one directorate can seriously affect another in clinical and financial terms. If a directorate should temporarily reduce its service commitment for financial reasons, e.g. closure of beds, there may be a considerable impact on other services if their patients overflow. Waiting lists may increase and cause these other directorates to fail to meet their contract targets. Operational policy should be discussed and decided at a council of all clinical directors. The overall financial position of the hospital would be considered on a regular basis, identifying by individual directorate the effect each is having on the overall financial position. Should a directorate regularly fail to meet its budgetary target, careful scrutiny is required to ascertain the reason or, more usually, the multifactorial causes, e.g. increased activity, unplanned equipment purchase, extra staffing or even, had the budget recognized all these financial pressures in the first place?

4.7 Resourcing general practitioner fundholders

Keith McLean and David Russell

Introduction

The general practice funding initiative element of the White Paper reforms (Department of Health, 1989) was designed to secure improvement in the quality of services for patients, to stimulate providers to be more responsive to the needs of general practitioners and their patients and to encourage the development of participating practices for the benefit of their patients.

In pursuance of the above objectives, participating practices were to be allocated funds in order to purchase certain hospital services, drugs and practice staff support. Hospital services covered by the scheme were the common elective procedures – whether on an inpatient or day-case basis – all outpatient services, all domiciliary consultations, most direct-access diagnostic testing and three direct-access treatment services (occupational therapy, physiotherapy and speech therapy).

In order to be eligible to exercise the statutory right to take a fund, practices had to have 9000 (now reduced to 7000) or more patients registered on their list, be able to demonstrate the ability to manage a fund (including the possession of adequate computer support), and to demonstrate the agreement of all partners to the venture.

The perceived benefits can be summarized as follows:

1 Improved quality of care.
2 More efficient use of resources.
3 Better integration of primary and secondary care.
4 Improved communication between consultants and general practitioners (GPs).
5 Better information systems.
6 Empowerment and development of primary health care.
7 More local decision-making.

There is no doubt that general practitioner fundholders (GPFHs) have stimulated improvements to the quality of provider services and in particular information systems. They have also acted as an additional impetus for district health authorities as purchasers on behalf of other GPs and have been used as a creative means of moving resources and activity from a secondary to a primary care setting.

Joining the scheme is entirely voluntary (and almost certainly will remain so) and this is seen as one of its strengths.

Allocation of funds to GPFHs

Each fund essentially covers the three main elements described earlier; prescribing, practice staff and a defined range of hospital and community services. The scheme is being extended with effect from 1 April 1993 to include community nursing, dietetics, chiropody and referrals in mental health and learning disabilities (see the section on what fundholders can buy, below, for further amplification of this).

In terms of the methodology for allocating funds, this is essentially based at present on historic usage of NHS services, including drugs and current practice staff costs.

Regional health authorities are formally responsible for establishing the fund, although in practice Family Health Service Authorities (FHSAs) are responsible for the prescribing and staff cost elements of the scheme, whilst the regional health authority has generally taken greater responsibility for determining the hospital services budget.

The prescribing element was agreed at FHSA/practice level using a standard approach which for 1993–1994 involved uprating each practice's 1992–1993 expenditure with a Department of Health uplift factor that covered both price inflation and product mix. FHSAs could then adjust this for practice-specific factors. The practice staff element was agreed at FHSA/practice level on the basis of the existing staff reimbursement position.

Most regions have established the hospital services element of the fund in reference to the practice's historic and current referral and treatment patterns for the services covered by the scheme (and provided by the NHS) and appropriate price information obtained from relevant providers. At its simplest therefore, the budget reflects agreed activity multiplied by the projected price, as given by the fundholder's historic and current providers. The basis for activity used by most regions has been a combination of prospective data collected by practices, validated by retrospective hospital-provided information. The latter however has generally been of poor quality.

This apparently straightforward approach to setting budgets for hospital services has therefore been beset by several significant practical problems:

1 Difficulties in establishing historic and current referral and treatment patterns. Most GPs traditionally did not have detailed records of treatment patterns and, where they did, they were often not recorded consistently with the way prices were made available.
2 Likewise most hospitals did not have (and many still do not have) data systems that record to practice level and good-quality outpatient systems have been even rarer. Where information systems do exist, they are still subject to the vagaries of the human factor.
3 Referral and treatment patterns vary enormously. There may be annual fluctuations at practice level which can have significant effects on activity which would tend to be smoothed out at a larger district health authority level.
4 In addition, the variations in referral and treatment pattern rates between GP practices make validation of data even more difficult. It may look odd but it could be correct!
5 The NHS has not traditionally needed to price its services in a sophisticated manner. Obtaining accurate prices has therefore been a major exercise which in turn has exposed major price variations between hospitals. These could arise from variations in clinical practice, the cost base of the unit or the method of apportionment and calculation used.
6 Other changes were being introduced simultaneously with GPFH. One significant example was capital charges. For the first time, hospital costs and therefore prices had to reflect the cost of capital assets in their charges. Capital charges vary greatly between hospitals and this not only adds a further complexity to the task of determining costs but also has the effect of being a further major variable that influenced relative costs.

It has to be remembered in all of this that GPFH budgets do not change the total resources available to the NHS or to regions. Fundholding changes the arrangements for allocating funds and can be seen as part of the wider process of separating purchasers from providers. However, any monies allocated to GPFHs for hospital services form a direct deduction from the district health authority from which the fundholder's patients are drawn.

The same budget-setting principles will apply to the extension of the scheme to community services, i.e. current levels of service will be used as the main baseline.

Summarizing the current position, budget-setting for GPFHs is very much an annual exercise. Until patterns have been established and some benchmark exists, fundholder budgets are essentially non-recurring.

In addition to the resources mentioned above, practices have available to them a management allowance which does not in itself form part of the GP fund. Clearly there are additional management expenses in practices to allow them to negotiate contracts and to run the relatively complex accounting systems necessary to manage the fund. Each participating practice therefore receives funding of up to £35 000 for those who are actual fundholders and £17 500 for those in the preparatory year (1993–1994 figures).

Future allocation strategies

What has been described so far has been the methods adopted in the first 3 years to setting and agreeing particularly the hospital services element of the budget. All regions have operated broadly similar approaches so far, although there have been differences in detail.

For example, a number of regions used price bandings whereby minor, intermediate and major procedures were priced for each specialty and these prices were multiplied by activity to determine the budget. One of these regions also set the inpatient budget on the basis of district average served population activity, adjusted where practice/unit information proved a higher level of usage.

However the variations which inevitably have arisen in terms of the *per capita* spend by GPFH practices has raised many questions around equity and has led in places to accusations of preferential funding of fundholders.

The NHS management executive has always clearly stated its objective to move towards a suitable capitation-based system for fundholding. Accordingly, with effect from 1993–1994, a national weighted capitation formula for inpatient and day-case services has been available as a benchmark in budget negotiations.

At this stage the capitation benchmark will be used to inform negotiations on budgets which nevertheless will still largely be based on historic activity and hospital prices.

Capitation-based systems can offer advantages in the systematic calculation of budgets and are regarded by some as being more equitable. Full capitation funding at practice level however will not be easy to establish because of factors such as:

1 The relatively small size of GP practices and thus the increased chances of statistical variation being significant.
2 The incidence of private patients within a practice that distort the demand for NHS resources.
3 Variation in the health care needs of different practice populations which ideally would need to be reflected in locally weighted capitation.
4 Allocation formulae do not increase total resources available and therefore for every gainer there has to be a loser. It is a well-recognized phenomenon that health authorities and others who gain under a particular formula support wish to see rapid implementation, whilst losers often believe the concept to be sound but the weightings inappropriate, with slow movement being necessary in any event. There is no reason to believe that fundholders will react any differently.

The whole issue of a move to a capitation-based system or indeed any other alternative resource methodology needs to be handled sensitively – not least because participation in the scheme is voluntary and fundholders who consider they are being disadvantaged may either withdraw and carry on referring at the same rate outside the scheme or simply overspend and seek to justify it on clinical grounds.

On the other hand, fundholding does greatly increase the opportunity to understand general practice level referral and expenditure rates, which in turn will increase understanding and potentially the ability to influence overall district health authority activity. It should become possible to identify inappropriate referral and treatment as practices that are above capitation levels are increasingly called upon to justify their position.

What can fundholders buy?

As has been referred to earlier, in the first phase of fundholding the GPs were enabled to purchase most outpatient attendances and investigations and a selected range of elective surgical procedures.

With effect from 1 April 1993, the scope of the scheme was extended to include a wider range of services:

1 District nursing.
2 Health visiting.
3 Chiropody.
4 Dietetics.
5 All community and outpatient mental health services.
6 Mental health counselling.
7 Health services for people with a learning disability (excluding inpatient care).
8 Referrals made by health visitors, district nurses, community psychiatric nurses and community mental handicap nurses for services covered by the fund.

It is envisaged that this extension to the scheme to include community nursing services will go some way to removing one of the historic barriers to the development of primary health care teams, i.e. difficulties in creating effective links between the GP service and the community health service. The inclusion of the costs of referrals made by community nursing staff also changes the focus of the initiative towards the wider primary health care team as opposed to the more limited GP partnership.

Where are fundholders able to purchase from and what if they spend more or less than their allocation?

Briefly, in the case of the extension of fundholding to community services, the 'where' question is relatively simple. Fundholders are required to place contracts for community nursing services with NHS providers and will not be able to employ these staff directly or use a private provider. They will, however, be able to use a different NHS provider than the one which currently provides services for their patients or use more than one NHS provider where practicable (circular EL[92]48).

In addition, to facilitate implementation of the scheme, fundholders will be limited to using fixed-price, non-attributable (i.e. not attributable to individual patients) contracts for community nursing services in the first year.

Fundholders are not however required to contract for mental health, learning disability, chiropody or dietetic services with NHS providers, and have the same freedoms to purchase from a range of providers as they do with hospital services provided the fundholders satisfy themselves that the provider is suitably competent to provide those services. Also, if the purchase of any service(s) is to be from a person or organization with which any member of the practice has a particular connection, the fundholding practice must obtain the consent of the relevant regional health authority.

Arrangements in this regard have tended to vary from region to region. In some cases regions in the first instance identified a maximum level of change which fundholders will be allowed; others left it to GPFHs and providers to negotiate. From a Yorkshire perspective, we wanted to encourage partnership between existing providers and the GPFHs and largely developed this approach, whilst not denying the opportunity for fundholders to change providers, where this was seen to be desirable and acceptable.

In practical terms, what could this fundholder freedom mean? They are free, subject to any regional agreements, to change NHS providers or to use private hospitals. They can employ certain staff, including consultants and other hospital staff acting in a private capacity (who must then include these earnings as part of their private earnings). They can employ physiotherapists and other professional staff and pay salaries direct rather than contracting with NHS providers.

Some of these freedoms can hold very real implications for providers, e.g:

1 GPFHs are funded at the full average cost of provision from their current NHS provider. They can therefore use this to exercise considerable influence and indeed leverage over providers. If a hospital were to lose the work formerly coming to them from GPFHs, they could find themselves financially squeezed as it is probable they will only be able to save the marginal cost of providing the service.
2 GPFHs may provide some services themselves to generate savings, provide a more local service, to raise income from other purchasers or to increase indirectly the income of the practice by seeking regional health authority agreement to charge the fund for a limited range of fundholder procedures where these are performed within the practice. The

regional health authority would of course need to look very carefully at the service quality and value for money offered by such arrangements.
3 By giving the fundholder considerable purchasing power, there could be arguments that this might put at risk some of the equity principles within the NHS.
4 Should GPFHs exercise in a significant way their freedoms to increase the number of staff they employ to provide services in-house rather than contracting with hospitals, this could have effects on certain services, e.g. pathology, physiotherapy, among those services vulnerable to change. It will however be particularly important to ensure that the quality of the service provided is monitored and controlled.

What can fundholders do with savings and what if they overspend?

Overspending in a sense is relatively simple to explain. If a practice overspends, the regional health authority must 'top up' the budget to leave the accounts in balance. Provided the overspend is deemed to be clinically justified, then no further penalty attaches to the practice. Ultimately, the regional health authority has the sanction under the GPFH regulations if it does not consider the overspend to be justified to remove GPFH status from the practice. The scheme is as yet too new for robust criteria for the demonstration of good or poor management of the scheme to have been developed. In particular, simple end-of-the-year accounts give no indication of the quality of the services provided to the fundholder patient population, so that no reliable judgement of clinical efficacy can be made. It is within this context that the development of population-based needs assessment and audit of practices becomes imperative.

On the question of savings, if the fundholders underspend their budget they retain the savings and can spend them on the range of services covered by the fund or on improvements to their practice premises. In other words, they could buy from their provider more elective surgery, etc. or develop the local service to their patients.

The savings must be spent to provide benefit to individuals on the practice list; they cannot benefit individual members of the practice directly. The term 'benefit to individuals on the practice list' is of course open to interpretation but nevertheless the intention is quite clear.

Savings cannot be spent until they have been established in fully audited accounts.

What next?

It is difficult at this stage to predict how far GPFH could/should develop. There is increasing interest in the extension of the benefits of GPFH to smaller (including single-handed) practices, either through the development of consortia (i.e. two or more practices joining together to reach viable practice population numbers) or through the FHSA acting as a management agent for groups of GPs, allowing the practices and their patients to benefit from the incentives of fundholding without the additional administrative burden.

Equally, many district health authorities have recognized the need to work closely with their local GPs and are therefore developing locality-based purchasing projects which enable many of the benefits of being a fundholder without necessarily the practice(s) managing the resources themselves. *Contracts for Health Services: Operational Principles* stressed that whilst district health authorities are responsible for securing contracts, GPs are best placed to represent their patients' views.

The likely pace of expansion of fundholding could therefore be influenced by a series of factors:

1 The willingness locally to develop district health authority purchasing which is sensitive to and meets the legitimate demands of local GPs.
2 How far practices and/or consortia are willing to join or indeed continue in the scheme.
3 Local arrangements for selection and ongoing recognition of fundholders, including views on de-registering if considered appropriate.
4 Support provided to fundholders and prospective fundholders from regional health authorities and FHSAs in particular.
5 The willingness of small practices to join together to form effective consortia which meet the standards and requirements laid down.

6 Any changes to the content or operational arrangements to the scheme nationally or regionally.

The other issue on the development of fundholding would be around other services which might be included.

The ultimate would of course be that all health care purchasing (i.e. for all services) is done through groupings of GPs. It is difficult to see this operating within the current definitions of practice size etc. for GPFHs. However, it would not be difficult to envisage a wider grouping of GPs, covering a population of say 50 000, operating as subcontracting purchasers on behalf of the local commissioning authority and within its health needs framework.

Other issues being addressed in various ways across the country include:

1 Linkage between GPFH purchasing intentions and district health authority overall health needs assessment role.
2 Development of GPFH business plans and linkage to some form of performance management/monitoring arrangement.
3 Linking GPFHs into the *Health of the Nation* and the health targets therein.
4 Development of local patients' charters outlining both rights of patients and their obligations – GPFHs are already required to include the national *Patients' Charter* standards in their purchasing specifications.
5 Clarification of the objectives of fundholding policy in relation to the level of fundholding penetration, i.e. is the policy maximization of numbers or maximizing the beneficial effects of fundholding?

Overall, the requirement has to be around achieving maximum health gain whilst retaining overall control and for the whole system to be health needs-driven.

Reference

Department of Health (1989) *Working for Patients*. HMSO, London.

4.8 Impact and future of general practitioner fundholders – two personal views

4.8(a) Overview

Howard Glennerster

I am currently monitoring the general practitioner (GP) fundholding scheme as part of a programme of research financed by the King's Fund on the NHS reforms.

When I began this research in 1990 I was basically sceptical of the contribution fundholding could play. Now I am convinced that fundholding is potentially the most important part of the reforms. It is already making its impact on the management of hospital care.

The origins of the fundholding idea

I think it is worth asking at the outset, as we did in our preliminary report, *A Foothold for Fundholding*, published by the King's Fund Institute in 1992: Where did this whole idea come from? The origins of fundholding predate the discussions on the White Paper *Working for Patients* by several years and have several sources. Professor Alan Maynard had suggested that GPs should be given the power to buy hospital services as far back as 1984. There were particular characteristics of the health care market, he argued, that did not lend itself to a full private market but that did not mean that the only alternative was that medical care must be provided in the style of a command economy. The family doctor was, in Britain, the patient's adviser and guide through the system of health care; why not give him or her the purchasing power to buy services on behalf of patients?

At the same time, and quite independently, the Department of Health or its predecessor in the early 1980s was looking with interest at American health maintenance organizations which purchased care from hospitals on their patients' behalf. Such a model would make possible a switch in funding from the top to the bottom of the service; it would force hospitals to compete for GPs' custom and would be a way of redressing the balance between primary health care and the hospital sector which had swung so far in the hospital's favour since 1948. The more one looks into the origins of this idea, the less it appears to have to do with some Thatcheresque vision of a privatized health care system and appears much more as part of a century-long battle between the hospital and primary health care or the consultant and the GP – a relationship that changed sharply in the consultants' and the hospitals' favour after the NHS was born.

Those working on the reforms for Mrs Thatcher's government had two models before them – a top-down model advocated by Alain Enthoven from the USA and others, in which the district became the purchaser, and this far more radical bottom-up version. As we now know, the government went for both at the same time, thereby giving us the rare chance of evaluating a social policy experiment.

Our study

Experiments are not much help, however, unless someone observes and compares the outcomes. We thought this experiment one of the most interesting and important of the whole 1990 Act reforms and were successful in getting the King's Fund to finance a reseach project beginning in January 1990.

We have regularly interviewed those administering the reforms, from the Department of Health, regions, Family Health Service Authorities (FHSAs), provider units, district health authorities and, above all, practices. We selected a sample who were thinking of entering the scheme. We finally narrowed down to follow in detail 10 practices in three regions, which represented a carefully chosen cross-section of GPs in the scheme in those areas. We also interviewed non-fundholders and are now following up a sample of third-wave practices.

The scheme

Originally practices of 11 000 or more patients could join. Then the limit was dropped to 9000 and then to 7000, with smaller practices let in too if they combined.

The budget fundholders are given, and taken off their district's budget, covers the purchase of inpatient services: ophthalmology, ear, nose and throat, thoracic and general sugery, gynaecology, orthopaedics, all outpatients and pathology, radiology and imaging. From 1993, community health services are also included.

The central questions

Enough about the detail of the scheme, which is discussed in our report. I want to concentrate instead on what I think are the central questions:

1 Is bottom-up funding by GPs an intrinsically better way of funding hospital services?
2 Can it work for everything or is the present balance of service provision incorporated in the GP budgets about right?
3 Can we universalize GP fundholding or is it destined to be at best a marginal activity for the best and largest practices?
4 What are the outstanding major problems?

Bottom-up funding

How successful have fundholders been in setting contracts and what does this tell us about contracts driven from below? Again one must enter caveats. The districts were, for the first 2 years, inhibited by central diktat from being innovative or ruthless in changing their providers, so the

first years may be unrepresentative. But they were instructive.

GPs were also advised not to change anything much. They showed tougher independence. Every GP in our sample had one or two hospital specialties where they felt they were getting a poor service and they sought to do something about it, shifting some of their custom to bring pressure to bear, taking all their custom and switching to a speedier or better and more co-operative consultant. They exercised the power of exit, as economists call it, and did so with considerable effect in those few key cases where dissatisfaction was high. That was almost universally true of hospital pathology testing. Yet this was an area where there was a real potential market. One practice got tests from several hundred miles away more quickly than from the local hospital. Virtually all our practices got a better deal by threatening to move, or by moving, custom. Most often this had a knock-on effect on services for other GPs.

I am impressed in our latest round of interviews at the extent to which fundholders are planning to extend that strategy in an even more tough-minded way.

Districts have not been so vigorous, nor have consultants felt the same kind of pressure. The key is that the incentives the two kinds of purchasers face are very different. In the end, district managers are sitting at desks thinking about broad health strategies. They are not dealing with hospitals and their irritations day by day. They are looking over their shoulders at politicians and up to the Department of Health. They ought to be concerned with the big strategic health issues.

GPs are faced with patients in pain who keep coming back, whom they know; they are professionally frustrated by not being able to get done what they know ought to be done. Their time is being wasted, at the very least. The price of inertia is very high. They have much more incentive to do the politically embarrassing thing and shift the contract. They also have a much more detailed knowledge of patient-relevant information – that consultant is rude, or you never see him, the journey to the hospital takes all day and there are no parking facilities. With the best will in the world, these are not the kind of things that can be easily discussed at district level. Information of this fine-grained variety gets lost as it travels up an organization.

Yet it was incorporated in the decisions our fundholders took on their contracts. Marginal decisions by fundholders to switch contracts began to act as a signal or a warning to sensible hospital managers. The district might be next to withdraw its custom. Indeed, some district managers told us they were relying on fundholders to make the running. A district would only be able to take major decisions to shift its contract in a limited number of cases each year.

In short, there are some good broader organizational reasons why one might expect GPs to be more effective purchasers of a range of services than districts and in the first and second round of contracts, and so far as I can see the emerging third-round contracts too, those theories do seem to have some support in the situations we observed.

The role of outpatient clinics is one of the most interesting examples of change. In one area our fundholders detect a sea change in the attitudes of consultants to visiting surgeries to see patients. The practices organize the appointments much more effectively than the hospital staff, and the patients come. The records are to hand and the tests are done and ready for the consultant. 'It was not on the agenda 2 years ago' one practice said, 'and now they are approaching us'. The contracts with hospitals are more innovative and demanding. Often there has been no absolute reason why some things could not have been done before, like employing a counsellor. Why refer the psychiatric outpatients to be seen by a junior doctor when immediate sessions with a counsellor in the practice would be much better than delayed outpatient visits to the psychiatric hospital? Now they have the freedom and the money to do so.

Criticisms

These are exceptional practices. Experiments always tend to work. You can't draw lessons from the first enthusiasts. All these comments have been made in the medical press. I think those points are fair. We need longer and more evidence.

The most frequent argument levelled against fundholding is that it is unfair and creates two standards. That is a joke. There is already an enormous variety in the standards of primary care in the UK. However, what fundholding does is to extend that inequality by enabling

large, well-organized practices to function even better. To me that is not a case for stopping the experiment. It is precisely because it seems a good idea that the inequity is arising. To stop it is rather like stopping the trials of a life-saving drug because it cannot be given to everybody immediately.

Moreover, it misunderstands the nature of competition. Sheer blatant favouritism by a provider is not likely to survive. Advantages won by one practice will be claimed by others. Second-round effects follow as the market adjusts to a new pattern.

Can the idea be extended?

I think it can. By 1994 a third of all patients will be in fundholding practices and in some areas most patients will be. There is considerable scope for practices to group together or use some management services in common. Even so, not all practices might want or be able to join up. In the interim I see these practices coming under the wing of the FHSA or some other umbrella primary care purchasing agency.

Extensive fundholding will destroy districts' capacity to plan, we are told. I would be more convinced if I thought districts had some crystal ball that told them how to measure health care needs in detail. I have no evidence they do. On the contrary, I think districts should welcome the extra information they will derive from GPs' revealing their and their patients' preferences, reached in the harsh light of a constrained budget. That is the way Sainsbury's or Marks & Spencer's head office works, after all.

We are told that GPs only respond to demand, not need. There are groups who never reach the surgery from an ethnic or social group, for example. That is the district's responsibility to research and to alert practices and devise services and incentives to change the situation in all practices.

Problems

What are the most important limitations and problems?

First, there is the way the budgets are set. The first-round budgets were set reasonably generously to avoid difficulties. There is considerable variability. Now the Department of Health is moving to formula funding, so much per patient on a practice's list. But then there will be the fear, justified by American experience, that incentives to turn away costly patients will grow. It is crucial to devise, as soon as possible, a formula-based funding system, that will reflect the differential costs that different kinds of patient may be expected to put on a practice.

That is easier said than done. It is what we have set ourselves to try to do in the next year.

The high standards set to enter the scheme and the varied managerial and computing capacity of practices have meant that most practices are concentrated in the suburban ring and in already effective practices elsewhere. This only adds to the social class inequities of the NHS. If the scheme is not to fall into disrepute on this ground, there should be ways to help practices in other areas with high morbidity and social deprivation, whether they join the scheme or not.

In short, the scheme has the potential to shake up the hospital system, to make it more efficient and consumer-conscious. It also has its dangers – but ones that are, I believe, possible to overcome.

References

Department of Health (1989) *Working for Patients*. HMSO, London.

Glennerster, H., Matsagonis, M. and Owens, P. (1992) *A Foothold for Fundholding*, Kings Fund Institute, London.

David Mathias

The concept of fundholding and the principles upon which it is based have been dealt with elsewhere. As with all innovative legislation, the interpretation of the statute depends to a large extent upon the individual interests and bias of those who are affected by it. In day-to-day terms the bodies involved are general practitioners (GPs), Family Health Service Authorities (FHSAs), district health authorities (DHAs), hospitals, be they district-managed or trusts, and the directorates within them.

The changes which have been brought about by GP fundholding affect the facets of health care in different ways, not only in respect of finance, but also in what is intended to be a shift in the overall control of resources away from the secondary and into the hands of the primary health care sector. This change has been best expressed as a move from the *provision of health care* by the hospital service to the *purchase of health need* by the general practitioner.

Aims of GP fundholders

It is the stated purpose of GP fundholders that they should create innovation with equity and achieve value for money. It assumes that the benefits obtained will outweigh the costs incurred.

The more simplistic rationale, expressed by some GP fundholders and by most DHAs, is that it is a means by which GP can protect their rights of referral. A more sinister interpretation suggests that it is a means by which the focus of health care can be switched towards the least expensive end of the chain.

The extent of GP fundholding

By April 1993, 24% of the population were covered by GP fundholders. With the advent of the third, fourth, and fifth waves of fundholders, the figure will increase to something in excess of 50%. It is unlikely that there will be any major expansion of the conventional fundholding scheme beyond this point, although it is now possible for GPs to form consortia of smaller practices under the umbrella of DHAs, FHSAs, or some amalgamation of the two bodies, and this may give a further boost to expansion.

Within an average health district and given the present limits on fundholders' ability to purchase health care, the proportion of the district financial allocation at the disposal of fundholders averages around 10%. This may increase to a maximum of 25% of the district allocation when the scheme has reached its full potential. Any further increase of the allocation to GP fundholders could only be brought about by an increase in their ability to purchase services such as emergencies and long-stay care.

The effects on hospital services

At directorate level there are considerable variations. Surgical specialties, particularly those with a low emergency admission rate, may depend on fundholding for much of their budget. By contrast, medical specialties are almost immune from its financial effects as far as inpatient activity is concerned. It must be added that whilst the overall proportion of the budget at risk may seem a small amount, in the context of a hospital budget of perhaps £70m with considerable fixed costs, this amount would be critical and might represent the difference between the success and failure of an institution or a department within it.

The views of purchasers

GP fundholders

Attitudes within the ranks of GP fundholders range from great enthusiasm for the benefits to be derived from fundholding to a feeling of neutrality. Many practitioners are willing to be convinced of the benefits that may accrue to their patients. The enthusiasts see an opportunity to induce changes in patient management through the proper use of the market economy, forcing the secondary sector to move away from entrenched attitudes and to provide what they see as a better and, in particular, more timely service. To date there have been numerous examples of shifts of contract, though these have been for the most part confined to diagnostic and elective surgical services.

Fundholding practices and FHSA's have, for the most part, stressed their unwillingness to obtain services for their patients which would be seen to disadvantage patients of non-fundholding practices. As the effects of the market place economy develop, there is every prospect that a more competitive attitude will emerge between practices and the honourable attitude that exists at present may well diminish.

Increased communication between consultants and GP fundholders has been quoted by many observers as an immediate benefit of the fundholding scheme. Examples have been given of hospitals contacting GP fundholders in order to attract more patients. Some GP fundholders have established minor surgical facilities and consultant clinics in their own premises from which savings have accrued. The establishment of limited companies has met with mixed feelings both within the ranks of GP fundholders themselves and others, although this is now controlled to limit any potential adverse effects.

One is conscious of a feeling of caution among GP fundholders at present. There is however an awareness of a potential for inducing change, particularly if the purchasing powers of GP fundholders were to be aggregated.

Finally, there is a noticeable distrust of directly managed units (DMUs) amongst GP fundholders. It is often felt that as the major purchaser within a district, the DHA may make contracts with its own hospitals which could limit the scope of the fundholders.

FHSAs

Whilst FHSAs do not play a direct role in the interrelation between fundholders and hospitals, they are intimately involved in the relationships between fundholding and non-fundholding practices. There is a general perception that if fundholding is perceived as beneficial, there will be a need for some form of closer relationship to be forged between DHAs and FHSAs. This prospect is further enhanced by the probability of changes at regional level. There is a possibility that the FHSAs may have a very limited tenure – a prospect unlikely to evoke feelings of enthusiasm among their members or employees.

DHAs

Although not overtly against the concept of GP fundholding, DHAs none the less exhibit some reservations. The uncertainty regarding the future of regional health authorities (RHAs) only enhances these anxieties. What are often regarded as innovations when perpetrated by GP fundholders are regarded as acts of irresponsibility when executed by DHAs. GP fundholders are perceived by the DHA as having insufficient accountability and a disproportionate amount of funds at their disposal. There is anxiety that GP fundholders may lack long-term perspectives and have an inherent capacity to destabilize the system. Furthermore, there is a danger of a loss of economy of scale which must ensue from the fragmentation of the total district allocation. This concept even threatens the maintenance of adequate reserves within a district.

Some concern has been expressed regarding what is seen as a lack of sufficient motivation for the furtherance of preventive medicine amongst GP fundholders. As the DHA will always pick up the bill for emergencies and the long-term sick, GP fundholders are seen to lack incentives in this field.

The views of providers

The effects of GP fundholding will be felt equally by providers, regardless of whether they hold trust status or not. There is an antipathy towards DMUs exhibited by trust hospitals because of the danger that district purchasers may show favour towards hospitals under their direct management. In common with other agencies, providers are determined to avoid what has been termed a two-tier service. This attitude stems, for the most part, from a desire to avoid a need to discriminate between patients but will inevitably impose restrictions on the ability of fundholders to alter current practice. Many provider units, aware of the need to attract patients from GP fundholders, have made approaches to fundholders and have set out their wares to an unprecedented extent. The risk of marginalization of departments due to shifts in contracts has been appreciated by contract departments, if not by all practising clinicians.

Whilst some consultants have agreed to undertake clinics in GP fundholders' surgeries, others have resisted such invitations both on the grounds of inefficiency and in some instances because of a fear of a diminishing outpatient resource.

Whilst GP fundholders and, for that matter DHA purchasers, may meet resistance in their attempts to change existing patterns of service, they have the right to transfer contracts to another provider unit. Some RHAs have acted to control the ability of purchasers to shift activity but it can be assumed that such restraint will not be applied indefinitely. It is probable that GP fundholders generally will exercise proper caution in their dealings with provider units but there have already been instances where fundholders have decided to obtain services at another hospital.

The net results of such activities could have a destabilizing effect on hospitals but there are some who would argue that the true benefits of the market place will not be realized unless fundholders are given every freedom to place contracts where they wish. NHS trust hospital rules prevent the overt cross-subsidization of departments which prove to be uneconomical and such departments would either be closed or be forced to undergo changes in organization, perhaps with the injection of more resources. Instances exist where major purchasers, unable to persuade providers to improve services, have injected money into more cooperative departments in other hospitals. In many instances alternative providers do not exist and some units,

responding to what they see as an opportunity, are seeking to set up new departments and to attract disenchanted purchasers. Whilst no single GP fundholding practice is likely to have the financial clout to make radical changes, consortia of practices will undoubtably bring pressure to bear on provider units, be they hospital, community or ambulance trusts. There exists a dilemma on the part of purchasers who, whilst wishing to provoke change in one aspect of the service offered by a hospital, would not wish to destabilize other services in the same hospital.

The present fundholder focus is on areas of extreme dissatisfaction with the delivery of secondary care. In order to soften the blow and to minimize the potential for rapid change, money has been poured into waiting-list initiatives. Such endeavours are to be welcomed but care must be taken not to risk throwing good money after bad and artificially propping up inefficient departments. In many instances the results of these measures have been increased numbers of patients waiting for operations, albeit for shorter periods. It has been argued that it doesn't matter how many patients are waiting, as long as the waiting period is not too long.

A similar argument may apply to the waiting time between referral and obtaining an outpatient appointment. Fundholders will rightly insist on shorter waiting times but it is argued that if they were achieved the inpatient waiting list would get longer. There is, however, little evidence to support this claim.

The Patient's Charter has already highlighted the need for patients to be seen by a doctor within 30 minutes of arrival at a hospital outpatient department. Whilst efforts could and should be made to minimize the waiting time without compromising the number of patients seen, it is virtually impossible to guarantee that all patients will be seen in this time scale.

4.9 Managing budgets in clinical service

4.9(a) Surgical specialties

Mark Harrison

Introduction

The Royal Hampshire County Hospital is one of the original six pilot sites for the Resource Management Project. Before being invited to join this project, plans were well ahead to involve medical staff in the management structure of the hospital. By late 1985 a clinical directorate structure had been agreed and eight clinical directors had been appointed. There are five ward-based directorates in general medicine, general surgery and urology, obstetrics and gynaecology and paediatrics, orthopaedics and special surgery (ear, nose and throat, ophthalmology, orthodontics and oral surgery) with three service-based directorates: anaesthetics (including all theatres, day surgery and intensive care facilities), pathology and diagnostic imaging. Clinical directors are members of the hospital management board with the unit general manager (UGM) as chairperson. The deputy UGM, the finance director, the director of nursing services and the director of human resources complete the board. Whilst all clinical specialties are represented within the directorates, other supporting services such as physiotherapy, hotel and catering services and the works department are not represented directly on the hospital board. Some of these hold district-wide responsibilities and report directly to the UGM. Others, such as hotel services and catering, report to the directorate nursing services.

Once the management structure was agreed, the directorates were given budgets. This is a personal account of accepting a devolved budget for the general surgery and urology directorate and of the problems and opportunities involved in the allocation, setting and management of such a budget.

Allocation of budgets

The Royal Hampshire County Hospital is the only acute hospital in the Winchester health district. It has 430 beds serving a population of 215 000. There are no regional services based at Winchester. The current annual budget of the unit, including capital charges, is £33m. Since 1985 the budget devolved to the surgical directorate has remained at about 5% of the total budget and currently stands at £1.8m.

This amount does not cover all the costs incurred but includes those readily identified as relating to clinical activity within the directorate and includes most costs than can be directly influenced by clinicians. There is no devolved budget for capital charges, electricity, water, heating or maintenance and repairs (except repairs towards furniture!). All major items of medical and surgical equipment have to be negotiated centrally at the hospital board to decide priorities across the unit. Small items can be purchased or replaced within the directorate budget. The anaesthetic directorate holds the budget for replacement and repair of theatre equipment up to about £5000. Items above this level and new developments such as laparoscopic cholecystectomy must have their funding agreed centrally.

The surgical directorate comprises five consultant surgeons and supporting junior staff, a senior nurse manager shared with another directorate, a business manager, three surgical wards and a surgical unit office which comprises secretarial, clerical and coding staff. Staff salaries, including all locum and temporary staff, account for 86% of the total devolved budget (£1.57m). Other devolved costs include drugs (7%), medical and surgical supplies (2.5%), surgical appliances and prostheses (3%), dressings (1%), stationery (0.3%), travelling expenses (0.4%), telephone calls (0.1%), family planning fees (0.1%) and central sterile supplies (0.1%).

Theatre costs are not allocated as part of the budget but are planned to be charged on a sessional basis. Theatre sessions are charged for a fully staffed theatre, which includes nurses, anaesthetists and all drugs and equipment. There is an additional charge for high-cost items such as vascular grafts and ureteric stents. Each session is 3.5 hours. There is a surcharge for over-running the session. (There will also be an allowance for emergency work.) If sessions are cancelled with at least 2 weeks' notice, the session is not charged and the onus is on the anaesthetic directorate either to reallocate the session or to rearrange staff rotas accordingly. Monthly information on theatre usage and its cost implications is circulated to clinical directors and discussion continues as to whether this is an appropriate way of handling the theatre budget. Currently this remains a paper exercise with the whole theatre budget still held by the anaesthetic directorate.

Other medical and paramedical services such as day surgery, X-ray, laboratories and physiotherapy are not currently charged to directorates but regular information about usage is circulated. Day surgery could certainly be charged in a similar manner to theatre sessions. X-ray and laboratories are more complex as there are large numbers of events involved. It is necessary to distinguish tests arranged by general practitioners from outpatients, from accident and emergency and to distinguish impatient and emergency investigations. The effort in staffing levels and computing to achieve this is not currently seen as a priority in terms of controlling costs.

Setting budgets

The initial budgets were set on a historical basis using those costs which could be identified. Each clinical director discussed his or her proposed budget with the finance director and, accepting that there would still be errors, these were adopted as the starting point of an evolutionary process. Regular discussions with the finance director clarified the accounting process and reports became more comprehensible to clinicians and more useful from a managerial viewpoint.

Before the start of each financial year, the budget was revised against the expenditure for the previous year and the budget was set at new levels. Significant areas of budget overspend were discussed at board level as they became apparent and, whilst the changes in the new budget were not dramatic, they took account of any significant developments or changes in activity. A small increase was made for inflation. Monies for pay awards were usually held at district level.

The management of budgets

For management purposes the budget was divided into three. The clinical director was responsible for medical staffing and held that budget. The nurse manager held the nursing budget and ran it in conjunction with the ward sisters. The business manager held the unit office budget. This triumvirate met weekly to discuss general management issues within the directorate, including the budget, and met with staff in the finance department three or four times a year for a formal review, although queries about monthly budget statements were dealt with as they arose. Major trends in overspending were often related to increased clinical activity or staff sickness, both of which required higher levels of agency or locum staff to maintain adequate staffing to cover annual leave, study leave and sick leave. Significant trends were discussed at board level as they became apparent.

Problems

The initial problems were those of detail. Budget statements are not friendly documents to read. Some of the budget headings were ambiguous and it was not always clear which items were included under which headings. Gradually both clinicians and finance department staff gained confidence and understanding of each other's problems and needs. A clearer understanding emerged of what information enabled budget-holders to manage.

More major problems became apparent slowly. Historically the locum budget for junior medical staff had been overspent. This budget was devolved on a proportional basis to the directorates according to their staffing structure but it was soon found to be inadequate in the busy clinical specialties. Moves to reduce junior doctors' hours, the cessation of prospective cover for leave, the reduced availability of student locums and the cost of agency locums have compounded, creating significant difficulties in containing this budget.

All nursing posts were budgeted at the mid-point of the salary scale for that particular post rather than the actual salary that the individual holding the post received based on her or his experience. The high cost of agency staff to cover holidays, sickness, study leave and staff leaving and who had not yet been replaced emerged as a critical issue in managing the budget.

We then started to look at how to control costs more easily. A common response to control escalating costs in clinical specialties is to reduce clinical activity. Beds are closed (and preferably whole wards) as the potential savings are greater. As nursing staff salaries make up such a large part of the total budget, unless there is a reduction in the total staffing or the need to employ agency staff the savings are not great. Staff must be relocated to other wards and if staff leave they are not reappointed or there is a significant delay in doing so. By such action the budget can usually be made to balance expenditure at the end of the year and then staff can be employed in the new financial year. This type of cost control is familiar to all in the NHS and was practised to achieve the 'level playing field' for the introduction of the NHS reforms in April 1991. Whilst this is effective in controlling costs, it is not efficient in providing quality care to patients. Elective surgical admissions are reduced and delayed, waiting lists rise and the pressure to discharge patients back into the community from the reduced bed complement is intense.

Opportunities

The new contracting process makes the above approach more difficult to follow as contracts have to be met within agreed limits. These are likely to become tighter as the process becomes more sophisticated and wild swings in clinical activity will be difficult to justify without very good reasons. Simply containing the budget is not enough and agreed levels of activity have to be met. Before April 1991 increased clinical activity in any given financial year was usually not funded and was often the primary cause of budget overspend. In theory this increased activity will now attract additional funding.

The ability to manoeuvre within the directorate budget is limited. Major influence on expenditure comes from political and managerial initiatives which are usually outside the control of the doctor as a budget-holder. If clinical directorates are to be successful it is important that clinical directors, as members of a hospital board with an executive rather than advisory role, should think and act in a corporate manner and not just as representatives of their department.

Good housekeeping, such as giving notice of theatre sessions that are not going to be used so that they can be reallocated to other specialties or used for waiting list initiative work, is important. Similarly, increasing the use of day surgery, which is widely advocated as a way of containing costs as well as providing treatment that many patients find more convenient and acceptable, helps the hospital to treat more patients within its total budget. However, in our directorate, as we did not hold the budget for day surgery, the loss of more minor cases from the wards put a greater strain on the ward staff and on the budget. Policies for cross-matching blood, for antibiotic usage, and for the management of common problems all have their place, but their influence on the surgical directorate budget is small.

We are likely to see more dramatic changes in nurse staffing as a result of changing demographics in the young female population, with the number of 18-year-olds available for training due to fall dramatically. Project 2000 will also have its effects, with fewer students on the wards during training. Increasing the proportion of nursing assistants and part-time nurses is certainly less expensive in budgetary terms and the setting up of local nursing banks for nurses who are not available on a regular basis (not in school holidays) has been helpful in reducing agency nursing costs.

The present drive to reduce junior doctors' hours will lead to a re-examination of the working patterns of both senior and junior medical staff. It is unclear what the effects will be on the budget of our directorate. What is likely is that fewer junior staff will be on duty at any given time than at present and that they will be working harder.

These changes in medical and nursing staffing put great pressure on staff, especially as clinical activity continues to rise each year and maintaining the quality of care given to patients whilst in hospital becomes increasingly difficult. If clinical activity cannot be reduced and staff are not to work excessively long hours, quality of care becomes a major area of concern.

Devolving budgets to the level at which decisions are taken and which affects those budgets does make people more aware of the budgetary consequences of their actions and does lead to better control of budgets. There is some limited flexibility to adjust staffing of the departments to the clinical need but this has to be set against the relentless rise in clinical activity which is not allowed for fully in allocations, and just how long cost savings can be made every year without adverse effects on the quality of care is unclear because the information available is limited. It is certainly easier to anticipate budgetary overspends at an earlier stage and to enable action to be taken at both a directorate and unit level to contain these overspends.

4.9(b) Medical specialties

John Meecham

Managing budgets in clinical directorates

Managing the budget can be considered at many different levels. From a hospital trust's point of view the total budget for the whole organization is of overriding importance – an overspend in one part of the budget, or in one directorate, can be balanced against an underspend in another.

Clearly a trust's budget can be broken down into progressively smaller blocks and budgets can be derived for hospital units, clinical directorates, subunits or subspecialties, departments and wards. In managing each of these a responsible person is trying to achieve a balanced budget against recognized workload and agreed commitments with appropriate targets and standards. I was Clinical Director in Medicine first at Arrowe Park Hospital and then at the Wirral Hospital NHS trust, and was concerned with the budget of the medical directorate, from 1987 to 1992.

Arrowe Park Hospital was one of the six original resource management pilot sites, and together with Clatterbridge Hospital became one of the first-wave trusts. During that period of development three changes occurred which were necessary to the creation of budgets and their devolvement to the directorates:

1 *Alteration of the management structure.* The hospital changed to a clinical directorate structure. Each directorate is headed by a clinical director, supported by a clinical nurse manager and a business manager.
2 *Development of hospital-wide information technology.* Relevant information has always been lacking in the NHS. At the Wirral Hospital we have installed progressively a hospital-wide computer information system. This purposely serves clinical needs first, as a patient care information system (PCIS). However it gradually serves more and more functions and interfaces with other systems providing information related to workload, throughput, demographic details, investigations, reports, staffing levels, drug usage, costs, finance, medical equipment, supplies, stores, repairs, catering, laundry, cleaning – in fact every area of hospital activity. Case mix details are also being developed together with planning of nursing acuity and skill mix, and planning of outpatients and theatre sessions. Prescribing of drugs through pharmacy pathways is to go live on the system shortly.
3 *Development of financial information and budgets.* Very early in my clinical directorship the treasurer and I realized that I could easily be submerged in the amount of detail that he could provide, which would make the exercise pointless from my point of view. We gradually developed a spreadsheet so that the majority of what I needed to know could be provided on one sheet – admittedly large – and assimilated within minutes. Each item on the spreadsheet could be broken down into finer detail if required. I believe this has been a major factor in my ability to keep pace with and manage the budget in the medical directorate.

The spreadsheet displays information divided into four main headings:
(a) Activity.
(b) Expenditure – staff.
(c) Expenditure – non-staff.
(d) Staffing levels.

Any heading or subheading can be expanded if necessary and others can be added. We have tried to have on-call costs as a separate heading but this has presented particular difficulties and at the moment is included in staff expenditure.

During this development the finance department has been restructured. There are now four teams of financial advisers. Each team is headed by a senior, well-qualified principal financial adviser who works with a particular group of directorates. This offers much more financial support to the directorates and gives a continuing close personal contact between the teams and the directorates to their mutual advantage.

The first budgets were issued to directorates on a purely arbitrary basis according to historical activity. There was an idea of what the hospital as a whole cost in a year, but very little idea of where the money went in various services. At first budgets were managed just in theory, termed shadow budgets, the responsibility remaining with the finance department. However 3 years ago the responsibility for running the budget was devolved to the directorates, and individual clinical directors became personally responsible, with a commitment to bring in a balanced budget at the year end. Directorates' budgets vary from about £1.5m to £6.5m. About 70% of the hospital budget is now at directorate level.

The clinical director as manager

Hospital-wide objectives are discussed at 'away days', once or twice a year, attended by clinical directors, the chief executive and the advisory team. Hospital and directorate objectives of course depend upon business plans and purchaser/provider contract agreements. Plans can be reviewed regularly in council meetings once or twice a month.

Individual directorates agree on objectives and budgets with the chief executive, and these are monitored at review meetings.

Managing the budget in the medical directorate

This depends upon receiving accurate data, which can be displayed in different sections of a spreadsheet.

Table 4.9.1 Activity details of the medical directorate: May 1992

	Plan/ Estab- lished 1992/1993	May	Year to date	Plan to date
Discharges	8000	687	1470	1333
Beds available	205	200.2	197.1	
Beds occupied		200.1	193.6	
Beds empty		0.1	3.6	
Inpatient days		6203	11 813	
Occupancy (%)		100.0	98.2	
Length of stay		9.0	8.0	
Throughput		41.2	44.7	
Outpatient dept clinics (including gastrointestinal)		44	90	
Outpatient dept total attendances		1201	2308	
Outpatient dept new attendances		144	308	
Adult day ward		0	0	
Day cases	660	183	356	110
Percentage day cases		21.0	19.5	

For example, information related to usage of beds in medicine for the month of May 1992 was

displayed simply as shown in Table 4.9.1. It can be seen that the occupancy rate was very high. In fact it was over 100%, for we often had 12–40 medical patients in beds in other specialties, which were often counted as occupied beds there rather than in medicine. It can be seen that the throughput figure was high also, even though the length of stay reflected the fact that many patients were ill.

These figures can be shown to vary month by month. If we look at the same figures for the month of June 1992 (Table. 4.9.2), we can see that length of stay was markedly shorter and throughput had dramatically increased.

Table 4.9.2 Activity details of the medical directorate: June 1992

	Plan/ Estab- lished 1992/1993	June	Year to date	Plan to date
Discharges	8000	771	2241	2000
Beds available	207	177.9	188.5	
Beds occupied		152.0	172.2	
Beds empty		25.9	16.2	
Inpatient days		4560	15 673	
Occupancy (%)		85.4	91.4	
Length of stay		5.9	7.0	
Throughput		52.0	47.6	
Outpatient dept clinics (including gastrointestinal)		63	153	
Outpatient dept total attendances		1741	4049	
Outpatient dept new attendances		246	554	
Adult day ward		0	0	
Day cases	660	239	595	165
Percentage day cases		23.7	21.0	

Activity has to be balanced against expenditure and this can be displayed in other parts of the spreadsheet. For example, expenditure on staff salaries for doctors, nurses, technicians, secretaries and clerks for the month of June 1992 was displayed as shown in Table 4.9.3. From this it can be seen that there is an overspend on staff salaries for that month of £17 111 but that this was mainly on nurses (£7752) and administrative and clerical staff. The cumulative overspend for the first 3 months of the financial year was £29 941 but the vast majority of this was in nursing staff – £27 586. As clinical director I receive statistics for staffing levels and details of nursing

Table 4.9.3 Medical directorate staff costs: June 1992

	Annual Budget	This period June			Year to date		
		Budget	Expenditure	Variance	Budget	Expenditure	Variance
Medical staff							
Senior medical staff	466406	38897	38917	20	116597	113916	2601
Other medical staff	37120	3095	2577	– 518	9279	8485	– 794
Junior medical staff	456678	35090	46100	8010	114170	118453	4283
Agency medical staff	33893	2826	1531	– 1295	8472	4323	– 4149
Medical staff total	994097	82908	89124	6216	248518	245177	– 3341
Staff							
Nurse – DNS and Assistant	28412	2418		– 2418	7166		– 7166
Nurse – Seniors	28450	2421	3687	1266	7175	11009	3034
Nurse – Sisters	413227	35163	24266	– 10897	104215	84431	– 19784
Nurse – Staffs	1454846	124010	123318	– 692	366978	373951	6973
Nurse – Enrolled	95920	10220	11996	1776	25873	32674	6801
Nurse – Auxiliary	307782	26361	29917	3556	78127	81071	2944
Nurse – Bank			15161	15161		33984	33984
Nursing staff	2330637	200593	208345	7752	589534	617120	27586
PHYS MEAS'T TECH'	85002	7090	8371	1281	20608	24201	3593
Professional/technical staff	85002	7090	8371	1281	20608	24201	3593
Medical Secretaries	12953	1080	1582	502	3140	1582	– 1558
Administration and Clerical (A&C)	24014	2020	26320	24292	5364	57694	52130
A&C Senior						2118	2118
A&C Middle grades	78064	6604		– 6604	19008	1180	– 17828
A&C Support	139772	11845	– 3989	– 15834	34046	2398	– 31648
A&C	254803	21557	23913	2356	61758	64973	3215
On-call payments	11834	970	476	– 494	2852	1739	– 1113
Other staff total	2682276	230210	241106	10896	674752	708034	32282
Total all staff	3676373	313118	330229	17111	923270	953211	29941

staff hours worked, sickness rates, bank nurses employed and similar figures for other grades of staff. Nursing staff figures are particularly important, of course, not just because of the work they do, but because they are by far the largest part of the workforce, and therefore the largest part of the budget. In any clinical directorate nursing staff salaries alone account for more than 50% of the budget.

Expenditure on things other than staff salaries is termed rather unsatisfactorily 'non-staff expenditure' and appeared in the June 1992 spreadsheet as shown in Table 4.9.4.

It can be seen that drug expenditure is the largest item here and was overspent that month by £3707, causing a cumulative overspend for the first 3 months of the financial year of £4366.

Any of the items can be expanded for a closer look if they seem to be running out of control. For example, the expenditure for drugs can be broken down by drug, or by ward, or by specialty, or by consultant. This enabled me to question the gastroenterologists about the comparative costs of various H2-receptor blockers, and the haematologists about the costs of various cytotoxic and antiemetic drugs, and more recently about new drugs for stimulation of the bone marrow.

Receiving the month's figures allows the director to get an early warning of overspends, or increasing overspends, so that he or she can take

Table 4.9.4   Medical directorate non-staff expenditure: June 1992

	Annual	This period June			Year to date		
	Budget	Budget	Expenditure	Variance	Budget	Expenditure	Variance
Non-staff							
Provisions	20394	1705	1123	− 582	5094	4671	− 423
Uniforms	1543	128	234	106	387	727	340
Patients' clothing	2940	255	578	323	738	1575	837
Hardware and crockery		1	5	6	1	20	19
Bedding and linen	6732	576	321	− 255	1699	723	− 976
Printing and stationery	12552	1134	1574	440	3132	5066	1934
Telephones			95	95			
Advertising	3200	266		− 266	798		− 790
Travel	29407	2833	2098	− 735	10204	5988	− 4216
Removal expenses			− 40	40			
Courses and travel	2865	238	275	37	714	1094	380
Transport			14	14		45	45
Cleaning materials	500	40	11	− 29	120	101	− 19
Furniture and equipment			588	588		2301	2301
Computer purchase/rental			544	544		574	574
Consumables not stat.						193	143
Contracts			13	13		13	13
Miscellaneous			252	252		1040	1040
Internal recharges	− 36550	− 3048	− 4866	− 1818	− 9138	− 13455	− 4317
Direct credits						− 101	− 101
Income	− 8822	− 734	− 1925	− 1191	− 2202	− 1925	277
Dressings	8800	675	777	102	2224	1592	− 632
Drugs	474637	43001	46708	3707	114661	119027	4366
Msse-labs			− 7	− 7			
Hire beds			78	78		423	423
Med & Borg Dopt & S	166651	15133	12969	− 2164	41673	42098	425
Msse-Occupational therapy						65	65
Total non-staff	684849	62201	61417	− 784	170105	171853	1748
Grand total	4361222	375319	391646	16327	1093375	1125064	31689

steps to recognize them and correct them. The problem for medicine, as opposed to other mainly surgical disciplines, is that the workload consists largely of emergency admissions rather than planned admissions from a waiting list. Medicine is constantly responding to immediate demand with little ability to cushion the load by varying planned admissions.

It just so happens that haematology has caused financial stress in medicine recently in several ways. For no apparent reason the workload, and inpatient throughput, has nearly doubled in the last 12 months. This greatly increases the drug bill for cytotoxics, antiemetics and antibiotics. But it also increases nursing costs for one may need extra staff to look after immune-compromised patients and they need to be trained staff. Extra locum doctors have been needed at times for similar reasons.

In order to balance the books the director needs to achieve underspends to balance overspends. It may be possible to avoid appointing a nurse or a doctor to a vacancy during the summer months when the workload may have eased. The trouble with overspending in the summer is that medicine expects to have a hectic workload and overspend in the winter. So it would be nice to be approaching autumn with a positive balance!

Costs of all kinds can be discussed with appropriate staff members or groups in order to agree a different, more economical usage. This can be encouraged by devolving parts of the budget further down the organization to ward level. In several directorates, including medicine, ward sisters have accepted financial responsibility for approved ward budgets. This includes ward staff costs.

In theory, the skill mix and seniority, and therefore salary levels, of staff can be varied, but in practice this can only happen slowly with retirements and resignations.

It is worth noting on the spreadsheets (Tables 4.9.3 and 4.9.4) that the total staff budget is almost £3.68m out of the total budget of £4.36m. In other words, 84% of the budget is staff salaries (and nursing salaries alone account for 53% of the budget).

The director has to manipulate as well as he or she can therefore within a relatively small proportion of the budget. It is to his or her credit, and that of the business manager and the finance adviser, that things work out as well as they do for most of the time.

4.9(c) Diagnostic services

Hugh Saxton

Although it is generally understood that a budget means a sum of money allocated to cover the running of a department, it is more fully defined as the expression in financial and other terms of an organization's agreed plans and objectives for a set period of time and the resources needed to achieve them. In current terms this is a service agreement and a budget is part of this agreement. The elements in the service agreement are:

1 Human resources – grades × wte.
2 Financial resources broken down in a standard way.

In today's environment there may also be:

3 Agreed output targets, e.g. examinations or tests performed.
4 Agreed quality pathways, e.g. maximum waiting time for routine appointment and so on.

In a few hospitals there may also be a system for charging part or all of the department's costs to user clinical firms, general practitioners, etc. When fully established, this system replaces a fixed budget with a flexible one but, as yet, it is so uncommon that a discussion here does not seem merited.

Problems in taking on a budget

Even though it may not be possible to avoid budgetary responsibility, it is important to be clear as to the drawbacks of holding a budget, if only because of the need for a tough stance in the preliminary negotiations. Apart from the additional work involved:

1 Thrifty departments start with a lower baseline and are worse off than if they had been careless over expenditure.
2 Unless all expenditure is fully covered in the initial setting of the budget, difficulty may arise, for example when lead aprons or cassettes or glassware need replacing.

3 Once a budget is held it is easier for the hospital management to apply fiscal pressure, removing funds at source.
4 Without a departmental computer it will be extremely difficult to monitor activity of various kinds, let alone achieve proper efficiency.

Agreements prior to accepting a budget

The consultant asked to take on a budget must negotiate very firmly with management who will, generally, be anxious to persuade him or her to accept the new responsibility. The following heads cover the most important issues and relate both to the initial desiderata and the rules under which the budget will operate:

1 *Management help*. A business manager is essential. This might be a senior medical laboratory scientific officer (MLSO) or radiographer with appropriate aptitudes and training, or a career manager. Smaller departments may have to share their manager.
2 *A computer*. The uses of a computer are less to do with direct financial control than with monitoring workload and its fluctuations; with recording the source of workload, i.e. by individual clinicians; with speeding the issuing of results/reports and simplifying record-keeping. In imaging departments it may be possible to record workload and service/repair costs by individual X-ray rooms. All these can help the department to be more efficient and hence to manage the budget more effectively.
3 *Establishing current expenditure*. Major costs like servicing, consumable expenditure and staffing costs will be relatively straightforward but problems may arise over items which are purchased intermittently. These are particularly important in imaging departments where they include such things as ultrasonic probes, X-ray tubes, vascular injectors, cassettes, lead aprons or film envelopes. In any department furniture, word processors, travel, subsistence, books, journals or teaching aids will be needed at some time. An appropriate annual budget should be negotiated for such items. Agreement is also needed on how items of major capital expenditure will be funded.
4 *Handling specific issues*. There are a number of items which are dealt with differently in different

hospitals and over which the rules must be clarified. In imaging departments contrast and drugs are an example. Will the budget stay with pharmacy or be transferred to the department budget? Similarly, rulings are needed over secretarial and administrative and clerical costs, portering, domestics, telephones, postage, laundry and so forth.

5 *Savings and virement.* The rules over the use of savings should be established. For example, it is usually possible to vire savings on the personnel account to buy equipment but not vice versa. Some hospitals distinguish between unplanned savings, for example if theatres closed for a month so reducing workload, and planned savings resulting from the department's management action. It is also important to determine whether savings can be carried into the following financial year.

6 *Overspending.* Will any overspending be carried forward and deducted from the following year's budget?

7 *Income.* If the department earns any income, how is that to be dealt with? In particular it is essential to make sure that it does not reduce the budget for the following year.

8 *The basis for next year's budget.* The way in which the next year's budget is arrived at should be made clear. It may well be the current year's figure with appropriate increments but the rules should be clear.

Running the budget

To those whose domestic budgeting is confined to looking at the final entry on their bank statement, a detailed departmental budget may seem alarming. This is one of the reasons for spending time on defining the elements in the budget in the phase of preliminary negotiations. However it should not be necessary for the consultant to monitor every line personally. The laboratory or radiographic staff costs will be monitored by the appropriate MLSO or superintendent radiographer who will also cover servicing, film and chemical costs. Secretarial, administrative and clerical costs, the running costs of the computer and the overall budget picture are likely to be the responsibility of the business manager while the clinical director covers medical staffing costs.

However, in general, the management of a budget is inseparable from the management of the department as a whole. Once the budget is established most departments will look for savings, so as to fund developments which are desirable. Making savings can be done in a wide variety of ways: among the more obvious ways are:

1 Shedding staff or at least maintaining vacancies for a period.
2 Using staff time more efficiently, e.g. matching staff rotas to work load.
3 Changing staff grades (hard to achieve because of grade drift).
4 Negotiating discounts with suppliers.
5 Applying guidelines/vetting requests.
6 In imaging departments, using protocols to reduce the routine views employed.
7 Trimming servicing routines.
8 Taking care over stocks, i.e. fewer types and fewer in number.
9 Income generation, e.g. through extracontractual referrals or work for fundholders.

Problems in running the budget

As noted earlier, the issues involved in keeping a budget under control are bound up in the management of the department. Any major action to create savings will have an effect on departmental staff so that their involvement is needed to make such plans effective.

The need for commitment accounting

A major problem in many hospitals is the lack of coordination between the finance department, the supplies department and individual budgetholders. For example, it is possible for an X-ray department to replace an X-ray tube in July and see no entry in their budget until late in the financial year or even in the following year. The best way to avoid this situation is for the finance department to offer some form of commitment accounting. In this the finance department is notified of the likely expenditure when the order is placed; it then shows a corresponding but approximate debit in the following budget statement. Failing this, the department should keep its own records and make provisional debits itself.

The need to check invoices

When a service is undertaken or repairs are carried out, the person who signs the job sheet will not know the precise charge being made.

The subsequent invoice may go direct to the supplies department and may contain items which are incorrect. Only someone in the department can verify the details but the supplies department is often unwilling to return such invoices for validation because of the time involved. Local arrangements are needed to enable checks to be made but it is important that they are done quickly in case any discount for prompt settlement is lost.

Problems of overspending

An overspend may be the result of central action by unit management imposing a cut but apart from this there are a number of problems to be considered:

1 *Recognizing the overspend.* As indicated, a lag in settling invoices may conceal an overspend.
2 *Ensuring that the expenditure belongs to the budget.* Misattribution can occur, especially in large hospitals or where there are shared facilities, e.g. cardiologists using an angiographic suite.
3 *Checking that the expenditure is correct.* This demands checks on invoices, as discussed earlier. It also requires careful checks on personnel statements; it is not unknown for staff who have left to continue to be paid. Equally, the effect of agency/overtime payments may have been overlooked.
4 *Dealing with the overspend.* Once it is clear that the overspend is genuine, action must be taken along the lines set out earlier. It is of course necessary to save at a rate which will bring the budget back under control within the time available before the end of the financial year and this often requires very harsh measures.

Problems of an underspend

It may seem paradoxical to describe an underspend as a problem but there are questions to be asked before an underspend is accepted at face value:

1 *Is it genuine?* Without commitment accounting it may be hard to be sure.
2 *Is it due to management action or luck?* The answer to this question reveals how firmly the budget is under control and whether the trend will continue.
3 *Will we be allowed to use the savings?* The answer to this question may depend in part on the under-

standings reached with central management when the budget was initiated.
4 *Will it affect next year's budget?* This too will depend on the prevailing rules.

Capital charges on major capital equipment

The broad principles of capital charging have been discussed in Section 4.3, where it is emphasized that hospitals now have to recover revenue to service the costs of their capital assets. Diagnostic departments, especially imaging departments, have equipment with significant capital values and they, in particular, have to consider as carefully as any hospital departments the effects of new capital purchases. As yet, relatively few diagnostic departments have been given much guidance on how to calculate capital charges on their equipment. This is probably because:

1 Few departments are charging directly for their services to other clinical directorates.
2 Asset registers are often incomplete, lacking such details as the date of purchase, cost of purchase and funding source. Without these fundamentals, any capital charge calculation is likely to be flawed.

None the less, it is likely that in time proper calculations will be made and pathologists and radiologists should at least understand the main elements which go to make up the capital charges on large items of equipment. The most important point to understand is the distinction between capital sums and the interest now charged on them and the capital charges which are an accounting concept, separately calculated and charged.

The aim of these charges is to make all concerned aware of the fact that capital has a cost and that this cost must be met in NHS transactions. A second reason is to bring NHS practices into line with those in the private sector. Capital charges therefore comprise an element for depreciation on the equipment concerned and an interest charge representing the interest payable on a real or assumed loan used to purchase the particular item of equipment.

The revenue costs of capital (see Section 4.3)

In a directly managed unit (DMU), the money provided to its purchasing authority by the region includes an element which corresponds to the perceived needs of the authority to meet the capital charges made by providers. The interest and depreciation payments derived by the DMU from such contracts and from extracontractual referrals (ECRs) are returned to the region – although the total derived from contracts, etc. and the total paid to the region may not be equal. The exact way in which capital sums for scientific equipment are made available to such hospitals is variable, but for the moment many still receive allocations through their regional scientific officers. DMUs do not pay interest on such capital allocations.

An NHS trust makes depreciation and interest charges in the same way, i.e. as part of the charges in its contracts with purchasing authorities and for ECRS; for trusts the term financial return target is used rather than interest, even though the figure is calculated in the same way as interest charges made by DMUs. To obtain capital for equipment and other needs, the trust must borrow, usually from the Department of Health. Such borrowing must be within the constraints of its external financing limit (EFL), negotiated with the Department of Health. (The EFL is intended to prevent trusts from borrowing excessive amounts.) The trust retains the money received for depreciation and interest charges. These surpluses are used for a variety of purposes, including new capital purchases, repayment of loans and payment of interest on such loans.

Interest charges and interest

It is important to understand the difference between interest charges as a part of the capital charges made by hospitals to purchasing authorities, and the actual interest paid on money borrowed by a hospital, the lender usually being the Department of Health.

The interest charge as part of the capital charge is intended, as discussed in Section 4.3, to provide a return on the capital used in purchasing the equipment, whether or not the equipment concerned was bought with borrowed money. Such a charge will continue to be made until the equipment has fully depreciated, even when the loan has been partly or wholly paid off. If the equipment was purchased with money given by a charity, depreciation will be applied as an internal accounting entry but, strictly, trusts are

not allowed to recover depreciation in health care contracts and ECRs on such gifted assets.

By contrast, when a sum of money is borrowed from the Department of Health, interest is charged at a rate determined from time to time, currently about 9.5–10% per annum. As the trust repays the loan, the actual interest payable will fall correspondingly. Thus, if half of a £400 000 loan has been repaid, the annual interest payment will halve. As explained above, this will not affect the interest charges made to purchasing authorities as part of the total contract price.

Calculating a replacement value

It is obvious that a unit costing £200 000 in 1992 will cost much more in 10 years, because of the effects of inflation. (This ignores a possible drop in prices due to changes in technology over 10 years.) So at present, every year, the replacement value of the unit is recalculated upwards by applying the annual rate of inflation to the original purchase price (see Table 4.9.1). Thus if, as shown, inflation is 8% per annum, each year the value rises, in the first year by $8\% \times £200\,000 = £16\,000$; in the next year by $8\% \times £216\,000 = £17\,280$, and so on.

Calculating and applying depreciation

Just as it is appropriate to index the replacement value to allow for inflation, so a similar adjustment has to be made to increase the sum charged for depreciation. Otherwise the total sum eventually charged would simply be the total of the original purchase price, insufficient to reflect the cost of a replacement machine. To correct for this effect, the sum calculated for depreciation is also indexed, as shown in Table 4.9.1.

The period over which depreciation is calculated will vary with the equipment. Sophisticated X-ray equipment will usually be written off over 10 years but it will be more usual to apply a 15-year period to a conventional X-ray unit. Some laboratory equipment may be depreciated over 5 years. Once the period has been determined, this will give the basis for the annual figure. Thus a £200 000 unit being depreciated over 10 years will show a basic depreciation of £20 000 at the end of the first year, i.e. one-tenth of the total. At this point indexation is applied and $£20\,000 \times 8\% = £1600$. At the end of the first year the accumulated figure is therefore £21 600. Table 4.9.1 shows how this indexation increases the accumulated depreciation total. The depreciation for the year is subtracted from the augmented replacement value and this gives the *net book value*. The net book value might be thought of as a fair price at which to sell an item of equipment at a particular point in time. It embodies an upwardly adjusted value to take account of inflation over the period since purchase, but it offsets this by subtracting the sums 'set aside' as depreciation which have also been increased annually in line with inflation.

Table 4.9.1 Capital charges on equipment with a useful life of 10 years. Value of equipment at 31.03.93 = £200 000; annual rate of inflation 8% (based on published indices)

| | Year ending | | |
	31.03.94 (£)	31.03.95 (£)	31.03.96 (£)
Replacement value			
Opening value	200 000	216 000	233 280
Indexation	16 000	17 280	18 662
Closing value	216 000	233 280	251 942
Depreciation			
Accumulated balance b/f	0	21 600	46 656
Charge for year	20 000	21 600	23 328
Accumulated total	20 000	43 200	69 984
Indexation	1600	3456	5599
Balance c/f	21 600	46 656	75 583
Year-end net book value (being replacement value less depreciation)	194 400	186 624	176 359
Interest charge – 6% (on purchase price in first year, then net book value)	12 000	11 664	11 197
Depreciation charge	20 000	21 600	23 328
Total capital charge	32 000	33 264	34 525

Charging interest

The interest charge is applied to this net book value, that is to a value which reflects both the upwards movement of prices generally and the fall in the residual sum owed as money is 'put aside' for depreciation. As shown in Table 4.9.1, over time the size of the interest payment diminishes somewhat as the net book value falls.

Total capital charge

Table 4.9.1 shows how the total size of the capital charge will rise because of the growth of the amount payable for depreciation. The adverse impact of this effect will, in general, be diminished by inflation. And it will be noted that within this overall figure the interest charge becomes progressively smaller as the net book value falls, even as the depreciation charge progressively rises.

It must be repeated that one of the purposes of the capital charging scheme is to make all prospective users think about the way in which they will use the equipment they wish to buy. For example, it is not unknown for a computed tomography scanner to be used for only 6 or 8 cases a day. This means that the impact of capital charges on the price charged for a scan will be over twice that for a scanner running nearer to a 'busy' usage, say 20 cases a day. This might point to the purchase of a cheaper scanner for a less busy department. (It hardly needs to be said that similar arguments apply to the cost of personnel employed in running the scanner.) Any department considering capital purchases will have increasingly to include such business projections in the case they make for capital to purchase a new piece of equipment.

Uses made of revenue from capital charges

It might be thought that the application of depreciation charges would, in time, provide a sum of money for the replacement of the equipment on which the charges were made. This is not the usual commercial accounting practice, nor does it apply in the NHS. The purpose of depreciation charges is to reflect the full economic cost of using the equipment but no money is actually put to one side. The sums received from capital charges as elements of a price will however add to a trust's year-end surplus. They might in fact be used to meet the latest pay award for nurses or some other purpose, but broadly they should contribute to the funds available for the purchase of new or replacement equipment or at least to pay interest and replacement on a capital loan. It is therefore up to pathologists and radiologists to point out to their chief executive the surplus accumulating each year and to negotiate an appropriate programme of replacement of equipment.

Conclusions

Running a budget efficiently is inseparable from good departmental management and requires the collaborative work of all within the depart-ment. While much can be done by delegation, it is important that the director of the department is sure that the systems in operation are effective and that everyone understands their responsi-bilities in helping to ensure that the budget is run efficiently.

Section 5

Building and capital equipment

5.1 Planning a new hospital building

Max Rendall and Sandra Carnall

Building schemes in hospitals never seem to be straightforward. Invariably they cost more than was budgeted, and take longer than was anticipated. The noise, the dust and the mud are tolerated with as much good grace as can be mustered, as being the price that must be paid for new facilities which will be ideal to allow medicine to be practised as it should be.

The outcome, sadly, is rarely as satisfactory as that, and there are many reasons why not. Some are financial, such as a decision to sacrifice the quality of finish and ease of maintenance in favour of a few more square metres of space. Some are contractual – delays, strikes, subcontractors going bankrupt and the like. Some are political. Yet others are because the brief given to the architects was not sufficiently considered, and the wrong building was designed and built.

Hospital building the world over does not have a very proud record. Even now huge hospitals are built which are not needed and can never be staffed – often monuments to political ambition. In the UK we have had our disasters – hospitals which we can never afford to run as they were designed, and buildings put up of defective design or materials.

Capital planning in health care is a complex process assailed by difficulties of all kinds – changing patterns of care, ever-advancing technology, altering public expectations, too little money, and the length of time between planning and commissioning new buildings. Although it might seem that NHS capital planning is an excessively bureaucratic system, the present planning structure is the consequence of many earlier errors.

As in medicine, a systematic approach is the only way to prevent mistakes and to ensure that nothing important is forgotten. Good planning is based on a number of simple principles:

1 Start from the beginning.
2 Set aside prejudices and preconceptions, and maintain an open mind.
3 Be certain what the objectives are.
4 Identify and examine all the constraints to see which are real and which can be changed.
5 Examine all the options, however unlikely they may seem.
6 Don't be afraid of uncertainty.
7 Remember always that you are planning for the future, not the present.

With these principles in mind, this chapter attempts to unravel issues in planning and construction, and to discuss the major contributions to health service planning which can be made by doctors.

The NHS planning system

Buildings cost money – to build, to run and to maintain. All monies taken for estate purposes come at the expense of direct patient care. Until the 1991 NHS Act there was no incentive to consider estate costs within the overall framework of health care delivery. Capital – the money required to build or convert buildings – came by a separate route from the Treasury, through the Department of Health and regional health authorities. It was effectively a 'free good' since no interest was charged, and building depreciation was not accounted for. Space to the user was part of their 'empire', and little thought was given to making it work more efficiently. There was little incentive to design buildings which were effective in use and easily maintained, so year-on-year estate revenue costs were often greater than desirable.

Capital will always be limited. The result is that departments within hospitals, hospitals within districts, and districts within regions have to enter a form of lottery. The winners in the past were usually the most politically aware and vociferous, but not necessarily those with the greatest justification in terms of patient need. Much time and money has been wasted on preparing plans for (and sometimes even building) developments which were not the most effective solution to a problem.

To establish order within the process of planning, and to assess demand on a structured, nationwide basis, the Department of Health devised its CAPRICODE system. It was introduced in the heady and optimistic days when Enoch Powell was Minister of Health, and money was being poured into hospital building. It is still in use today and, despite its deficiencies, it is a sensible process based on sound logical principles. It defines a number of stages through which the potential health builder has to pass. Each stage is a necessary step towards designing a building which will be fitted to its *future* use, rather than recreating the past.

The first CAPRICODE stage (stage A): obtaining approval in principle

Large hospital buildings are extremely expensive, and by far the largest contribution to their cost comes from the public purse. Rightly, therefore, the need for new facilities has to be most closely examined and persuasively argued. The feasibility of building on the available space must be determined, and all the other ways in which the required services might be provided examined, so that a preferred option can be chosen and justified.

Establishing the need

The first formal step is to decide what is needed and why. The answer must be honest and sound, for it will be the intellectual foundation of the building, which will be energetically and expertly assailed. It is a process of information gathering, consultation, predicting the future and rethinking. It is of course influenced by politics, and it cannot be done too quickly because time invariably throws up previously unconsidered issues and solutions. It must take account of scores of considerations, among which these are the most important:

1 The present and future population and its age/sex structure.
2 Deprivation and other local social factors.
3 Local prevalence of disease and standardized mortality ratios.
4 Catchment population and extraterritorial referrals.

5 Location of other services in the vicinity.
6 Travelling times and lines of communication.
7 How medical practice and service delivery are changing.
8 Lengths of stay, turnover intervals, etc.
9 Cost per case.
10 Market viability – who wants the service and at what cost?
11 Research and teaching issues.

The outcome of this step is in effect a business plan for the future. It should incorporate an assessment of strengths, weaknesses, opportunities and threats (SWOT analysis) for each service proposed and, to a greater or lesser extent, for the hospital itself. The final product will allow an objective assessment of where money should be invested for greatest benefit.

Clinicians have a major role to play in this process since it is they who determine the future face of medicine. They will have a particularly important and difficult task in trying to predict how practice will have changed when the new building is in use. They will need some guidance, for gazing into the future is famously unreliable, but there are techniques, such as a Delphic study, which can help to make predictions workably robust. The planning clinician not only has to analyse how the *practice* of medicine in each specialty will change; he or she also has to make a realistic assessment of quantum and cost. In other words, consideration has to be given to the hard truth that the ideal may not be affordable.

What must emerge from this stage is a detailed *functional content* – that is, a statement of the number and quantum of functions to be undertaken, and the facilities needed to accomplish those. This will set out the numbers of beds, day-care places and outpatient sessions per specialty, and a quantification of all the support service facilities required.

Site factors

At the same time as the functional content is being established, technical experts will be examining a number of physical issues, such as the capacity of potential building sites, planning constraints, the adequacy of power and drainage, existing boiler capacity, and the like. A combination of this analysis and the required functional content will generate a list of possible building options. Most will have to be carefully considered, and clinicians have an important task in advising on such issues as the desirable physical relationships between different departments, the sharing of certain facilities, patient access, and so forth.

The option appraisal

All schemes costing more than some £5m require an option appraisal of the possible solutions which are capable of providing what has been defined as the need. Too often, apparently cheap solutions can seem desirable which, on further analysis, can be more costly or constraining in the longer term. Conversely, expensive new building is not always the best way to provide what is needed.

An option appraisal is a way of quantifying considerations which should properly be taken into account in identifying a preferred solution, and setting them against capital and revenue limits. These might, for example, be travelling times for patients and staff, effects on service delivery, the effects of teaching and research, phasing of the building project, and how effectively the hospital could be run during the construction of different alternatives. Once the list of issues to be considered is complete, each can be given a relative weight. The list of possible building options can then be reduced to a short list of three by testing them all against the criteria identified. The three remaining building solutions are then examined in detail, including an assessment of their physical and cost characteristics. The best performing option against each criterion is given a score, which is multiplied by the weighting assigned to each of the test criteria. This process is repeated until all the options have been tested against all the criteria, and a numerical score will then identify the preferred option.

The clinician working with the planning team must be involved in helping to determine both the test criteria and the relative weight which should be attached to each.

The approval in principle document

The preferred option is therefore the one which performs best in service and financial terms. The arguments for reaching this decision are then written up in detail and submitted to the Department of Health, in a document applying for approval in principle for the building scheme it describes.

This document also has to present the best estimate of the capital cost of the competing options. This is done using the Department of Health's CONCISE method, which gives departmental and equipment cost allowance guides (DCAG and ECAG) based on building schemes around the country of a similar nature. To these CONCISE DCAG and ECAG costs is added what is known as an 'oncost' (normally between 65 and 95%) to reflect the particular difficulties of building in the proposed location. These might be a very constrained city site, a sloping site or poor ground conditions, additional building transport costs, differences in the local labour market, and other such issues.

Approval in principle, if granted, is given to the expenditure of the stated amount of capital, which must not vary by more than 10% during the process of design and building. If these limits are breached, the approval in principle lapses and the project must be represented for secondary approval.

The second CAPRICODE stage (stage B): planning and design

Most people imagine intuitively that the first thing to do if you want to build is to find an architect. In fact, it is only some way into the second CAPRICODE stage that an architect and other professional advisers (quantity surveyor, structural and services engineers) are selected, after competitive fee tendering. There will probably have been 2 years of hard work before this stage is reached.

Management control plan

The first task after receiving approval in principle is to set a timetable for the project, and a date for completion and commissioning of the building. This must be realistic and take account of the often very intricately interrelated tasks. The programme should be as robust as possible so that the inevitable delays do not have a domino effect upon the whole programme.

Preparation of whole hospital and departmental operational policies, and schedules of accommodation

It is in these tasks that doctors have their second major contribution to make. Before becoming involved in a mass of detail, it is important to think through and define exactly what the role, philosophy and requirements of each department should be in the future. Whole hospital functions are such things as the main entrance and commercial areas, computing, works and supplies, fire and health and safety, and the like. At this stage the current *modus operandi* of all departments should be challenged and reassessed. For example:

1 Food may have been delivered to the wards in bulk. Should there not be a change to plated meals or a cook/chill system with regeneration at ward level?
2 Instead of weekly sessions in a remote outpatient department, is there a case for some departments to see smaller numbers of outpatients everyday actually in their departments, where the necessary investigations can be done?
3 Secretaries may have been housed in a central secretariat. Would they be better working within the clinical department whose work they do?
4 Statutory regulations may have changed since the establishment of an existing department. What physical and operational changes are needed to conform to the new requirements?

The doctor on the planning team may have a difficult time with colleagues who wish to maintain the status quo, but his or her job is to ask 'why?' and 'what if . . . ?' and to challenge assumptions. He or she should involve junior consultants and senior registrars who may have come from places where practice and organization are different. He or she might organize visits to hospitals where innovative thinking is working well. Above all, he or she should never allow a senior and perhaps intimidating figure to recreate an outmoded department in which that person will never work and which will need radical change to bring it up to date.

It is also important to recognize at this stage that the detailed design will be done by architects and engineers who, however skilled in hospital design, cannot fully understand the complexities of each hospital's way of working or the evolving changes in medical practice. The clinician on the project team must ensure that clinical practice, which may seem self-evident, is clearly and fully explained to professional advisers. Departmental operational policies go some way towards doing this for they are documents which lay out in a fixed format how each department will work. It should not simply be a paper exercise because the new departments will be designed to facilitate their working as described in the operational policies. The policies should consider everything about the departments: name, objectives, the services provided, cost per case, security of referrals, staffing, management arrangements, flows of patients and supplies – where they come from and where they go – and identify other departments and services upon which each department depends.

The end-product of this great body of work is a book of whole hospital and departmental operational policies, which becomes the essential reference work and forms the basis of all future planning.

Having established *how* each department should operate in the future, the planning team will then prepare schedules of accommodation. These convert the broad policies for each department into a list of the appropriate numbers of rooms of the required size to fulfil the stated functions. The Department of Health produces health building notes for each department as a guide to this process. However, it is important to recognize that:

1 Building notes give generous-sized rooms, and all the facilities required in a 'standard' department. They do not however describe an entitlement. The use of space has a direct effect on the cost per case in each specialty, and space may therefore have to be reduced to meet the capital and revenue available.
2 They are often out of date. Departure from the building note provision therefore can be justified on the grounds of changed practice, but only within the finance available.
3 Building notes do not exist for a number of specialized departments normally found only in teaching hospitals. In these areas greater justification may be required; comparison with precedents elsewhere can be helpful.

Room data sheets and sketch drawings

The architect will take the schedules of accommodation and convert them into preliminary layouts for each department, which must then be taken back to the staff. At this stage there must be an opportunity for all concerned to comment (nurses, paramedical staff, technicians, secretaries, clerks, cleaners and others) – not just the clinicians – for they will all have valid and useful points to make.

At the same time room data sheets are prepared which list exactly what the requirements for each room are. They identify:

1 All the activities to take place in each room.
2 The number of people who will work permanently in the room or who may be present temporarily at any one time.
3 The temperature and lighting levels required.
4 Number of socket outlets, telephone and computer points, etc.
5 Ventilation and fume extract needs.
6 Wall, floor, ceiling and window finishes.
7 All the furniture and equipment which will stay in, or move in and out of each room, and the consequent power requirements and heat gain.

These sheets are the basis of the final design. If they are wrong or inadequate, the building will also be wrong. The ability of all the users, prompted by the planning team, to identify what may seem to be so obvious as not to be worth mentioning is the key to success. For example, a common problem is that rooms in new buildings overheat because the brief did not identify the heat gain from equipment such as freezers or personal computers.

Major equipment schedules

From the room data sheets is derived a full list of all the furniture and equipment required. This can then be specified and costed. The doctor should ensure that specifications for equipment are appropriate for the task to be undertaken, and advise on standardization, the use of one or more suppliers, and so on.

Final drawing approval and briefing information: 'Freezing the brief'

Sketch layouts are gradually converted into final drawings. The doctor will be responsible for seeing that all drawings are 'signed off', after final consultation with the future users, as being the best design solution possible in the circum-

stances. It is important, at this stage, that the end-user understands fully what will be the end-product since, at this point, the plans are 'frozen'.

The design team will all have large teams at work on drawings. Changes at this stage will cost time and money, and will necessitate space reductions elsewhere. At the end of this stage bills of quantity are prepared; this is a detailed specification of the building, against which competing building and engineering contractors can tender.

Construction

Once tenders have been received and analysed, the construction work will be awarded to one company, usually the lowest tenderer. A contract is entered into whereby the builder agrees to provide the building to the tendered specifications for the price and to the programme agreed. Work starts immediately; plant and equipment are ordered, labour and materials arrive on site, and subcontractors are appointed.

There are today many different types of contract. The traditional approach is to design the building, then build it. It is now however common practice to start construction before design is complete, and there are variations on these themes. Broadly it can be said that the traditional method makes costs easier to control, but takes much longer. The design-and-build type of contract delivers a finished building quicker, but cost containment can be a problem. For that reason they have not been seen much in NHS building but this is changing, and it will have an impact on the CAPRICODE system.

From the time that building starts, change is extremely costly, for a number of reasons:

1 Contrary to common belief, contractors make a low profit margin on major projects (usually well below 5%). To win the contract in competitive tendering they have to reduce their bid to the lowest they think possible. Any unilateral variation to the contract by the client breaks the legal contract, and allows the contractor, now that the client is effectively locked into a relationship with him, to renegotiate the price quoted. Contractors know there will be variations of this kind, and make their money in this way.
2 Although it may seem that nothing much is happening on a building site, every day in a tight programme counts. Client change can negate much of

what has gone before, and create the need for more labourers, more time, changes in plant or materials already delivered, and so on.

While the building is going up the planning team has three important tasks:

1 To ensure that no change occurs unless absolutely essential. It is usually cheaper to change a building after take-over than to run a building contract with continued argument between builder and client over the cost of change.
2 To maintain constant contact with existing hospital staff, particularly when building is going to cause noise, dust or other interference with normal working. Discussion before the nuisance occurs will obtain maximum cooperation.
3 To plan the commissioning of the new building when it is handed over.

Commissioning

New buildings require a lot of work to bring them into use. A doctor is an essential member of the team planning and undertaking this work. Among the tasks involved are:

1 Training staff so that everyone knows the layout, access routes, fire escapes and the like, and can operate all the systems provided.
2 Organizing a programme of commissioning, department by department. This will be a compromise between getting it done quickly, and too much interference with existing work.
3 Arranging for furniture and equipment delivery on time, and unpacking, checking and putting each item in the right place.
4 Arranging for departments to move into their new accommodation, either during a weekend (when less back-up is available), or during the week, which may involve cancelling clinics or ceasing to provide a service for a short time.
5 Decommissioning vacated buildings.
6 Keeping the organization informed.

The project team and the role of doctors

As soon as approval in principle to a major building scheme is granted, a project team will be brought together. It will be responsible for the day-to-day management of the scheme. Its membership will vary from one project to another, but it will always have on it the profes-

sional advisers (architect, quantity surveyor, structural and services engineers – collectively also called the design team) and the projects director of the hospital. A separate commissioning team, reporting to the projects team, will be composed of a planning nurse, representatives of the regional health authority (unless the project is for an NHS trust) and a clinician. There may be, in addition and when necessary, the hospital works officer, and representatives of finance and local medical school. Both teams will usually meet monthly.

It is usual to select a member of the consultant medical staff to represent the clinical point of view. He or she is there not as a delegate, but as a member of the team to which he or she can bring knowledge of the processes and needs of clinical medicine. The clinician must be selected for his or her interest in the project, and should be of an age which will mean that he or she will practise in the new building. He or she must have a professional and emotional stake in the building and its success. There will be stages when it will take a lot of time, and others when involvement will be nominal only. He or she should be a negotiator, but also be prepared to resolve conflict by decision. Certain tasks for which he or she will be responsible can be delegated to other members of the team, probably to the planning nurse, who will also have responsibility for representing the nursing interest in its own right. It is an interesting and rewarding role for the right person.

The new building can and must be shaped to a considerable extent by the clinician on the team. He or she will quickly learn to whom to go for advice. Seniority does not necessarily equip someone to know how a new department should be planned; in fact the contrary may be the case.

During the preparation of the approval in principle document there is also a most important contribution to be made by the medical staff. A clinician, and preferably the one who will join the project team when it comes into being, should chair a group to look at the future requirements of the hospital, and how it will be affected by changes in practice. This team should be composed of predominantly younger consultants, whose minds are as open and fair as possible. They will perhaps have seen or be aware of different thinking and its effect on hospital buildings elsewhere.

Conclusions

Hospital buildings in the UK have a planned life of 60 years (although the engineering services within them will require replacement two or three times in that period). It is a happy thing that the Victorians took a more confident and optimistic view of the future, for many of their buildings are still in use today, and most of ours are likely to be showing their age in 60 years, and equally likely to have to give service for twice that time. This underlines the importance of building for the future, and getting as much right as possible. This, as we have seen, depends on a systematic approach, attention to detail, involvement and consultation, and choosing the right people to do the job. Amongst them practising clinicians have a crucial part to play, and the ability to make the jobs of the others involved easier or more difficult.

5.2 Buying capital equipment

Hugh Saxton

At the time of writing there are indications that current systems for capital allocation may be changed. The long-standing arrangement whereby all equipment costing more than a certain sum – currently £20 000 – is paid for by the regional health authority has already been changed in respect of NHS trust hospitals. These hospitals have, or are said to have had, the capital previously held by regions devolved to them. Departments which previously had at least some chance of obtaining capital which was earmarked for scientific equipment now have to persuade their trust that their need is greater than that of other elements within the trust: earmarked capital no longer exists. Even for those districts which have not moved towards trust status the future is uncertain; it is even possible that the Department of Health will take control of certain purchases. So it may be that in the next few years the routes by which capital for major equipment reaches the ultimate user in a hospital department will vary both from region to region and from time to time.

Whatever the method of allocation, there will in the future be an increasing emphasis on a full justification for proposed purchases and also on getting the best value for money once purchase has been approved. Whether justification is by means of a formal business plan, showing how the equipment will earn an income sufficient to cover its running costs and its depreciation, or by some other method, doctors must expect more and more searching questions about their needs. This section therefore considers the justification, selection, purchase and installation of equipment from the standpoint of the clinician and his or her colleagues.

Initial considerations

The choice of major equipment, like the choice of a car, can have psychological overtones. The boost to an ego given by a BMW or Mercedes on the drive has its counterpart in the acquisi-tion for one's department of the latest piece of impressive technology. But while it is reasonable to spend more of one's own money than is strictly necessary, this is not so with NHS purchases: here it is essential to obtain value for money. On the other hand it is very important to be clear that durability, reliability and low servicing costs are also prime considerations. As with cars, a low purchase price may not represent the best value for money.

Multiple purchases and competitive tendering

When purchase of a new item of equipment is contemplated it is natural for the clinicians concerned to want to have an unfettered choice. This may be possible if they are buying to equip a new hospital or buying highly specialized equipment for a unit taking tertiary referrals from a whole region. It may also be possible for the entrepreneurial consultant working in a trust which is prepared to give him or her freedom of manoeuvre to negotiate highly favourable terms with suppliers: this may even become common as doctors take the opportunities available with greater enthusiasm. But for those in a more conventional environment wishing to purchase units which are in widespread use, it may well be that the purchasing authority will expect to obtain the economies which can come from buying a number of units from a manufacturer after a process of competitive tendering. Provided this is done with due regard to the views of the clinicians and others involved, the balance of arguments is in favour of this process. The prime desiderata are:

1 That all concerned are able to contribute to the preparation of a detailed specification, as discussed below.
2 That the importance of durability, good service quality and user-friendliness is accepted by the purchasing authority.

Such an arrangement does mean a loss of choice for the individual hospital or department but if it makes it possible for six units, meeting an adequate specification, to be bought instead of five different units, this should be acceptable to most people when capital is desperately limited.

Justification

The rigour which the capital depreciation system and external financing limit rules were expected to bring to the NHS has not yet been fully realized. Nevertheless, the clinical team who seek to replace an ageing item of equipment or to purchase something with new attributes will make their task less difficult if they prepare a case under the following headings:

1 *Clinical need*. This would include the current relevant workload, together with any expected increase, e.g. under proposed agreements or contracts. Alternative means of meeting the demand should be reviewed; for example, two hospitals 4 miles apart may not both justify a computed tomography scanner unless the anticipated workload on both is sufficient or if there is a particular clinical case load which makes it necessary to have an instrument on both sites, e.g. a heavy trauma load in one and an oncological unit in the other.
2 *Clinical staffing*. It is important to show that clinical capabilities exist to make proper use of the new equipment, both in the service department – if that is where the instrument is to go – and in the clinical units with whom they will work. The units who are to operate the equipment should also be able to show that they have, or will have, sufficient trained staff to run it effectively.
3 *Priority*. The degree of priority will be dependent on many factors – the age and condition of existing equipment, the needs of particular clinicians or the need to meet competition from equipment in nearby hospitals. Many regions now expect, and trusts will probably expect in future, a list of items for replacement in the current and in subsequent years.
4 *Business plan*. This will look at the proposal in terms of the way the equipment will be used; for how long each day; for how many days a week; what arrangements will be made for emergency work – if appropriate. The staffing, servicing, depreciation and consumable costs set against this anticipated load will give the expected unit costs for an average workload. An indication of the likely competition from nearby hospitals may be needed in some situations.
5 *Location*. Alternative sites may be considered, though in most cases there is little question as to the most appropriate location for the equipment.

Specification

Whatever the means of purchase, a careful specification is essential, both from the standpoint of the clinical team and of the purchasing authority, e.g. a region through their scientific officer. The initial drafting may be undertaken by either group, but it should be agreed by all involved before a tendering process is undertaken. If the clinical side has particular requirements it will, clearly, have to argue for them. The medical equivalent of 'go-faster stripes' is unlikely to be acceptable but there may well be features which can be fully justified either in terms of a special case load or an anticipated improvement in patient throughput.

The specification has a number of distinct functions:

1 It will be used by the purchasing agent, e.g. the regional scientific officer, in negotiating with the manufacturers, possibly in the context of a multiple purchase. Here a precisely drawn specification helps to ensure that the manufacturers really offer what is needed.
2 The discipline of drawing up or checking the specification is invaluable in ensuring that future users think really carefully about their needs. They should bear in mind that once the specification has been accepted they may have to accept whatever equipment fits with its provisions. Because of this, the more detailed the specification, the better.

Looking at the equipment

However exact the specification, it is essential that future users should visit hospitals where they can see the proposed equipment in use. The main reasons for this are:

1 To ensure that the specifications are met: manufacturers can be somewhat relaxed in their interpretation of details in the specification.
2 To learn about unexpected problems in discussion with users and to see the equipment in action.

The final selection

The fact that at present capital for equipment purchase does not come from the same purse as the running costs can have a distorting effect on the final selection. It is obvious to those who have struggled with unreliable equipment that a high level of breakdowns or poor servicing or higher service costs can very soon lead to a greater level of expenditure than would occur with a more reliable, even if more initially expensive, installation. This point may not be acknowledged by those responsible for the final decisions, especially if they take the view that their function is solely to husband scarce capital resources. The point is none the less valid and must be urged very firmly by doctors involved in the discussions about which equipment is to be chosen. In this regard the argument is likely to be more easily accepted by the local management when capital has been devolved to a district or a trust.

A similar point arises in relation to the characteristics of the proposed machine in terms of its operating behaviour. At a time when patient throughput is seen as a vital aspect of the operation of any hospital unit, it is clear that equipment which is easy to operate will reduce the time taken for each procedure carried out on the instrument. This also saves on staff time and so on staff costs.

All these matters will be discussed in relation to the final selection as well as more obvious questions about the performance and technical specifications of the units under review. The influence of doctors will be in proportion to the force and clarity of their arguments and these will be most effective when they have a complete mastery of the specification and have seen all the units at work.

Installation

There are a number of points to be resolved concerning installation of the equipment, once it has been ordered:

1 *Installation costs.* The costs of installation vary enormously, from a few hundred pounds for some units which need little more than plugging in, to many thousands for major imaging units such as computed tomography or magnetic resonance imaging scanners. These costs will often fall on the district or trust and must, of course, be considered in advance of the purchase. In the past it has been common for clinicians to get agreement for a particular purchase by region and then present their district with a *fait accompli*. This kind of 'foot-in-the-door' approach may be less successful today

and it is probably best to acknowledge the problem at an early stage. If the 'foot-in-the-door' technique is used its risks must be accepted by all involved.

2 *Installation team.* For any significant installation it is advisable to form a management team. Their function will be to coordinate any necessary design work, to oversee the building work involved, to prepare plans for utilization of the new equipment, and so forth. Membership will vary but may include representatives of the purchasing body, the manufacturer, the contractors, the hospital works department, possibly the hospital physics department and members of the department concerned.

3 *Design aspects.* For any major installation it may be necessary to undertake some design work in and around the room where the equipment is to be housed. This will often be initiated by the manufacturer's design department but the local installation team must take a close interest, particularly the members of the department concerned. Without going into detail, the design must look at the room itself as well as at the surrounding area. Some of the points for consideration are:
   (a) *Overall environment* – including air-conditioning or magnetic shielding.
   (b) *Traffic flows* – covering the movements of patients and staff, remembering the need to allow for wheelchairs and trolleys.
   (c) *Supporting functions* – chemical stores, processing facilities, sterile preparation and storage, drug storage, wheelchair/trolley store, recovery and resuscitation area.
   (d) *Waiting area* – changing cubicles, toilets with wheelchair access, public telephone, public address system, amusements, toys, refreshments, etc.
   (e) *Office accommodation* – if this is not provided elsewhere.

Details of the room design are too numerous for discussion here, but it should be emphasized that attention to details of room layout are vital if the room is to work really well. If, for example, it takes time to get a patient on a trolley up to an X-ray table or if it is not possible for staff to see the patient clearly during examination, something needs to be changed. A cardboard mock-up can be useful for those who have difficulty in reading plans. Another helpful check is to write down all the functions which will be carried out in the room. Thus, if cardiac physiological measurements are to be undertaken, this demands space for the equipment and power sockets. Regular use of anaesthesia will demand piped gases and suction, and so on.

Conclusions

If the process described here from justification to installation seems long and tedious, it must be remembered that much can be delegated to others. But just as the farmer's foot is the best manure, so the clinician's involvement at every stage is an important element in ensuring that the right equipment is selected and the most effective installation is achieved.

5.3   Finance of capital equipment by leasing

Paul Eldridge

Traditionally, capital equipment has been obtained in the NHS by purchase. The Treasury discourages alternative financial arrangements and this is reflected by finance departments at hospital, district or regional level. However, as a result of the reforms within the NHS, these can be attractive options providing care is taken to enter into the correct type of contract. They are now accepted by finance departments when a good business case is presented. The purpose of this article is to outline the pros and cons of lease deals. For full details of the complex financial rules the reader is referred to a standard accountancy text (*The Accountant's Guide*, 1990).

A lease is a contract between a lessor and a lessee for the hire of a specific asset. The lessor retains legal ownership of the asset but conveys the right of use of the asset to the lessee for an agreed period of time in return for the payment of specified rentals. The lease may be defined as either operational (rental) or finance (purchase). In the former contract there is no transfer of ownership or bargain purchase option at the end of the lease term, the term is for a period substantially less than the asset's useful life and the total lease payments excluding interest should be less than the asset's fair value. If any of these conditions is not met, the contract is a finance lease. Deals in which the capital value of the equipment is not declared but included within the price paid for revenue items used are frequently found in laboratories and termed reagent rentals.

Lease contracts directly with the equipment manufacturer are preferred to a lease from a finance company. The interest rates tend to be lower. The manufacturer, as legal owner, is more likely to ensure reliable operation of the product in order to maintain the company profile and win the subsequent replacement deal. In contrast, finance companies are unlikely to know about the equipment and are only interested in their profit.

It has proved difficult to obtain funding for capital equipment in most hospitals. High-value major items such as X-rays, computer systems and laboratory analysers above a certain cost, typically £20 000, are usually funded from regional budgets, with lower-cost items funded from district or hospital. In health trusts capital for major equipment is borowed from the Treasury as external financing limit (EFL) money. Typically, the budgets available are limited so that equipment has to be used well beyond realistic lifetimes, often with consequent inefficiency, low-quality service and poor staff morale. This particularly affects capital equipment used in service departments such as pathology, which tends to be considered lower priority than that providing front-line patient care. Obtaining additional equipment is more difficult than replacement. The total cost of senior staff time spent preparing bids, lobbying and in committees competing for a share of the equipment budget is substantial.

Advantages of leasing

Capital outlay is spread over several years, improving cash flow. This can be of benefit where several major items need to be purchased within a short period of time and enables new or replacement equipment to be obtained when needed.

If the the lease of replacement equipment can reduce revenue costs above the cost of the lease through increased efficiency, then the business case is easily justified. Many laboratories have funded replacement major analyser systems directly from revenue budgets by savings on staff costs. This reduces demands on and competition for limited capital budgets. If the new or replacement equipment can generate additional income, this can be used to fund the lease partly.

In a lease contract directly with a supplier or manufacturer, it may be possible to renegotiate the lease for more suitable equipment if the workload changes substantially within the period of the lease. Similarly, if technological change is rapid and there is a financially or clinically sound case for updating equipment, this is more likely to be possible via a direct lease with a supplier. This is particularly attractive where the equipment provides a service which generates income on a volume basis.

Where the lease includes service provision, typically a maintenance contract and reagents for a laboratory analyser, it is often possible to obtain VAT exemption for the total cost of the deal, depending on the local VAT inspector's interpretation of the tax laws. This can offset or exceed the interest charge built into the lease.

Where an operating lease is established, there is no capital value assigned to the lessee, no capital commitment to the lessor and hence no capital charges.

Disadvantages

The total cost of equipment obtained via a lease will be higher than by direct purchase because of the interest charge. This could be substantial for long-term leases.

Within a health trust a finance lease is taken to be gain of ownership and thus EFL money has to be committed to the total capital value, whereas this is not the case with directly man- aged units at present. Thus, as both EFL interest charges and capital charges are applicable, purchase is the best option if an operational lease cannot be established.

A reagent rental may represent an expensive option in the long term. The contract must have agreed prices for the reagents and other revenue items which decrease appropriately with increasing volume and have a realistic element for inflation for the duration of the contract. The supplier will have based the cost of the revenue items on an agreed workload in order to fund the equipment and obtain a working profit. If the workload increases substantially, along with a proportional increase in use of supplies, the supplier's profit margin will escalate. Typically, the workload on major laboratory equipment increases by 50% over 5 years.

In summary, an operating lease provides an attractive method for obtaining equipment where cash flow is a problem; the costs can be offset against revenue savings; the interest charge of the lease is low; VAT savings are possible and exemption can be claimed from capital charges. Finance leases are less attractive but provide benefits where cash flow is a problem.

Reference

The Accountant's Guide (1990) *A Handbook of Standard Statements and Rules for Professional Accountants.* Section 4.21, Certified Accountants Educational trust.

Section 6

Managing people

6.1 A framework for studying human resource management

Roger Dyson

Introduction

The body of knowledge that is referred to as the social or behavioural sciences offers an important framework for analysing the behaviour of people at work. Its value to a manager is not only as a guide to understanding how and why colleagues and staff behave/work as they do, but also as a framework to assist with the introduction of change. However, knowledge of the framework does not itself guarantee success. Managers who operate entirely by instinct can be successful and those who fully understand the intellectual concepts that guide their actions can fail. Other things being equal, though, change is more likely to be successful if managed by someone who understands and uses the analytical framework offered by the behavioural sciences.

Each of the main academic disciplines has made its contribution to the understanding of workplace behaviour by individuals and groups, primarily in analysing what motivates people. At the risk of generalization, there has been a broad historical sequence from economics to sociology, psychology and political theory when applied to the study of people as workers. A second aspect of the study of workplace behaviour is the regulation of behaviour within sets of rules of varying precision. Employment law and industrial relations each have their own analytical concepts with which to study rules and the control that they exert. There are also rules determined by the employer that are separate from and addi-

tional to this legal and collective bargaining framework and these are often the least precise and the most significant in the implementation of change, as are the separate and almost entirely unwritten rules of employees. Table 6.1.1 lists these different disciplines.

Motivation

In studying motivation, it is important to remember that using the concepts of one behavioural discipline and ignoring the rest is likely to have unforeseen consequences. This is because of their interrelationship in determining the overall pattern of motivation in any given workplace. It is like balls in the bottom of a bowl: if one is moved, the others will adjust to the movement. The unique contribution of each discipline and their relationship to the others is considered below.

Economics

Economic man responds to an economic incentive. His or her working time and working effort are aimed to maximize his or her income within a personal balance of income and leisure. In a large and tightly regulated workplace, e.g. a hospital, the perceived relationship between income and time (hours) can seem much more real than the relationship between income and effort (personal performance). This produces a perverse economic incentive to reduce effort in order to maximize hours and therefore income, balanced only by the degree of importance attached to leisure. For the employer, however, this results in higher costs and lower productivity. As a result, employers have traditionally resorted to performance-related pay systems. These range from the basic piecework systems of factory

Table 6.1.1 Behaviour at work

Motivation	Regulation
Economics	Employment law
Sociology	Industrial relations
Psychology	Employer regulation
Political theory	Employee regulation
Philosophy/ethics	
History	

production to sophisticated profit-share schemes; but to be worthwhile in economic terms, they need to sustain a clear relationship between effort and income in the mind of the worker. If they lose that, they lose their economic *raison d'être*.

This analytical framework also has a clear explanation for trade unions. Their purpose is to control the supply of labour in order to increase the price when bargaining with employers. If the supply can be controlled, e.g. through an arduous craft training system or by introducing a pre-entry (pre-employment) closed shop where only union members can be employed, it becomes more likely that demand for labour will outstrip supply and prices will rise.

Assumptions about economic man dominated the industrial relations debates of the 1950s, and a classic statement of this approach can be found in Hare (1954).

Sociology

Sociology has become a less popular discipline in industrial relations. Its heyday was in the late 1960s and early – mid 1970s when it challenged the relevance, or at least the completeness, of the concept of economic man as an explanation of the way people behaved at work. In terms of industrial relations, the most widely read text at the time providing a clear exposition of the alternative to economic man was that by Fox (1968).

Sociologists could demonstrate by research that workers did not respond to economic incentives in the way many economists believed. An individual piecework incentive in a factory could lead to standard output across the work group and sometimes tickets for work completed were destroyed rather than cashed. This was explained as due to the strength of work-group loyalties with their unwritten rules and codes of behaviour that were more compelling to the individual than an economic incentive. The desire to protect the weakest in the group from failing to achieve and losing employment and the desire to stop the employer taking too much out of the group in effort are illustrations of the motives of such group behaviour. The less creditable side of this illustration is the fear engendered in the individual by the severity of the retribution occasioned by the breaking of these codes.

Sociologists can see work as a pluralistic rather than a unitary society. In the latter, the workers and employers share the objectives of the organization whilst in the former their objectives overlap to a greater or lesser extent but are not identical. Central to the overlap is the wish for the organization to continue in order to keep providing wages and profits. Outside the overlap, workers have collective objectives to enhance the authority of the trade union and extend collective bargaining to all aspects of decision-making, in effect to give the work-group a veto on all decisions, not just economic ones, that affect themselves. A typical illustration of a unitary society is one in which there is a single team leader, the manager analogous to a rugby team captain. In a pluralistic society the work-group see their union steward as perhaps a more important leader, but in the same 'team'. Managers were claimed to like the unitary analysis because it legitimized their authority.

Psychology

Psychology did not appear and blossom and fade in the same chronological way as sociology's popularity in industrial relations, but its application to the general debate about workplace behaviour and industrial relations was, in the main, subsequent to the first impact of sociology. Psychology is concerned with the individual rather than the group and provides an analytical framework to explain why a particular person chooses to react this way rather than that, respond to this stimulus rather than that, depending upon states of mind and personality. This is pursued in more depth by Baron and Greenberg (1990).

Contrary to the views of many mainstream as well as Marxist sociologists, managers today tend to view the workplace as a unitary society and increasingly use psychological testing as a part of the interview process to try to ensure that the person to be appointed has the personality characteristics identified as appropriate for the job. The claim to seek round pegs for round holes is perceived widely as a beneficial objective of employers in contemporary society. Potential employees can be identified as possessing drive, loyalty, etc., but in many posts it is often felt that someone who will not question the objectives of the organization is a high priority. The science involved is not yet precise and there is both controversy about its use and about the ease with which potential employees can produce what they believe to be the desired test results.

Another very specific use of the analytical tools of the psychologist is in negotiating skills training. Negotiating skills were first developed in the workplace as an adjunct to collective bargaining, but they have been increasingly extended to all aspects of team and individual interaction inside and outside the organization, ranging from effective interpersonal skills to the conduct of large set-piece negotiations. In the broader arena, as employers have moved from task training to quality of performance, they have relied more upon the analytical framework of psychology.

Political theory

Political theory, in the context of the workplace, provides a framework for analysing power in the organization: who wields it, what is its source and the pressures that lead to its redistribution? This also includes the rules that legitimize power, the rule-making institutions and the rule-making process. An important text for the study of power in organizations is *The Bureaucratic Phenomenon*, by Crozier (1964).

To the student of politics it is no surprise that some workers may seek goals that are wholly contradictory to those of the organization in which they work. Their motivation is to weaken the organization in pursuit of some wider goal to which their employment is subservient. It was noticed in the first widespread strikes in the NHS in 1973 that several individual strike leaders took employment just before the action and left immediately afterwards (Yorkshire Regional Health Authority, 1974).

Throughout the history of industrial society, however, the role of political agitators or extremists has often been exaggerated and it is only necessary to recognize the possibility that from time to time individuals and groups can be motivated by purely political goals inimical to the interests of the organization. What is much more important to doctors as managers is the changing distribution of power within the hospital, the structures and systems which give it effect and the way in which the search for power and authority, or its rejection, motivates people as employees. Since the Griffiths Report of 1983,

uniform authority structures have become more diverse, with sometimes considerable redistribution of power at the head of the local organization. The same has happened to the traditional relationships in multidisciplinary clinical teams at the level of service provision to the patient and this aspect of change is analysed in much more depth in Section 6.6.

Philosophy/ethics

The humanities play a less dominant part in the general analysis of what motivates workplace behaviour, but the study of ethics as a branch of philosophy has an important contribution. There is a strong collective professional ethic which to a greater or lesser extent sets limits to the behaviour patterns of doctors and nurses. The Hippocratic oath or its equivalent is enshrined in professional codes of conduct which constitute powerful external rules, frequently sanctioned by statute, which shape the behaviour of individuals as professional workers. For those who wish to pursue the intellectual debate more rigorously, consult White (1991).

The problem for the manager, doctor or otherwise, is that codes of conduct can easily become weapons in a conflict that owes its primary motivation to objectives that are more the province of sociology and political theory.

Finally, there are general ethical standards that help shape the conduct of all individuals. The particular relevance of this to health care is the often stated but only anecdotally based view that employees choose to work in the health industry because of a strong sense of personal commitment to caring and a relatively weak attraction to the motivations of economic man.

History

History's only relevance to this study is in the extent to which it shapes particular patterns of behaviour. The sense of history possessed by the individual or group does not need to be accurate or balanced. It may be highly partisan or even largely mythological; its relevance to this study is merely its ability to exercise a strong influence on workforce behaviour. Religious, trade union and even professional loyalties can be influenced by a sense of history; and protecting traditional ways of working from the threat of change can take on a wider symbolic role by appealing to a sense of continuity that draws on sometimes powerful historical imagery.

In industrial relations, if a factory or hospital has a history of bad manager – employee relationships, this can prove very difficult to remove, despite continual changes in key personnel, during which period neighbouring hospitals doing the same work can exist in relative harmony. In these circumstances researchers have claimed that a strong historically based sense of injustice can continue to force new workers to identify with sides, despite their personal motivation and antipathy to such behaviour (Dyson, 1971). History and sociology interact as key disciplines in the analysis of this phenomenon.

Regulation

The regulation of workplace behaviour may be analysed in a series of levels of declining formality.

Employment law

Employment law now constitutes a wide-ranging framework which gives statutory authority to sets of rules which govern the relationship between employers and employees. These can be divided between a number of key statutory objectives.

Health and safety

The health and safety of the worker have been the subject of much legislation since the industrial revolution. This framework continues to strengthen and its penalties become more severe as society seeks greater relative protection for workers. It also grows as science opens up new processes and new materials.

Contract

The basic contract between employer and employee gives statutory rights to both, and in health care has been extended to cover such things as the employment of consultants and their dismissal. Statutory rights to payment, periods of notice, compensation etc., are included here.

Discrimination

The law seeks to proscribe unfair behaviour by an employer who may seek to discriminate in employing, in disciplining or in dismissing staff on grounds of sex, race, religion or just on the grounds of arbitrary behaviour against a particular employee. Appeals to industrial courts against such discrimination can produce fines or the requirement to reinstate/cease discrimination.

The protection of the customer/patient/society

This covers substantial legislation which regulates the way employers and employees behave.

This framework is now being enlarged by the growing role of the European Community, which extends to each of the branches of employment and protection law listed above. The importance of employment law in the way workplace behaviour is regulated seems set to grow in the 1990s.

Industrial relations

Industrial relations draws widely upon the various behavioural science disciplines, but at its core is the study of the rule-making process between employers and trade unions, and the structure of the rules themselves (Flanders, 1965). It is concerned with the voluntary framework of rules in collective agreements – both their substantive content about pay and conditions and their procedural content dealing with such things as the appeal processes for staff and the roles and rights of union stewards, etc.

In the NHS the part of this framework covered by national Whitley Council regulations has so far been given formal support by statutory instrument, although this is now diminishing. This has never extended to local agreements, that have always been purely voluntary. This is developed further in Section 6.3.

Employer regulation

In the early 19th century all rules were imposed by employer regulation. Working times and output targets were imposed by employers and often supported by employer-regulated fines. In the last 200 years the territory of employer regulation has declined due to legislation and collective bargaining, but issues such as the strategic objectives of the company and how they are to be fulfilled leave a core of employer regulation in even the most strongly trade union-dominated industry.

Employee regulation

This goes back to the content of industrial sociology. Some work-groups make unwritten rules which limit what employees may do despite employer inducements or which permit behaviour which is formally barred by employer regulation, e.g. types of 'theft/perks', or 'Spanish customs'. This contradiction in the structure of rules can lead either to collusion or conflict or both.

Influencing behaviour

The potential value of the structure shown in Figure 6.1.1 is that it provides a means of altering behaviour by altering the balance of motivation and regulation. Every workplace has a complex pattern of motivation which includes all the individuals and groups within it. One can show empirically that if this pattern of motivation does not match or balance the pattern of regulation, there will be overt and/or covert conflict whenever the rules in question are brought into play. Thus, before the law on unfair dismissal, managers insisting on the right of foremen to use summary dismissal could be faced with strikes demanding that union stewards should be allowed to argue the individual's case before the dismissal was decided. Alternatively, a new manager changing rules unilaterally could be faced with a strike or more covert reactions to reject the new rules or render them impotent.

The substantial body of empirical evidence to support this cause and effect has led to two general conclusions:

1 If managers wish to reduce conflict within the organization in the short term, they should change the pattern of regulation to match the pattern of motivation. This can be interpreted as simply giving in to trade union or employee pressure but the issue is often much more complex than this win/lose image. Nurses are currently seeking to change their perceived image as handmaidens to doctors and

have come to reject more and more of what they see as medical primacy. Their changing motivation requires changes in the rules about professional tasks and responsibilities. Without change there can be and has been conflict, but often the changes have been achieved gradually, with both the doctors and nurses involved viewing the changes positively.

2 The second and more controversial conclusion is that when motivation and regulation are out of balance it is possible to change the patterns of motivation within an organization, if managers wish to retain a particular regulatory framework. If managers have a clear perception of the strategic objective of the organization and if these are not open to negotiation with employees or their representatives, there could be conflict because this fails in some degree to match the pattern of employee motivation. In these circumstances the managers may prefer to change motivation rather than change their strategic objectives – in the language of the sociologist, to move towards the concept of the organization as a unitary, rather than a pluralistic society. In the short term such a move is high-risk and will engender conflict. An industrial example would be Michael Edwards at British Leyland. In the longer term, if time and objectives permit, such a change could be more systematic and less traumatic.

In what is now often seen as the mistakes of the 1960s and 1970s, there was a tendency to regard this pattern of motivation as being outside the influence of managers. Marxist academics endowed its natural direction with an almost religious sense of mission – as something that was strictly out of bounds for managers with their outdated unitary philosophies and their desire to play team captains. What this meant in reality was that external influence was permitted (of the sort analysed by the student of political theory) in an attempt continually to reduce the area of shared objectives between manager and managed, whilst managers were trapped in a culture that rejected their right to exercise their own influence.

The 1980s have seen a sharp reaction, as a new breed of managers has increasingly realized the value and importance of the unitary framework for the health, success and well-being of the organization in economic terms. These managers have begun to change what they view as inappropriate patterns of motivation as part of a long-term policy to secure wider acceptance of the strategic objectives of the organization, using economics and psychology as the key tools of change. This has been assisted by a broader political culture that accepted short-term conflict as legitimate when unavoidable. In Section 6.6 this framework is applied to the management and leadership of clinical services in the NHS.

References

Baron, R. and Greenberg, J. (1990) *Behaviour in Organisations*, 3rd edn.

Crozier, M. (1964) *The Bureaucratic Phenomenon*. Chicago University Press, Chicago.

Dyson, R.F. (1971) The development of collective bargaining in the cotton spinning industry 1893–1914. Unpublished PhD Thesis, Leeds University.

Flanders, A. (1965) *Industrial Relations: What is Wrong with the System? An Essay on its Theory and Future*. Faber and Faber.

Fox, A. (1968) *Research Paper 3 of the Royal Commission on Trade Unions and Employers Associations*. S.O. code 73–42–3. HMSO, London.

Griffiths, R. (1983) *Report of Management Inquiry – The Griffiths Report*. HMSO, London.

Hare, A.E. (1954) *The Economics of Industrial Relations*. Leeds.

White, J.E. (1991) *Contemporary Moral Problems*, 3rd edn. West Publishing, St. Paul's, MN.

The Ancillary Staff's Industrial Action in the Spring of 1973 (1974). Yorkshire Regional Health Authority.

6.2   The management of change

Robin Gourlay

Introduction

This section explores the nature of leadership, differentiating between two approaches that have been identified by researchers (Bennis and Nanus, 1985; Ticky and Devanna, 1986; Kotter, 1988).

Organizations need leadership, otherwise they wither and fail to meet the needs of their customers, be these clients, patients or whatever. Organizations are collections of people who work with resources to achieve some results. One form of leadership welds the people and resources together by defining the objective and results to be achieved. It is a different form of leadership that keeps the organization on track once the direction has been decided.

The first type of leadership has been defined as *transformational*, the second as *transactional*. Both types are necessary for a healthy organization. Transactional leadership is what most managers do. Their skills are to manage the internal and external organization pressures so that progress in the right direction is maintained. They are involved in transacting with the internal and external environments to achieve short-term objectives.

The elements of transformational leadership

Put crudely, transformational leaders forge a long-term strategy for their organization, and through the process of doing this, and through its implementation, garner the commitment of people to do their part in making the strategy work. The thinking model used for shaping and positioning the organization in its market place is straightforward. It involves an analysis of the present – both the internal capabilities of the organization as well as its external environment – an analysis and forecast of the future looking at factors that will influence the success of the organization; then an analysis of the gap be-tween now and then, resulting in the development of strategies to bridge the gap. Each of these elements will be taken in turn to show what a transformational leader will do to make the organization successful.

Transformational leadership and the present state

Mission

Organizations are successful when they have a clear purpose on which they concentrate. Unless there is such a clear purpose or mission, then energies and resources may be devoted to activities which deliver marginal benefits to the consumer – whether patient or client. Transformational leadership is about gaining clarity of such purpose through debate and eventual decision on what needs to be done for the organization to be successful. For example, Drucker (1990) quotes the work done by an accident and emergency unit in determining what its core purpose was. After much debate initiated by the leader and after analysing what the department did, the staff came to the conclusion that their core purpose was 'to give assurance to the afflicted'. This may sound obvious or even trite, but the staff found that eight out of 10 casualties only needed to be told that they would be OK after a good night's rest.

The department now gives effect to its core purpose by ensuring that any casualty is seen within 2 minutes of entering the department by a professional who will reassure the patient by explaining what will or should happen next to him or her.

Values

A second key aspect for the transformational leader is that of values. Values are the principles which influence the way people behave. Clearly articulated values are influential and inspirational. Perhaps a value about which many people know is one of Anita Roddick. In building up her Body Shop she has made clear her own beliefs about the environment and the protection of the species. This value attracts customers and is one to which her employees readily subscribe.

Values are what you live and manage by. If you have explicit values about how customers/patients and others should be treated, you empower your staff. As Nelson said, 'They know what is expected of them; they do not need telling how to fulfil such expectations'. This can be left to their initiative and enterprise.

SWOT analysis

Values may be 'soft' but experience shows that genuine attempts to get these right is highly inspirational. However, the hard facts of the present cannot be ignored. A useful technique for analysing the present and starting to move towards the future is a SWOT analysis. This analysis considers what the organization's current strengths and weaknesses are, and what are the opportunities and threats posed by the environment. From this analysis the transformational leader starts to construct a vision of the future.

The future state

The vision

By definition a transformational leader is one who is constantly thinking about the future and how well-positioned the organization is to survive and grow. Just as the mission is an essential prerequisite in examining the present state, then so is the concept of the vision critical to the future state.

A transformational leader is one who can describe the vision for the organization in terms of both a dream and a practical reality. Visions should have elements of a dream because at first acquaintance, they may appear unrealistic. Visions describe what the organization will be in the future, and how it will be relating to its customers and how its management and staff will be behaving towards each other. But visions

must be tested against practical reality. They must be seen as possible even though their achievement may require great transformations in the way things are currently done.

President Kennedy had a vision of getting 'a man on the moon by the end of the decade'. At the time of articulation, in the early 1960s, this sounded impossible. But the stimulus it gave to NASA to get itself organized was extraordinary. And, of course, the vision was realized. When people see how what they do is contributing to the achievement of a well-formed vision, the effect is one of engendering cooperation through team-working, as well as enhancing individual motivation.

The vision will be informed by careful analysis of the opportunities and threats posed by the social, technological, economic and political environments in which the organization has to function. It requires transformational leadership to bring all this together and be debated in a frank and open way. For an excellent example of these processes at work, see *Making it Happen* by John Harvey Jones (1988) who describes how he undertook this task as chairman of ICI.

The gap

Once the future vision has been described, and the current capability of the organization ascertained, there is likely to be a gap between aspirations as defined by the vision and what is currently being done. There are likely to be many strategies that are necessary, requiring changes in, for example:

1 Organization structures.
2 Profiles of the labour force.
3 Human resource policies.
4 Financial and investment strategies.
5 The work being done.
6 Capital assets.
7 Marketing.

The transformational leader's task is to ensure that there are the functional and professional skills to bring about these changes. But, just as importantly, the leader has to be able to manage the processes that will bring commitment and support to the achievement of the vision. The transformational leader is as concerned with the 'how' of the change as ensuring the 'what' gets done by others.

The 'how' includes strategies on communications, gaining commitment or, at the minimum, acquiescence to the changes, and building trust: the key one is communications.

Communication strategies

Much is written, and moaned, about organization communications. Commitment to visions and objectives will come about only when people understand where the organization is going, and why; and what their part is in achieving objectives. Such understanding does not come from dictates handed down from the top, but from involvement in the processes that result in the vision and objectives. Essentially there are two vital elements to a communications strategy. The first of these is to do with the systems; the second with the culture.

The second element is often overlooked, reliance being entirely placed on the system and procedures. The systems element addresses the problems of getting messages into the organization fast and accurately, and just as important are the problems of getting honest messages into top management from the body of the organization. There are many systems that are used to solve these problems. Perhaps the best known is the cascading communication system known as briefing groups, developed by the Industrial Society. In this system, top management briefs those below them in a short session, setting out the key points management wants to get across. Second-level managers then brief their subordinates and so on throughout the organization. The system must also provide for lower levels of management and staff to feedback their views to the senior levels.

Communications can be open and honest, in which people feel free to say what is on their mind; or secretive and closed where they fear retribution if they make any critical comments. Unfortunately, in too many organizations which are riddled by hierarchy and bureaucracy, the latter culture is much the most pervasive. Changing such a culture is hard work. It begins with the transformational leader being open in his or her own team meetings and encouraging and rewarding others to make proposals on how things can be improved.

This demands of the leaders a well-developed set of interpersonal skills. The main one of these is that of listening to others without distorting what they say. Indeed, Peter Drucker (1990) argues thus:

> As the first such basic competence, I would put the willingness, ability and self discipline to listen. Listening is not a skill; it's a discipline. Anybody can do it. All you have to do is to keep your mouth shut.

Transformational leadership and managing change

The transformational leader has two concerns – forging the direction, and then ensuring that everyone is working in harmony with that direction. This may mean that people have to change their behaviour or acquire new skills, or develop different attitudes.

Ideally the aim is to achieve absolute commitment to the proposed direction and objectives. However the ideal cannot always be achieved. The next best thing would be for compliance to the changes. This is where there is an acceptance by staff of the need for change and the approaches to achieving it, but it falls short of active promotion of the change – on the other hand, attempts to scupper the change will not be made. The least desirable state of mind is brought about when coercion has to be used to make people change. This approach acknowledges that individuals may resist the change so strongly that they will – if they had their way – try to prevent the changes happening.

The transformational leader will aim to get commitment but will also be able to deploy approaches that may lead to compliance or compulsion if commitment is impossible to achieve in some staff.

The following paragraphs describe the sorts of approaches a transformational leader may use.

Integration approach

The essence of the integration approach is that of belonging through meaning. The aim of the approach is to facilitate the integration of individuals' goals and needs with those of the organization; to gain, in other words a personal identification from all individuals to what the change objectives are. Two key ingredients will make this approach work. The first is that of communication so that people understand what has to be done and why. Discussing with people the development and promotion of mission and vision statements is a way of doing this. The second ingredient is that of participation. There are two results from participation that create integration. The first is that there is more commitment from people to objectives that they have played some part in shaping. The second is a group dynamics phenomenon. If individuals find their colleagues in the group or team to be congenial, then the group itself can exert influence over the individual member and gain his or her commitment to what group members agree. This approach often appears almost evangelical in practice.

Educational approach

Underlying this approach is the belief that if people are educated about the need for change and the reasons for it, then they will accept that they themselves have to change to adapt to the new order. This approach is appealing because of its inherent rationality. But it does not always follow that understanding of itself leads to changes in behaviour. However, with the possible exceptions of brainwashing and other compulsory change approaches, understanding does at least need to precede change.

Contextual change approach

This is another well-tried approach based on the assumptions that if you change the context in which an individual is behaving, the behaviour itself will ultimately change. There is certainly considerable evidence to support this view (Milgram, 1974). It is the rationale for organizational restructuring. The argument is that forced changes in relationships created by changed organizational positions will lead to behavioural change. Regrettably, often too much weight is attached to this approach and organizational restructuring is seen as sufficient – and often as an end in itself; it gives the appearance of change, even though all that may have happened is that the chess pieces have altered their positions.

Confrontation approach

Using the word confrontation implies aggression. It can be aggressive but it does not have to

be. CND and Greenpeace have used aggressive confrontation on occasions to challenge current views and achieve change.

On the other hand, particularly at an individual level, confrontation can be non-aggressive. It holds up to the individual the potential consequences of current and predicted behaviour patterns and engages the other in a discussion about the acceptability of these. Such analysis can generate other options, leading to ultimate changes in behaviour.

Negotiating approach

Like the confrontation approach, this can be seen in aggressive win/lose terms or in more integrative win/win terms. The essence of this approach is that of doing deals. Those who may be reluctant to change agree to the changes on the understanding that they gain some benefits to themselves – either from the change or from something else. Where there are genuine differences in objectives or interests, this strategy can be very successful. It does not necessarily create whole-hearted commitment, but it does guarantee that once an agreement has been reached, changed behaviour will follow (Gourlay, 1987).

Political approach

This approach is to do with mustering power and then deploying it to force change. It is an approach used by many individuals who create a power base through control of resources, or through the creation of a network of power people. The downside of this approach is that those subject to it feel manipulated and may resist by building up their own power base and then engaging in 'warfare'.

Threat approach

This approach works in the short term, particularly when organizations are in crisis. The rationale for this approach is that, unless individuals change, they will disappear from the organization – or the organization itself will disappear.

For the approach really to have an effect, the threat has to be plausible. This can be engendered by implementing the threat against one or two individuals – a symbolic indication of the reality of the new world. However, organizations cannot be really effective if under constant threat. It becomes too uncomfortable. Further, the approach will only work if individuals are clear what changes are required of them and have the competence to put these into practice.

Composite approach (or behavioural science approach)

This is an approach based on an amalgam of the approaches described above, informed by an understanding of the psychological and sociological dynamics of people in their organizational setting.

Achieving change in complex organizations demands that a variety of strategies be employed. The overall approach is conditional upon a diagnosis of who and what has to change.

A key question in this approach is: What part of the organization would give the most leverage to make change happen? This results in a critical mass of people being identified who, if their support were forthcoming, would act as 'spreaders of the word'. Once the critical mass has been identified, the transactional leader will deploy a number of approaches to win their commitment – or at the minimum, their compliance – to the change objectives and processes (Beckhard and Harris, 1969; Gourlay, 1992).

Transactional management

This section has concentrated on transformational management because this is less frequently found in organizations. For doctors who are leading clinical directorates, the most appropriate approach is that of the transformational leader. The day-to-day business can then be managed by a transactional leader. This is much more akin to a traditional management role, leaving the clinical director to concentrate on the future strategy free of the day-to-day problems.

Conclusion

By way of a summary it is interesting to contrast the transactional leadership with transformational leadership.

- Transforming leaders inspire others by their vision and values.
- Transactional leaders gain commitment through discussion of objectives and personal development plans.
- Transforming leaders are interested in the whole person, both at work and at home.
- Transactional leaders tend to separate work and home.
- Transformational leaders create trust so that there is implicit understanding of what has to be done.
- Transactional leaders get work done through explicit deals and contracts.
- Transformational leaders stir up people in the organization.
- Transactional leaders fix things.
- Transformational leaders have a long-term focus.
- Transactional leaders have a short-term focus.
- Transformational leaders challenge people and encourage risk-taking, accepting mistakes.
- Transactional leaders provide shelter and coaching.
- Transformational leaders reward informally.
- Transactional leaders reward formally, often with money.
- Transformational leaders like argument and debate.
- Transactional leaders prefer conformity.
- Transformational leaders are turbulent and appeal to the emotions.
- Transactional leaders are orderly and appeal to rationality.

References

Beckhard, R. and Harris, R. (1969) *Organisation Development – Strategies and Models*. Addison Wesley.

Bennis, W. and Nanus, B. (1985) *Leaders*. Harper & Row.

Drucker, P. (1990) *Managing the Non Profit Organisation*. Butterworth-Heinemann, Oxford.

Gourlay, J. R. (1987) *Negotiations for Managers*. Mercia Publications

Gourlay, J. R. (1992) *Handling Difficult Colleagues*. Mercia Publications.

Harvey Jones, J. (1988) *Making it Happen* Collins.

Kotter, J. (1988) *The Leadership Factor*. Free Press,

Millgram, S. (1974) *Obedience to Authority*. Harper & Row.

Ticky, N. M. and Devanna, M. A. (1986) *The Transformational Leader*. Wiley, Chichester.

6.3 Terms and conditions of employment

Nigel Brunsdon

Machinery for determining pay and conditions

When the NHS was established in 1948, the (then) Minister for Health was placed under a statutory obligation to take into account the views of NHS staff before determining pay and other conditions of service (NHS Act 1946). This was done by establishing Whitley Councils, based on the model first proposed by the Whitley Committee in 1919 and already in use in the civil service and local government (Connah and Lancaster, 1989).

Each council covered a specific staff group, and operated at national level. In total, these functional councils covered the great majority of staff in the NHS. By the end of 1950 there were seven functional councils and a general council (McCarthy, 1976).

The first significant change to this system occurred in 1962, when the Review Body for Doctors' and Dentists' Remuneration was established following the report of a Royal Commission (1960). The task of the review body was – and still is – to consider evidence and then recommend to the Prime Minister of the day the appropriate levels of remuneration for doctors and dentists. This model was to be adopted later for other groups of staff.

The Whitley system came under review in 1975, when Lord McCarthy was appointed by the Secretary of State to 'review the workings of the NHS Whitley Council machinery'. The resulting McCarthy Report (1976) contained a wide-ranging set of recommendations to improve the working of the Whitley System. These recommendations were designed to:

1 clarify the influence of central government and NHS employers respectively on the bargaining process;
2 improve NHS management commitment and influence on the process;
3 improve secretariat support to the system;
4 extend bargaining machinery to regional level or below;
5 stimulate a review of the use of third-party involvement (e.g. ACAS) to resolve disputes;
6 encourage more joint consultation on non-pay issues;
7 reduce the number of recognized staff organizations.

Whilst some improvements to the working of Whitley resulted from the review, any historical analysis must conclude that little significant change emerged. This was no fault of Lord McCarthy. Any substantive change required joint agreement, and this (with minor exceptions) was not forthcoming.

The next significant development came with the extension of the pay review body model in 1983 to cover nurses and midwives; unqualified nursing staff; and most of the professions allied to medicine: physiotherapists, radiographers, occupational therapists, orthoptists, chiropodists and dieticians. (Speech therapists were not included, at their own request.) The respective Whitley Councils for these groups (nurses and midwives and PT'A') were abandoned at this stage, and replaced by central negotiating committees to deal with matters other than pay (Commons written answer, 1983).

Although the great majority of staff have their pay and terms of service determined through Whitley Councils and/or pay review bodies, there are some important exceptions. The first is maintenance staff, where negotiations take place directly with the appropriate trade unions at national level through a maintenance staff management advisory panel. This covers craft grades and the associated semiskilled and unskilled workers. Second, there are some *ad hoc* grades which are very small in number and pay is determined by direction of the Secretary of State. In addition, new arrangements were introduced in 1986 for general managers, consisting of a pay spine linked with administrative and clerical conditions of service. This spine is determined by direction of the Secretary of State and is thus not subject to collective bargaining. A very similar arrangement was extended to other senior managers from 1987 and for senior nurse managers from January 1991. Finally, for ambulance staff, in addition to negotiations in the Ambulance Whitley Council, the Association of Professional Ambulance Personnel (APAP) has been recognized by the Secretary of State in a separate ambulance negotiating body.

Whitley Councils and review bodies relate to staff in the UK.

Structure – Whitley Councils

Each of the functional Whitley Councils comprises a management and staff side. Much of the detailed work takes place in joint negotiating meetings, but for an agreement to be valid it requires ratification by the full council, and then to be approved by the Secretary of State and implemented by way of a Direction.

The management side of each council comprises representatives from the Department of Health, Scottish Home and Health Department and Welsh Office, together with NHS management members. The staff side consists of those trade unions and staff associations recognized for collective bargaining purposes for the staff group in question, with seats allocated approximately proportionate to the membership strength of the organization. Details of the constitution of the staff sides are given in Table 6.3.1.

The General Whitley Council (GWC) which negotiates conditions common to most staff groups, also comprises a management and staff side, with membership drawn in each case from the respective sides of the functional Whitley Councils. It operates in a similar way to the functional councils in determining agreements.

Structure – pay review bodies

The pay review bodies operate quite differently to Whitley. The pay review body members are appointed by government but are independent both in the manner of working and nature of recommendations made. They are given secretar-

Table 6.3.1 Staff side composition of Whitley Councils

	Members
Administrative and clerical council	
Association of NHS officers	2
Confederation of Health Service Employees	4
General, Municipal, Boilermakers and Allied Trades Union	1
National and Local Government Officers Association	19
National Union of Public Employees	4
Transport and General Workers Union	1
Ambulance staffs council	
National Union of Public Employees	8
GMB	4
Transport and General Workers' Union	4
Confederation of Health Service Employees	4
Ancillary staffs council	
Confederation of Health Service Employees	4
GMB	4
National Union of Public Employees	4
Transport and General Workers Union	4
Professional and technical B council	
Confederation of Health Service Employees	3
Electrical and Engineering Staff Association	2
Manufacturing, Science and Finance	3
National and Local Government Officer's Association	3
National Union of Public Employees	3
Supervisory, technical, administrative managerial and professional section of UCATT	3
Union of Shop, Distributive and Allied Workers	2
Scientific and professional council	
The staff side composition of this council remains unagreed at 1.9.92 (see text)	

iat support by the Office of Manpower Economics, and in practice work by taking evidence from staff and management side interests, as well as carrying out such investigations of their own which they may regard as appropriate. Their task is to advise the Prime Minister of the day (normally by way of a report) on the appropriate levels for remuneration for the staff group in question. The government is free to accept, reject or modify this advice. Most commonly it is accepted, occasionally with a staged implementation. In 1970 the government of the day announced its intention only to implement half the recommended increase for career grades of hospital doctors, and this prompted the resignation of the review body. The matter was resolved after a general election in June 1970 and a new review body appointed, with a government commitment that recommendations would not subsequently be rejected unless there were obvious compelling reasons to do so (Report of the Review Body on Doctors' and Dentists' Remuneration, 1971).

General Whitley Council

The GWC deals with a range of conditions of service which are of common application to NHS staff (and thus not covered within individual functional councils). There are some exceptions to this, where only specified elements of the GWC agreements apply to certain groups. The exceptions apply to:

1 Hospital medical and dental staff.
2 Doctors in community medicine and community health services.
3 Administrative dental and community clinical dental officers.
4 Works maintenance staff.
5 Ancillary staff.
6 Certain senior managers.

The extent to which GWC provisions apply to these groups is indicated in the appropriate functional council handbook (where relevant) or in the text of the GWC handbook itself. The introductory section to the GWC handbook gives details of the application of agreements, together with other definitions of terminology.

The areas covered by the GWC provisions can be broadly categorized as follows:

1 Leave provisions.
2 Expenses.
3 Enabling agreements.
4 Protection and redundancy.
5 Employee relations.
6 NHS reorganization provisions.
7 Miscellaneous.

In the following description of these provisions, reference is made to the appropriate section number of the GWC handbook. These references are subject to annual review.

Leave provisions

Annual leave entitlements are determined by functional councils, but the GWC (S.1) deals with proportionate allowances during the first and final year of service; arrangements to carry forward from one leave year to the next; and sickness during annual leave.

Arrangements are also set out (S.2) for statutory and public holidays, and the 2 'extra statutory' days for NHS staff, the designation of which must be the subject of joint consultation. There is provision for these 2 days to be converted to additional annual leave by local agreement.

Provision is also made for granting special leave (S.3). Whereas there is a general discretion to employing authorities to grant unpaid leave, the granting of paid leave is confined to the express Whitley provisions or other guidance given by the Secretaries of State. The GWC specifically enables paid leave to be granted for candidates applying for NHS posts; compassionate leave; leave for domestic, personal and family reasons (see also the section on enabling agreements, below); maternity (S.6); contact with notifiable disease (S.7); jury service (S.8); witness in court (S.9); magisterial duties (S.10); parliamentary candidates (S.11); local government activities (S.12); training with the Reserve Forces (S.13); Whitley Council meetings (S.14); witness at appeal hearings (S.15); health authority membership (S.16); and membership of community health councils (local health councils in Scotland; S.17). In each case, maximum limits apply to paid leave.

At the time of writing, the GWC was revising parts of sections 3, 4 and 7 to 17 into a single and largely discretionary agreement.

Expenses

The provisions regarding reimbursement of expenses contain considerable detail, and include specific rates which are regularly updated. There are subsistence allowances, designed to cover costs of meals and/or accommodation when working away from one's normal place of work. Travelling expenses cover the use of public transport and use of a car (S.23), and provision is made for employers to provide 'crown cars' for staff who need transport to do their job (S.24). The broad scope of this GWC agreement has encouraged many employing authorities to introduce innovative and attractive car lease schemes (covering private and business use) which help with the recruitment and retention of staff. Provision is also made for the payment of removal expenses for staff (S.26). The GWC agreement covers considerable detail, but broadly the scheme provides for the payment of removal expenses both for staff moving from one NHS post to another and, in certain circumstances, for staff newly recruited to the NHS where it is agreed that removal of the home is required. The extent to which payments can be made is considerable, and this facility can be a powerful aid to recruitment, but equally it can be very expensive. It is therefore important to clarify in any particular case the extent and scope of the entitlement, and make decisions about the discretionary elements. The GWC Handbook includes a useful checklist of eligibility. Negotiations are fairly advanced in the GWC to deregulate section 26, which will leave the decision about scope and level of removal expenses to the employing authority and the individual concerned.

To complete the expenses section, provision is made regarding reimbursement of telephone expenses (S.27) and payment of lecture fees (S.28).

Enabling agreements

There are a number of GWC provisions which are not substantive in themselves, but commend to employing authorities the development of their own substantive local agreements. In most cases the GWC agreement sets out some principles to be incorporated into local agreements. The provisions of this type cover:

1 Leave for domestic, personal and family reasons (S.5) – providing for paid leave for a broad range of domestic responsibilities.
2 Disputes procedures (S.33) – providing a procedure for the resolution of disputes between the employer and employees (normally collectively).
3 Facilities for staff organizations (S.38) – providing for agreed facilities for recognized staff organizations to carry out their role.
4 Joint consultation machinery (S.39) – providing for the establishment of machinery to encourage proper consultation with recognized staff organizations on all matters affecting the interests of employees.
5 Harassment at work (S.48) – providing a national framework for local agreements, affirming that harassment at work in any form is wholly unacceptable and encouraging employing authorities to create a working environment where the dignity of the individual is respected.
6 Retainer schemes (S.50) – providing a scheme to encourage (particularly) skilled staff to return to work following a prolonged career break, e.g. to fulfil domestic responsibilities.
7 Child care (S.49) – providing for the development of local facilities to assist with child care, e.g. nurseries, child care vouchers.
8 Counting of previous service (S.61) – providing discretion to employing authorities to count previous service in determining annual and sick leave allowances for new staff.

It is significant that four of the above enabling agreements have been made since 1990. This reflects a trend to move away from prescription to the establishment of principles with flexibility at local level to incorporate these into locally determined agreements.

Appeal arrangements (S.32)

The GWC provided a procedure for staff to pursue any difference they may have with the employing authority on the application of terms and conditions of service, including matters of grading. (The most prominent use of the section was the numerous grading appeals lodged by nurses and midwives following the introduction of a new clinical grading structure in 1988.) Such appeals had to be heard by (or on behalf of) the employing authority and could be pursued to a regional appeals committee comprising three staff side and three management side representatives. Where the committee could not reach a decision, it could be referred by either party for hearing by the appropriate Whitley Council.

In an unprecedented move, the Secretary of State for Health revoked this agreement with effect from 30 March 1992. This followed lengthy attempts to reach a negotiated settlement to change the agreement. In place of the agreement, employing authorities were required to introduce new procedures at local level, subject to consultation with staff organizations. This change provided employing authorities with an ideal opportunity to introduce a single procedure to deal with all grievances, and to contain the process of resolving such matters within the organization.

Redundancy, premature retirement and protection

The GWC sets out the arrangements for staff who are dismissed by reason of redundancy (S.45), and premature retirement on grounds of organizational change. The agreement sets out the qualifying conditions for entitlement to a redundancy payment (based on length of service and contracted hours) and the payments to be made. The latter are based on length of continuous service, earnings and age. Loss of entitlement to a redundancy payment can occur where an employee is dismissed for reasons of misconduct or refuses to apply for or accept 'suitable alternative employment' – a term the GWC broadly defines. Appeals concerning eligibility for or amount of a redundancy payment can be taken direct to an industrial tribunal under S.112 of the Employment Protection (Consolidation) Act 1978.

Premature retirement provisions apply separately from GWC provisions in circumstances of redundancy and in the interests of the efficiency of the service. The GWC agreement (S.46) adds to these circumstances by providing for premature retirement 'where in contemplation or furtherance of organizational change (statutory or managerial), the premature retirement would be in the interests of the service'. The scheme applies to staff aged 50 or over with at least 5 years' service, and the member of staff must agree to the arrangement. On premature retirement (where eligible) the individual can receive immediate payment of pension benefits as well as a redundancy payment.

Protection of pay and conditions in circumstances of organizational change is also provided for (S.47). This covers short-term and long-term protection of earnings, and protection of specified conditions of service. In each case protection applies for specific periods of time, depending on the length of service of the postholder.

Taken together, the GWC agreements on redundancy, premature retirement and protection provide a comprehensive package of safeguards for staff. It is common practice for employing authorities to have a local policy/procedure on

dealing with the staffing aspects of organizational change, and for the GWC provisions to be incorporated together with local arrangements.

Miscellaneous

There are a range of other GWC provisions covering the following areas:

1 A statement of commitment to equal opportunities in employment (S.51).
2 Disciplinary procedures (S.40). The principles are almost invariably incorporated by employing authorities into locally agreed procedures.
3 Position of employees elected to parliament (S.52).
4 Membership of local authorities (S.53).
5 Payment of annual salaries (S.54).
6 Preparation for retirement (S.55).
7 London weighting (S.56) – this sets out the rates of the allowance and the geographical areas covered.
8 Statutory sick pay – qualifying days (S.57). (The full sick pay schemes are determined by the functional councils.)
9 NHS reorganization 1974 – continuity of employment (S.58).
10 NHS trusts – continuity of service (S.59).
11 Minimum periods of notice (S.60).

Summary of national arrangements

The long-term future of both the Whitley system and pay review bodies as mechanisms for determining pay and conditions has been thrown into some doubt following the NHS and Community Care Act 1990, which provides for the establishment of NHS trusts. These trusts will have complete freedom to determine pay at local level and the implications of this are dealt with in the section on moves to flexibility, below. The position at March 1993, however, can be summarized as follows:

1 *Whitley Councils.* There are five active functional councils:
   (a) Administrative and clerical (including the ambulance officers' joint negotiating committee).
   (b) Ambulance staff.
   (c) Ancillary staff.
   (d) Professional and technical B.
   (e) Scientific and professional staff (*note*: the staff side composition of this council has not been agreed. In practice, the council functions by meetings between management side and staff

side representatives, based on old Whitley groupings).

In addition, there is one general council.

2 *Pay review bodies*. There are two:
   (a) Doctors and dentists.
   (b) Nurses, midwives, health visitors and professions allied to medicine.

3 *Other arrangements*. These apply to:
   (a) Maintenance staff.
   (b) General managers and senior managers.
   (c) Small groups not allocated to a Whitley Council.
   (d) New staff groups, covered by local determination (see the section on moves to flexibility, below).

Individual staff groups – terms and conditions

The detailed rates of pay and terms and conditions of service for each staff group are determined by the appropriate functional Whitley Council (with the exceptions described earlier) and published by way of formal letters to employing authorities. For nearly all groups a handbook of these terms and conditions of service is published and kept updated by amendment sheets. These are the key source of up-to-date information for managers and staff alike at local level.

The diverse and detailed nature of terms and conditions of service is illustrated in Figure 6.3.1, which summarizes the annual leave allowances just for scientific and professional staff.

For all scientific and professional groups there is now employing authority discretion to vary these allowances between the minimum and maximum during the first 5 years of service (10 years in the case of hospital chaplains).

In general terms, the determinant of all terms and conditions is the grade of a post, as salary and other allowances will depend on this. Each Whitley Council incorporates in its agreement some description of the duties and responsibilities of the grade, though since 1990 the management side policy within Whitley Councils has been to move away from detailed definitions of grade to broad grading indicators in order to encourage local flexibility in application.

In very general terms, the reward package for an individual will comprise all or some of the following elements:

1 Wage or salary scale, with incremental progression.
2 Premium rates, for overtime, weekend/bank holiday working.

3 Premium rates for night duty.
4 Allowances for on-call or standby.
5 Allowances for items such as qualifications, acting up, etc.
6 Annual and sick leave schemes.

The amounts and conditions relating to eligibility are set out in the appropriate agreements. In some cases these can be very complex and require careful reading. Personnel officers normally provide expert advice on all these matters. It is increasingly the case that there is local flexibility – rather than national prescription – on these issues, and this is considered below.

Pension arrangements and retirement

With few exceptions, all staff working in the NHS are eligible to join the NHS pension scheme, irrespective of hours worked. The scheme is funded by contributions from members of 6% of salary (5% for manual workers) and a contribution from the employer. Membership is not mandatory.

The scheme does not come under Whitley arrangements, but is governed by the NHS (Superannuation) Regulations 1980 (as amended) and run by the Department of Health on behalf of the Secretary of State.

The pension scheme provides a comprehensive range of benefits which can be summarized as follows:

1 A pension and lump sum on normal retirement.
2 Pensions which are increased after retirement by index linking.
3 Lump sum and family benefits in the event of death.
4 Immediate payment of benefits in the event of retirement on grounds of ill health (subject to a minimum of 2 years' pensionable service).
5 Immediate payment of benefits in the event of redundancy at or after age 50 (subject to minimum of 5 years' pensionable service).

The retirement age for NHS employees is a matter of policy for determination by each employing authority and will apply irrespective of whether or not the member of staff belongs to the NHS pension scheme. On the basis of case law, the 'normal' retirement age for men and women must be the same and is invariably at age 65. In practice, of course, the actual age at which employees will retire will be based on a number of variables. Members of the NHS pension

Speech therapists	
Spine points 18–29	5 weeks
Spine points 18–29 (with 5 years' service)	5 weeks + 3 days
Spine points 30 and above	6 weeks
Speech therapists' assistants	
With up to 5 years' service	5 weeks
After 5 years' service	5 weeks + 3 days
Scientists and optometrists	
Spine points 00–12	5 weeks
Spine points 00–12 (with 5 years' service)	5 weeks + 3 days
Spine points 13–36	6 weeks
Hospital chaplains:	
Under 5 years' service	5 weeks
Over 5 years' service	5 weeks + 3 days
Over 10 years' service	6 weeks
Clinical psychologists	
Spine points 12–29	5 weeks
Spine points 12–29 (with 5 years' service)	5 weeks + 3 days
Spine points 30 and above	6 weeks
Child psychotherapists	
Basic and senior grades	5 weeks
Basic and senior grades (with 5 years' service)	5 weeks + 3 days
Principal grade and above	6 weeks
(new agreement pending for child psychotherapists)	
Pharmacists	
Preregistration	4 weeks
Spine points 00–08 (up to 5 years' service, no emergency duty)	5 weeks
Spine points 02–10 (up to 5 years' service, with emergency duty)	5 weeks
Spine points 00–08 (after 5 years' service, no emergency duty)	5 weeks + 3 days
Spine points 02–10 (after 5 years' service, with emergency duty)	5 weeks + 3 days
Spine points 09–32 (no emergency duty)	6 weeks
Spine points 11–34 (with emergency duty)	6 weeks

Fig. 6.3.1   Annual leave: scientific and professional staff.

scheme, for example, may take their retirement benefits at age 60 (age 55 for special classes, i.e. those working in the field of mental health or learning disability, female nurses, midwives, health visitors and physiotherapists) and may therefore decide to retire at these ages. The actual date of retirement is a matter that is effectively decided by individuals on the basis of their personal circumstances, including the benefits payable to them from any pension scheme. In practice, therefore, an employing authority's retirement date amounts to an upper age limit beyond which continued employment is at the employer's discretion.

Pay comparisons

Whatever the machinery, the outcome of the determination process is the various rates of pay and conditions of service for over 1 million NHS employees. How do these terms compare with one another, and with external comparators? Statistical data abound, and the production of appropriate evidence – by both the management side and trade unions – to support a case is at the heart of the pay determination process. Avoiding great detail, however, it is possible to deduce some general points about pay trends in the NHS.

Table 6.3.2 shows changes in real earnings for a variety of public sector groups.

Table 6.3.2 Earnings changes for specific occupational groups 1979–1989

	Change in real weekly earnings (%)	
	1979–1981	1981–1989
Medical practitioners (M)	55	26
NHS nurses (F)	57	38
Ambulancemen	25	11
NHS ancillaries (F)	11	8
Primary teachers	36	17
Police constables (M)	34	26
Local authority administrators (M)	21	9
Private sector		
Accountants (M)	47	38
Finance specialists (M)	68	54
Whole economy – all employees	24	25

(Extract from HMSO: New Earnings Survey, 1990.)

There are two key conclusions about NHS pay that can be drawn from this figure:

1 Staff whose pay is determined by pay review bodies have done better than those whose pay is determined by Whitley Councils.

2 With the exception of top trained nurses, however, NHS pay has risen by less than the average for all non-manual workers.

Any general conclusions may, of course, depend on the base year chosen, and the period over which comparisons are drawn. Nevertheless, the two conclusions above are borne out by almost every set of reputable data available. Figure 6.3.2 provides more detail.

A third general conclusion can be drawn from this figure: NHS pay has kept ahead of the retail price index – i.e. in the periods in question it has increased in real terms, with the notable exception of administrative and clerical staff.

Moves to flexibility

For some considerable time there has been pressure from NHS managers to introduce more local flexibility into NHS pay and conditions. The arguments have centred on the fact that Whitley (and pay review bodies) is centralized, common across the whole NHS, and highly prescriptive. This leaves no room for employers locally to adapt to the labour market and prevailing local pay levels, and little room to design local jobs for local needs because of national grading definitions.

DNO – DHA 1 (T)	267	All industry female non-manual average 241
RNO – RHA 1	260	
Senior I chiropodist	231	
Maximum full-time consultant & A +	230	All industry male non-manual average 237
Basic speech therapist	227	
Staff nurse	225	
Radiographer	225	
Sister II	223	
DA – DGM + DISC. + PRP	216	All industry manual female average 216
Basic full-time consultant	215	
Registrar	213	
Regional scientific officer	208	
Scale 29/senior manager 6	206	
Nursing auxiliary	201	All industry manual male average 206
Lowest ASC scale	197	
Senior/clinical psychologist	195	
Third-year student nurse	194	
Highest ASC scale	191	Retail price index 190
Administration and clerical scale A	162	
23	162	
SAA	162	
HCO	162	

Fig. 6.3.2 Comparison of the NHS with all industries/services and the retail price index. 1987 shown as a percentage of 1979.

The publication of *Working for Patients* (HMSO, 1989), outlining the government's proposed reforms to the NHS, signalled the first significant moves to introduce local control of pay and conditions of service. The proposals – since enacted in the NHS and Community Care Act 1990 – included the right for NHS trusts to be completely free of central pay bargaining and determine pay and conditions for all their staff. But *Working for Patients* also stated the intention to increase pay flexibility in the whole NHS, not just in the special circumstance of trusts. The stated government purpose was to give managers greater control over the resources for which they are responsible (pay accounts for over 70% of all NHS expenditure; HMSO, 1989), to allow managers to relate pay to local labour markets, and to reward individual performance. This flexibility was to extend to conditions of service as well as pay.

Since 1990 this increasing flexibility has been very evident, particularly in Whitley agreements, as opposed to pay review body-related terms. Recruitment and retention supplements, determined at local discretion, have been introduced for many staff, together with freedom to determine starting salaries, discretionary points on salary scales, flexing of annual leave allowances and broader grading definitions. The significance of these changes cannot be overstated: after a 40-year history of being implementers of pay agreements, managers now have to really manage what is often their largest resource.

A further, and in many ways even more fundamental, change was introduced in 1990 when authority was given to NHS employers to determine the entire reward package for new staff groups, i.e. any new type of worker not currently covered by Whitley or other arrangement. The most significant new group is the health care assistant/support worker, and the most obvious of these is the health care assistant in nursing. The need for such a support worker has been driven by the introduction of new training arrangements in nursing and midwifery – Project 2000. Implementation of Project 2000 training requires a fundamental review of skill mix in nursing, with different levels of health care assistant to support the trained professional nurse.

For NHS trusts, there is complete freedom in matters of pay and conditions, subject only to the exception of junior doctors. In practice, the speed with which the first trusts were established has meant only limited immediate change, with the majority of them keeping Whitley/pay review body terms and rates within a trust employment contract, whilst they develop a longer-term strategy to deal with the enormous task of developing local reward arrangements. Such changes raise fundamental industrial relations questions, including that of trade union recognition, the development – or otherwise – of local bargaining arrangements, and the establishment of completely new local procedures for local control of pay.

As the development of trusts continues, it is clear that significant variations will emerge between them as far as pay and conditions of service are concerned. In the longer term, this is likely to raise questions about the continuing need for Whitley and pay review body machinery, if more and more staff opt to accept locally determined reward packages.

References

Commons Written Answer 27.7.1983. Hansard vol 44, no. 31, columns 461–462.

Connah, B. and Lancaster, S. (eds) (1989) *NHS Handbook*, 4th edn. National Association of Health Authorities. MacMillan Reference Books.

McCarthy, (1976) *Making Whitley Work – A Review of the Operation of the NHS Whitley Council System*. DHSS, London.

Report of the Review Body on Doctors' and Dentists' Remuneration (1971) Cmnd 4825. HMSO, London.

Royal Commission on Doctors' and Dentists' Remuneration 1957–1960 (1960) Cmnd 939. HMSO, London.

Working for Patients. (1989) White Paper on the NHS. HMSO, London.

6.4   Training staff in the NHS

John Rogers

Introduction

This section describes the arrangements for the education and training of NHS staff. It also touches briefly on the mechanisms for registration and discipline in some of the health care professions, because these are often the responsibility of the same bodies who regulate education. The format is that of, first, a general overview of education and training, followed by greater detail for selected staff groups and professions.

Part I

There is a multiplicity of professions and occupations in the NHS and in health care generally. The arrangements for education and training are similarly complex. It is possible, however, to group these occupations in two ways – first, by the mode of regulation of education/nature of resulting qualification and, second, by funding regime.

Mode of regulation/nature of qualification

Regulated health care professions

Education in a number of professions is regulated (as to standard and content) by statutory bodies established by Act of Parliament. These bodies are as follows:

1 General Medical Council (GMC).
2 General Dental Council.
3 General Optical Council.
4 UK Central Council (UKCC) for Nursing, Midwifery and Health Visiting, together with four national boards for each of the countries of the UK.
5 Council for the Professions Supplementary to Medicine (CPSM; covering chiropodists, dieticians, medical laboratory scientific officers (MLSOs), occupational therapists, orthoptists, physiotherapists and radiographers).

In addition, there is a group of professions whose regulatory bodies have statutory recognition (e.g. by royal charter or by statutory instrument restricting NHS employment to those with a professional qualification issued by the body concerned).

1 Royal Pharmaceutical Society of Great Britain.
2 College of Speech Therapists.
3 British Psychological Society.

'Unregulated' health care professions

There is a small number of health care occupations or professions which are not statutorily regulated but which have been seeking some form of statutory recognition. Among these are psychotherapists, operating department assistants, health promotion officers, art, music and drama therapists. In 1992 the osteopaths achieved statutory recognition after a campaign lasting more than 50 years. In addition, the NHS employs a wide range of scientists with a specific health care-related training and qualification (e.g. clinical biochemists, cytogeneticists, microbiologists, medical physicists, bioengineers).

Generic professions

A large number of NHS staff possess professional qualifications, whether or not statutorily regulated, which are not specifically health care-related, e.g. architects, engineers, surveyors, accountants, personnel staff. Specific to the health care sector are the professional qualifications awarded by the Institute of Health Services Management.

Vocationally trained and untrained staff

There is a further wide range of staff who receive a formal vocational training. Among these are ambulance personnel, dental hygienists, dental technicians, dental surgery assistants, pharmacy technicians, hearing therapists, audiological technicians, medical physics technicians (MPTs) physiological measurement technicians (PMTs) cardiographers, cytology screeners and medical laboratory assistants. There is often no clear dividing line between some of these groups and those identified above, other than such factors as size of the profession/occupation or length of time it has been established. For some of these groups, qualifications within the National Vocational Qualification (NVQ) framework are being developed (e.g. ambulance personnel, PMTs MPTs). A further group of staff possess vocational qualifications which are not specific to the health care sector, e.g. craft workers, some catering staff. Finally, there are staff groups, mostly working in support of those delivering patient care (but in some cases delivering it themselves) who traditionally have had little or no formal training, such as nursing auxiliaries, the helpers to the professions supplementary to medicine, porters, clerical staff, domestic staff, etc. However, a formal training and qualification as a health care assistant is being developed within the NVQ framework, which may ultimately embrace many of these staff.

Funding regime

The education and training of NHS staff may also be categorized by funding regime. There are three broad groupings, although the boundaries are not exact. First, there are those trainings where most of the cost is borne by the education sector (usually higher education: HE). Among the health care professions these include pharmacists (although the NHS bears the training costs of those who undertake their preregistration year in hospital pharmacy), speech therapists, dieticians and most chiropodists. Second, doctors' and dentists' education costs are shared, albeit on an uncosted basis, between the NHS and the HE sector. Third, there are those staff whose training is predominantly NHS-funded. Overwhelmingly, the largest group is nurses, midwives and health visitors. Others include occupational therapists, physiotherapists, radiographers, orthoptists, clinical psychologists and MLSOs. Most vocational training is funded by the NHS. The costs of in-service training and development for all groups of staff are borne predominantly by the NHS.

The costs involved in professional education alone are substantial. Table 6.4.1 shows the approximate numbers and costs of some key groups. Although these figures are slightly out of date, the numbers involved have not changed substantially in subsequent years.

Table 6.4.1

Profession	Training intakes (1988)	Approximate cost of training per cohort (£m) (1988 prices)
Medicine	3752	236*
Nursing and midwifery	20 267	280†
Radiography	532	10
Physiotherapy	811	15
Occupational therapy	714	13
Orthoptics	39	0.7
Chiropody	346	5
Dietetics	125	2
Speech therapy	317	6
Pharmacy	297	2‡
Clinical psychology	156	5

* Excludes postgraduate medical education.
† Net costs, excluding proportion of salary attributable to in-service contribution during training – gross costs over £400m.
‡ Preregistration year in NHS only; total costs include initial pharmacy degree; other pharmacists undertake their preregistration year in retail pharmacy or in industry.

The NHS reforms resulted in some changes to the previous funding arrangements for education and training. For undergraduate medical and dental education, the excess costs incurred by teaching hospitals continue to be recognized by formula-based additional funding – the service increment for teaching and research (SIFTR). Rather than forming an addition to the general allocations to ditrict health authorities, SIFTR is now the subject of separate contracts between regions/districts and individual hospitals. The funding for postgraduate medical education now takes the form of top-sliced regional funding, administered by the postgraduate dean(s). Continued medical education (CME) for consultant staff is the responsibility, in terms of funding, of individual trusts or directly managed units (DMUs). All NHS-funded non-medical professional education is now funded regionally through what is generally known as the Working Paper 10 budget (so called after a working paper issued as part of the series which followed up the White Paper *Working for Patients* in 1989). These arrangements involve regional health authorities (or, in some instances, local consortia of trusts and DMUs) collecting forward estimates of demand for newly qualified staff from employers, and contracting with HE institutions or NHS-based colleges for the appropriate number of students to be trained. Most regions also fund some forms of management development for professional staff (especially doctors) as well as managers. All other forms of training and development are the responsibility of individual trusts and DMUs.

Professional registration and conduct

All professional bodies, statutory or otherwise, have as part of their functions the regulation of the professional conduct of their members. Statutory professional bodies (e.g. the GMC, the UKCC or the CPSM) also have the function of entering appropriately qualified individuals on a statutory register. Maintenance of an individual's name on that register usually involves payment of a periodic fee. Doctors will be familiar enough with their own professional code of conduct (the GMC's *Blue Book*); a significant difference of emphasis in the nursing equivalent (the UKCC Code of Conduct) is the importance the latter attaches to the nurse's role as the patient's advocate, including taking action on poor physical conditions or inadequate staffing levels. This may lead, and indeed has led, to conflict between nurses and management where nurses have considered that their code requires them to speak out publicly about these issues.

Part II

This section describes the arrangements for education and training of selected staff groups in more detail. It aims to highlight some of the issues which may confront doctors in management.

Doctors

Under present arrangements it takes at least 15 years to train a doctor from entry to medical school to the point where he/she is competent to perform as a consultant.

Undergraduates are trained over a period of 5 years. The course is divided into 2 years for basic medical sciences and 3 years for clinical study. There are 27 medical schools in the UK, with a high concentration of schools in the London area – nearly half of all medical students are educated in London. Decisions on student numbers are taken nationally, based on the recommendations of the Advisory Committee on Medical Manpower Planning (representatives from the profession, universities and Department of Health). One significant trend is the increase in the number of female undergraduates – in 1991, for the first time, just over half the intake was female.

Postgraduate medical education is provided over a period of approximately 10–12 years. Training is provided through experience in a series of rotational posts in the doctor's chosen specialty. In addition, the junior doctor studies for the membership examinations of the appropriate Royal College.

Concern has been expressed that the NHS reforms will make the interface between medical schools and hospitals more difficult to handle. A major problem, for example, relates to financial arrangements. Currently there is no financial adjustment made in respect of the cost which a hospital incurs in providing services for the medical school or vice versa. It is possible that more explicit charging for services will result in pressure for this informal arrangement to end, although the 'knock-for-knock' principle remains enshrined in policy at present. Teaching hospitals may also be affected by changes in the undergraduate curriculum, with possibly a greater emphasis on experience of general practice and community settings.

There will be major changes to the number of doctors in postgraduate education over the next decade. The report *Achieving a Balance: A Plan for Action* published by the Department of Health in 1987, identified serious career blockages in the training grades. The report recommended that the numbers of consultants should be expanded as a proportion of the total workforce, with parallel reductions in the training grades. This process is in hand, but the 1991 agreement between the Government and the profession to reduce junior doctors' hours of work may produce demands for more junior staff, not fewer. Meanwhile, the employment of junior doctors is a major exception to the general freedom of trusts on pay and conditions of service; this group of staff, who may rotate through a number of different trusts and DMUs during the course of their training, are subject to national pay and conditions and trusts are obliged to cooperate with rotational schemes.

Trusts and DMUs are responsible for funding the continuing medical education of consultants, but their plans are subject to guidance and approval from postgraduate deans. It is, however, far from clear what would happen in the event of a major dispute between a trust and a postgraduate dean over the quality or quantity of its provision for CME.

Nursing, midwifery and health visiting

Traditionally, basic, preregistration nurse education was provided on two levels – registered nurse education and a lower-level qualification, enrolled nurse education. The periods of education were 3 and 2 years respectively. Most preregistration education was provided separately for three main specialties – general, mental illness and mental handicap nursing. The major proportion of education was located in NHS schools of nursing, but since the 1970s an increasing number of universities and polytechnics have provided nursing courses leading to a degree. However, NHS-based education still accounts for over 90% of the total.

Paediatric nursing and midwifery education were generally provided as post-registration qualifications, although in both cases there were a handful of direct-entry basic courses in these fields. Health visitors, district nurses, school nurses, occupational health nurses, community psychiatric nurses and community mental handicap nurses were, and are, mostly educated in the HE sector, via year-long, off-the-job courses. Other post-registration qualifications for specialist areas of work (e.g. renal services, operating theatres, intensive care and accident and emergency) were provided by NHS-based schools. Possession of such qualifications is, however, not compulsory for work in these areas, except as part of a local management policy.

Fundamental changes have been implemented in nurse education. The changes as they affect pre-registration education were outlined in a report, *Project 2000* published by the UKCC in 1987. The main changes are:

1 A new single level of nurse, known as a registered practitioner, replacing the present registered and enrolled nurses. Enrolled nurse training has, as a consequence, virtually been phased out.
2 A new course takeing 3 years and consisting of a common foundation programme of 18 months, followed by a branch programme in one of four areas – mental health, learning disabilities, nursing of the adult and nursing of the child.
3 That students make a substantially reduced contribution to the provision of service during training.

The first Project 2000 courses began in 1989 and were introduced in stages. Part of the reason for this was the question of cost. This arose primarily because of the loss of students' contribution to rostered service during their training. For example, students in general nursing were rostered as part of the workforce for approximately 60% of their 3-year training period. Under the new arrangements, only about 6 months of the third year will be spent in rostered service. Although additional central funding meets the net additional cost, there is a challenge for management in redeploying the workforce to take account of the loss of student labour, determining the appropriate skill mix and training non-professionally qualified staff (health care assistants).

The other major change in nurse education over the last few years has been in the management and status of NHS-based schools of nursing. The Project 2000 qualification is validated at HE diploma level. This has necessitated much closer links between NHS schools and HE institutions. In many cases, this has led to moves to incorporate hitherto NHS-based education in HE. Those schools which remain in the NHS are now frequently part of multidisciplinary colleges of health, organized and managed completely separately from trusts and DMUs which provide patient services. When the government, in England at least, set its face against trust status for education providers; the consequence was to accelerate the move to a merger with HE.

At the time of writing, the UKCC is in discussion with the government over the Council's proposals for post-registration education for nurses, midwives and health visitors (PREPP). These involve a framework for mandatory updating and further training if professional registration is to be maintained. Even if the question of cost can be resolved, there will still be implications for management in providing access to continuing education for nurses.

Pharmacy

Entrants to the NHS must have completed a degree course in pharmacy. These courses are funded through the HE sector. Before achieving professional qualification, however, pharmacists must undertake a year's preregistration work experience in the hospital sector or in community pharmacy. Salaries for the preregistration year in hospitals are borne by regional health authorities as part of the Working Paper 10 arrangements. There are proposals that a preregistration year should encompass both hospital and community experience. This will entail establishing formal rotational programmes.

Other NHS-funded training

This section covers education for those professions where the NHS has responsibility for both numbers and funding. These are physiotherapists, occupational therapists, radiographers, chiropodists, orthoptists and clinical psychologists.

To take the first three professions first, education was in the past in a mix of NHS schools and HE. Within HE, funding was either via the UFC/PCFC or, in a few cases, paid for by the NHS. The position has now been rationalized, with a transfer of the funds from the education sector to the NHS, so that the NHS now bears the whole cost, together with, in most cases, location of courses in HE at degree level. With these relatively small professions, there is a particular necessity for trusts and DMUs to get their estimates of forward demand for newly qualified staff as accurate as possible; there have been significant shortages in these professions for some years, but it would be easy for the pendulum to swing the other way.

Chiropody education is extremely complex. It takes place in NHS or private schools or in HE or further education(FE) institutions. Responsibility for planning numbers is diffuse, with no one agency having overall control. Funding is from the health sector in respect of a small part of the costs of clinical placements and of NHS schools, but is mostly from the education sector in respect of course costs, *discretionary* local education authority awards and some of the costs of clinics attached to HE and FE institutions which provide treatment to NHS patients. On the whole, local NHS management has little influence over chiropody education.

Orthoptists are unique in that they are the only profession whose education is centrally funded by the Department of Health, which funds two degree courses. An issue for management in places geographically distant from the two courses (Liverpool and Sheffield) may be the future supply of newly qualified orthoptists.

Finally, clinical psychologists undertake an initial psychology degree in the HE sector, but thereafter undertake a 2- or, more usually, 3-year course of in-service training as NHS employees. The training is intensive, and costly in terms both of trainee salaries and academic (HE) staff.

Scientists

The NHS recruits a number of science graduates – e.g. chemistry, biochemistry, physics, (micro)biology, genetics or engineering graduates – who then receive further in-service training to become clinical biochemists, cytogenetecists, microbiologists, medical physicists or bioengineers. The numbers in any one of these groups are extremely small, which again points to the need for local management to get estimates of future demand as accurate as possible.

Speech and language therapists and dieticians

These two groups are educated in HE, and the numbers in training and funding are an HE responsibility. The NHS is, however, involved in providing clinical placements during educational programmes. These can have significant management and cost implications, but are vital if education is to remain vocationally relevant.

MLSOs, MPTs and PMTs

Training for these groups takes place on an in-service basis, with off-the-job training provided mostly in FE. Planning of numbers and funding are mostly a local responsibility of trusts and DMUs, although in many cases consortia of pathology departments (or staff of regional training departments on their behalf) negotiate jointly with educational institutions. Some course costs are met by the education sector. A proportion of MLSOs are science graduates who undergo shortened training. Some regions fund supernumerary training posts for MPTs and PMTs.

Other staff

Space precludes a detailed description of the training arrangements for the many other occupations within the NHS. Some mention, however, should be made of operating department assistants who are usually locally trained, often in conjunction with the education sector. As with some of the technician groups, consortia of employers often negotiate jointly with FE colleges.

Main implications for doctors in management

Doctors in management will need a working knowledge of most, or all, of the following issues:

1 The implications of achieving a balance and the agreement on reducing junior doctors' hours. There may also be implications for teaching hospitals in proposed changes to the medical undergraduate curriculum, with more emphasis on experience in the community (not just general practice); and the implications for the nursing workforce of implementing Project 2000. The changes are extremely difficult to manage if the opportunity is not taken to review student numbers, the matching of staffing to workload, the mix of skills in the workforce, and the training of non-professionally qualified support staff.
2 The need for local management to play a full part in the Working Paper 10 arrangements for the education of most of the non-medical professions. Accurate and well-founded workforce planning is essential at the local level; if the view is taken that these issues can all be sorted out by the region, the

likelihood of significant over- or undertraining is significant.
3 Local management in provider units still has an essential role to play even where education is based in the HE sector. All the health care professions require extensive clinical experience during training and most units will be involved in supplying this. There is a cost, in terms of extra supervision and on-the-job training, which, at present, is in most regions not met as part of the Working Paper 10 arrangements. But it would be short-sighted to take a narrow financial view on this; there are less tangible benefits of better staff morale and improved future recruitment to set against the costs which may be incurred.
4 The impact of the NVQ framework should not be underestimated. Better-trained support staff should, at the least, provide greater-quality assurance; while in some cases it may be possible to make significant financial savings by adjusting the skill mix within the profession.
5 Although this section has concentrated primarily on professional education, the need for management education and development for many professionals should not be underestimated. In hospitals, for example, the ward sister is a crucial part of front-line management; without investment in these and other staff, the aspirations of management to provide a high-quality, cost-effective service will be frustrated.

References

Achieving a Balance: A Plan for Action. (1987) Department of Health, London.
Working for Patients. (1989) White Paper on the NHS. HMSO, London.

6.5 Being a good employer in the NHS

Alison Brunsdon

Introduction

Being a good employer makes good economic sense; treating employees properly in the way that they are utilized, developed and communicated with, produces a skilled, informed and motivated workforce. The opportunity now exists for trusts within the NHS to reassert themselves as good employers. Two important factors giving rise to this opportunity are:

1 *Increased freedoms*. Changes in national agreements give trusts complete freedom to determine their management style, culture and employment terms and conditions.
2 *Demographic changes*. Current levels of unemployment are temporarily masking the long-term demographic trend of a decrease in the numbers of people available for work. The labour market will become increasingly biased in employees' favour, making it important positively to attract and retain the right people. Another factor is that women will make up an increasing proportion of the labour force, which will cause organizations to examine traditional working patterns, which tend to be based on full-time working.

Although it is up to the trust to determine the overall policies and procedures, the responsibility for making good employment practice work lies with line managers and supervisors – the people who deal with staff on a day-to-day basis.

The aim of this section is to set out the principles of good employment practice in the organization, focusing responsibility on the line manager. The chapter adopts a sequential approach, from advertising a vacancy through to the end of employment.

The role of personnel

The NHS reforms have enabled the personnel function at trust level to change from a largely administrative role to a proactive role in developing policies and agreements designed to maximize the extent to which the human resource contributes to the achievement of the trust's objectives.

In order to implement the NHS reforms successfully, the government recognized the need to strengthen specific functions, particularly at local level, to fulfil the new roles that would be required. The personnel function, along with finance and information technology, has received extra funding to recruit additional personnel staff and provide development activities for members of the function.

The move to a more proactive personnel function has been accompanied by the increasing devolution of budget and the responsibility for decisions about staff to the line manager, in line with the increasing emphasis on allowing managers to manage.

Recruitment and selection

The selection of the right people is always important to an organization but is paramount when an organization is as labour-intensive as the NHS. Although proper selection can be costly in terms of time and money, selecting the wrong person increases the cost and disruption to the organization. Also, a job that has been properly thought through, when care has been taken in the selection process, sends the message that 'we think carefully about the people we want' to both existing and prospective employees.

The recruitment process for consultants is set out in a statutory instrument which must be followed (Statutory Instrument, 1982). For senior registrars the process is summarized in a Department of Health Circular (1982). For other staff, local procedures will exist.

Generally the selection process can be thought of in four stages:

1 Examining the workload.
2 Defining the requirements.
3 Attracting candidates.
4 Selecting the candidate.

Examining the workload

A vacancy or the creation of a new post offers the opportunity to examine the current division of work in a department and decide if the job is needed in its present form. The job now required may be different to the work undertaken by the previous incumbent, as most jobs evolve over time and are often built around the strengths and weaknesses of the incumbent. Alternatively, the work could be divided up in a different way to create development opportunities for existing staff and a vacancy of a very different type to the original job.

Defining the requirements

Armstrong (1984) states that: 'A job description defines the overall purpose or role of the job and the main tasks to be carried out'. He emphasizes the importance of the job description to the selection process since it forms the basis for the person specification, the advertisement and the interview.

Usually there are standard formats for the job description, which will cover the purpose of the job, the main responsibilities, reporting lines and relationships.

The person specification is derived from the job description and defines the main characteristics needed to fulfil the job requirements. It will normally include the level of attainment, experience and personal qualities. Standard methods exist for drawing up the person specification, such as the seven point plan (Roger, 1952) and the fivefold grading system (Munro-Fraser, 1954).

Attracting the candidates

In most cases the vacancy will need to be advertised to offer an equal opportunity for anyone to apply. In the case of consultant appointments it is a statutory requirement to advertise all vacancies (Statutory Instrument, 1982). For other posts, local policies will apply, but generally vacancies will be advertised. Recruitment consultants can often be used in addition, particularly for executive appointments; however, the local personnel department can advise on the most appropriate sources of recruitment.

Selecting the candidate

A short-list is drawn up by matching candidates' details to the job and person specifications and the short-listed candidates can then be assessed using a variety of methods. The interview is still the most popular and is most effective when properly structured (Purseu et al., 1980). Armstrong (1984) describes the purpose of the interview as to 'obtain and assess information about a candidate which will enable a valid prediction to be made of his future performance'. Interviewing therefore involves processing and evaluating evidence about the capabilities of a candidate in relation to the job specification (Armstrong, 1984).

For the appointment of consultants, statutory regulations set out who should be on the appointments committee for the interview, the terms of reference of the committee and the respective roles of the committee members (Statutory Instrument, 1982). The external assessor represents the respective Royal College or Colleges to assess whether or not the candidates meet the requirements of the College and are therefore acceptable for appointment as consultants. After this has been assessed, the whole committee will then decide on the best candidate.

For senior registrar appointments, the Department of Health has issued guidelines (1982) on the interview procedure, membership and role of the appointment committees. For all other vacancies local procedures will exist on the composition of any interview panel.

Psychometric tests are being used increasingly in selection and there are two main types – ability and personality. Ability tests are used to test for a specific skill or aptitude, such as numerical ability, whereas personality questionnaires examine personal qualities such as leadership style and anxieties. Both types of test can provide useful additional information about candidates that cannot readily be obtained from any other source. Ability tests are predictive in that doing well in the test indicates that an individual will do well in that aspect of the job.

When using these tests, they must be reliable; that is, produce consistent results, and valid; that is, measure a skill or attribute that is required for the job.

Controversy has raged over the use of tests, particularly in the area of equal opportunities, and guidelines have been drawn up for the use of selection tests (Equal Opportunities Guidelines, 1991). For ability tests, it is important to ensure that the particular skill measured is required at the level tested. There is no point testing for graduate-level numerical reasoning ability if it is not required for the job; indeed it can leave the way open for discrimination claims.

For personality questionnaires the information should be used to build up a general picture of the applicant and open up areas for exploration at interview. The danger with these questionnaires is to try and 'clone', which again may lead to discrimination claims. Overall, these tests can be very useful as part of the selection procedure but they should be used in conjunction with other selection methods and in line with existing codes of practice.

Other methods, such as group discussions and exercises or presentations, can also be very valuable in selection and often it is useful to combine a number of methods. References may provide useful information as to the past performance of candidates and usually these are taken up after a decision has been made on the candidate but before an offer is given. For doctors and dentists, guidelines on the procedure for the use of references is set out in a circular (Department of Health, 1982). The overall aim of the selection process is for both the organization and the candidates to find out as much as possible about each other to decide who best fits the job requirements.

When offering the job it is important to be clear about the terms of the offer and generally advice can be sought from the personnel function.

Equal opportunity issues arise throughout employment but particularly in the selection process. It is unlawful to discriminate on the grounds of sex, marital status (Sex Discrimination Act 1975), colour, race, nationality, ethnic or national origins (Race Relations Act 1976). Discrimination can be either direct where, for example, a woman is treated less favourably than a man, or indirect, where either one sex or an ethnic group is less able to meet an unjustifiable requirement. Therefore, all criteria throughout the selection process should be objective and justifiable to comply with legislation. In terms of good employment practice it makes sense not to exclude unjustifiably groups of people who would be perfectly capable to do the job required.

There have been increasing efforts to bring together the worlds of work and education through the use of training schemes and work experience, to enable educational institutions to equip individuals with relevant skills and knowledge and for young people to have the opportunity to assess a wider choice of careers. Given the potential shortage of school leavers, these schemes can be a useful way of attracting potential candidates. The NHS has an added advantage that young people are exposed to the organization through the school nurse and doctor, which can also be useful for attracting potential recruits.

Induction

Induction is the process by which an individual is brought into the organization. A well-planned induction is important to ensure that the employee becomes familiar with the organization and is therefore effective as soon as possible. It will also give a positive message about the organization to the new starter.

The induction process should be systematic and may involve different stages, including general information about the organization's aims and structure and more detailed information about the role of the specific department, its structure and departmental rules and procedures.

As well as understanding his or her individual role and how it fits into the department, a new starter will need to know relevant personnel policies such as training, health and safety, and organization rules and procedures, employee involvement, e.g. trade unions, and employee facilities.

In addition most employees* have a statutory right to receive a written statement of the main terms and conditions of employment (Employ-

* All employees who work at least 8 hours a week and where employment lasts for at least one month.

ment Protection (Consolidation) Act 1978 and Trade Union Reform and Employment Rights Act 1993) within 2 months of starting work. A contract of employment exists when an employee accepts an employer's terms and conditions. The contract of employment contains four main categories of terms:

1 Expressed terms – those clearly written.
2 Implied terms – those which are obvious, or custom and practice.
3 Incorporated terms – collective agreements or documents which are incorporated into individual contracts.
4 Statutory terms – imposed by law.

When a person is appointed he or she will receive a letter of appointment which will form the contract of employment. Collective agreements and other documents such as staff handbooks, rules and procedures will usually be referred to in this letter and also form part of an individual's employment contract.

The precise format of the letter of appointment will differ between different trusts; some may produce a letter of appointment containing full details of terms and conditions, whereas others may send a short individual letter with standard terms and conditions in a separate document.

It is important that contracts of employment are flexible to allow employers to introduce reasonable changes as the workload changes. (Any alteration to a contract must be by agreement.) However, getting the contract correct is not only important from a legal point of view; it also clarifies the role of the individual in the organization.

Employment packages

Increasing freedoms in remuneration in the NHS have led to the development of imaginative employment packages, particularly for those staff groups that are difficult to recruit and retain.

It is important to note that the NHS has always offered benefits to staff but generally, unlike private companies, these have not been marketed. Current benefits in the NHS include a generous superannuation scheme, subsidized canteens and access to discounts at stores or on insurance. Many authorities are using car lease schemes, formerly crown cars, as recruitment

and retention tools, by subsidizing the contributions made by the individual. Crèches, child care voucher schemes and playschemes are being increasingly introduced as the number of women in the workforce increases.

There has been debate over an idea to allow NHS employees preferential access to NHS facilities in the same way that many private-sector companies offer this facility in terms of services or products to their employees. This debate will almost certainly rage for a while as many feel that this would amount to little more than queue jumping, whereas others argue that by allowing NHS employees preferential access it will enable these staff to be back on their feet in the shortest possible time, and able to care for the patients. Whatever the outcome of this debate, certainly staff on site may be able to attend the beginning or end of clinics to minimize the time away from work.

Some trusts and authorities are examining a 'cafeteria-style' approach to employment packages, particularly for more senior appointments which allow an individual an element of choice in how the remuneration is comprised. The attractiveness of this system to employees is that it allows them a degree of choice over their benefits.

Benefits which are on offer in this system in the private sector include:

1 Higher levels of contribution to lease cars.
2 Additional annual leave.
3 Child care vouchers.
4 Mortgage subsidies.
5 Private health insurance.

An individual can opt for salary only, or a lower salary plus one or more of the benefits on offer.

This area is very new to the NHS and many authorities are still experimenting with the use of cafeteria style. It can be extremely complicated to administer but it offers a good opportunity to attract good individuals. Therefore, if it is established it could well be extended to all groups of staff.

Working patterns

Although the standard 'nine to five' working day has never been a reality in the NHS, there are benefits to both staff and managers in examining flexible working patterns. There are different options to a standard full-time working week.

Annual hours

This is a system whereby the number of hours to be worked is defined over a whole year. The hours are usually distributed in a schedule. It has been defined as:

> a contract which enables the employer to vary the number of hours worked in a defined period (daily, weekly, quarterly, yearly) within a context of the agreed standard working hours for the year. (Brewster and Connock, 1985).

Generally annual hours allows the employer to reduce overtime and provide greater employee flexibility to cope with peaks and troughs, as employees can be asked to work extra hours at short notice. However, this can reduce the freedom of employees to plan their leisure.

Flexible working hours

This system allows employees some freedom over their working hours. Generally the schemes have a core period when people must be in work but the starting and finishing times are within flexible bands and employees can choose as long as they work an agreed number of hours each week. Often these schemes allow for employees to work longer hours and 'bank' these to work a shorter week or take an extra day's leave.

A flexible working scheme has many advantages for employees, particularly with domestic commitments or travelling arrangements. For employers it can reduce paid overtime, as employees may 'bank' extra hours instead; it can enable people to attend clinics or appointments without reducing hours and can allow for greater cover as people may be available right through the whole period, including the flexible bands. However, it is important that the system is managed to ensure there is full cover for a department and it should be recognized that staff will need to take time off in lieu of any extra hours worked or receive overtime pay. This will need careful management, particularly during busy periods, otherwise staff costs will be high.

Part-time working

This system is where an employee works less than the full-time hours in a standard week. It has the advantage of opening up an alternative pool of labour as it allows an easier combination of work and domestic commitments. Part-time workers can provide additional cover for peak times and can provide out-of-hours working.

Part-time work is often an ideal method of attracting women back into work after career breaks and many companies offer returner schemes where women are offered part-time work plus training to build up their confidence and ease them back into the world of work.

Job sharing

This is an extension of part-time working where a single full-time job is divided between two people who share the responsibility, pay and benefits. It is ideal for jobs which are not easily split, such as managerial jobs. The work can be split on a daily basis with one partner working mornings and the other afternoons, or with the week split between two people. The advantage of job shares is that it allows for the recruitment of skilled and experienced workers who may not be available for full-time work.

The Employment Department job share scheme offers grants for the creation of part-time work or job shares and Job Centres are able to provide further information.

Flexibank/locums

The use of locums and flexibank nurses has been widely used in the NHS. It allows for short-term cover at short notice whilst allowing individuals who are not available for regular employment to keep updated with their profession.

The use of flexible working patterns can attract and retain employees as well as providing the most efficient staffing arrangements.

Supportive culture

This can be examined in terms of welfare services and communications. Employee welfare encompasses the work environment as well as an individual's general health.

Health and safety

The Health and Safety at Work Act 1974 places overriding duties on employers for the health and safety of all people at work. Individuals as well as employers can be prosecuted for failing in their duty and European Community proposals will place a greater burden on employers to demonstrate clearly the health and safety aspects of any changes to the workplace. Generally an employer must produce a written health and safety policy (where there are five or more employees) and recognized trade unions have the right to appoint safety representatives.

As well as being desirable to maintain a safe place of work, the legal implications of failing to do so are far-reaching. The Health and Safety Inspectorate can serve improvement notices on a person contravening the statutory provisions, requiring him or her to remedy the situation within a given period, or issue a prohibition notice which requires the activity to cease either immediately or after a period, as the inspector believes that there may be risk of serious personal injury.

Employees have a duty not to endanger themselves or others and so health and safety issues are a joint responsibility.

Occupational health programmes

These can serve a wide range of needs and are usually based on an occupational health department with assistance from the personnel function. Occupational health departments can offer such services as pre-employment health screening, regular voluntary health checks, screening and stress counselling. Such facilities show a general concern for an individual's welfare which can attract and retain individuals as well as lowering absence rates.

Providing a safe and healthy atmosphere and the opportunity to remain fit and healthy is an important aspect of valuing employees. In addition to these activities, managers have a role to demonstrate a place for caring management and an interest in an employee as a whole person.

Communication

Employee communication is important for a number of reasons:

1 to provide accurate instructions;
2 to exchange ideas and views;
3 to reduce misunderstandings;
4 to help to make staff feel part of a department and organization (*ACAS Employment Handbook*, 1990).

There are a number of useful methods of communications, such as team briefings, department meetings, regular presentations, staff handbooks, staff magazines, noticeboards and suggestion schemes. Any method needs to be monitored to ensure that it is effective both up and down the organization and across staff groups.

Most organizations also have formal employee involvement schemes, either with trade union and/or staff organization representatives. Where unions are not recognized, an individual may represent a department or working group. Formal communications can take the form of consultation or negotiation: consultation is where management will listen to the views of employees' representatives before making a decision. Negotiation is where a joint decision is reached by management and representatives.

The most effective communication strategies usually have a mixture of both informal and formal schemes.

Reprofiling the workforce

The increased devolution of responsibility for staff-related issues to line managers is a recognition that they are best placed to know the numbers and type of staff required for that department to undertake its role.

Information is available on the effectiveness and efficiency of departments which can prompt managers to examine how work is undertaken. For example, a national report by the NHS Management Executive's Value for Money Unit (1990) examined the staffing levels and the composition of the workforce in outpatients departments. It concluded that the existing skill mix was inappropriate to the tasks required and that qualified staff were being underutilized. The report went on to recommend the steps to achieve a more appropriate balance of qualified and non-qualified staff.

The Audit Commission has produced a report (Audit Commission, 1991) reviewing the use of ward nursing resources and conclude that it is possible to improve patient care and create more satisfying jobs for nurses at little or no extra cost by examining, among other things, skill mix issues. With staff budgets increasingly being devolved as complete budgets rather than linked to specific posts, this will allow managers flexibility in determining numbers and type of staff they need to fulfil the departmental requirements.

Changing working patterns, particularly the increased use of part-time workers, mean a more flexible workforce, allowing an imaginative use of time to provide the service required.

Changing technology and changes in the education of health care professionals have encouraged an examination of the way staff are utilized, not just in terms of numbers and type, but in the tasks they perform, with particular attention to demarcations between professionals. Professor Dyson (1990) states:

> Changing skill mix is essentially about changing the boundaries within the intricate network of Health Service demarcations either by moving a boundary marker or by subdividing an existing boundary or by merging boundaries to create broader skill or task competences.

Any examination of the way people work appears threatening, as it is often perceived as deskilling. However, examining roles to remove mundane tasks will mean that a higher proportion of a professional's time is spent on those tasks for which he or she was trained, thus increasing job satisfaction and motivation. Cutting down on duplication will increase the efficiency of the service offered to patients (Dyson, 1990).

This is a sensitive issue and it is important to keep staff informed right from the start. By offering these skill mix studies as an opportunity to increase job satisfaction, managers can gain the commitment and the ideas of their staff.

Training and development

The development of an individual to attain the skills, knowledge and experience necessary both to fulfil the requirements of the job and to progress should be regarded as an investment rather than a luxury. It is important that development is systematic rather than haphazard and reactive.

An individual's development needs should start with an examination of the aim of the department, which in turn is related to the business plan of the unit. The process can be summarized as shown in Figure 6.5.1.

The examination of an individual's skills and abilities is effectively achieved through a performance appraisal system. An appraisal usually comprises an interview on a regular (often annual) basis between an individual and his or her appraiser, usually the line manager. The appraisal interview is a two-way process to discuss past performance, to review strengths and weaknesses and to set future objectives. From this interview, an individual can develop a personal development plan which outlines the activities he or she will undertake to improve performance.

The performance appraisal system can provide valuable information about the current and future skills of the workforce. This information can be used for succession planning, which is a process of matching internal candidates to future vacancies.

Training and development can be carried out in a number of ways, including on-the-job training, planned work experience in the form of secondments and/or projects, courses including open learning or distance learning packages.

Management development is concerned with the development of capabilities required for management positions. These capabilities generally need to be developed over time and are not just for those with 'manager' in their job title. Most people in all the professions take on managerial responsibilities as they progress.

There has been an increasing emphasis on management development in the NHS with the launch of a management development strategy (NHS Management Executive, 1991) which sets out the national policy of the NHS management executive for management development in the NHS.

Development centres are increasingly being used (as part of management development); these offer individuals who fulfil a management role in any discipline the opportunity to assess their current and future management skills. Although the trend is for cross-functional centres, development centres have been used for specific functions such as nursing, finance and personnel managers.

Management of absence

Any absence can cause problems for managing workloads. If the absence is planned, then

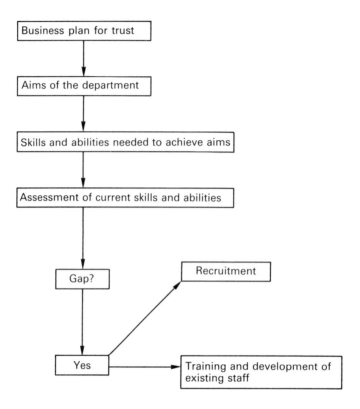

Fig. 6.5.1 Diagram to show how recruitment, training and development relate to the business plan for the unit.

these difficulties can be reduced by rearranging the workload or bringing in temporary assistance.

Planned absences include:

1 Maternity/paternity leave.
2 Special leave.
3 Career breaks.

Maternity/paternity leave

Under the Employment Protection (Consolidation) Act 1978, women who have fulfilled minimum service requirements are entitled to up to 29 weeks' maternity leave (the level of pay will depend on the length of service; employers can extend this provision) and have the right to return and so plans should be made to cover their work on a temporary basis during this absence. Some units have negotiated more generous packages for maternity leave and re-

turning mothers, such as guaranteed crèche places.

Increasingly, fathers are being offered 'paternity leave' to attend the birth, undertake domestic commitments during confinement or even an extended period to assist in the care of the child. It is interesting to note that the European Community is proposing in its Social Charter to make paternity leave a right for all fathers. (Industrial Relations Legal Information Bulletin, 1990).

Special leave

This type of absence is usually unplanned and will cover extenuating circumstances which require time away from work, such as domestic crises, bereavement and family sickness. Increasingly employers are also allowing time off for people to spend with a newly adopted child. Special leave is usually at the discretion of the manager within guidelines and allows for a sympathetic response to an individual's need.

Career breaks

Increasingly people are looking to take a break from work for a number of reasons:

1 to raise a family;
2 to care for a dependent relative;
3 to follow a course of study.

As this becomes more acceptable, employers are developing career break schemes which are a powerful retention tool. These schemes will include methods of keeping in touch with ex-employees to encourage their return. Employers may send newsletters, offer a few weeks' employment each year and pay subscriptions to professional bodies providing the person returns, guaranteeing a position for when the individual is looking to return to work.

Poor attendance

Poor attendance can be due to sickness or just a failure to turn up for work. The latter is clearly a disciplinary matter.

An individual who has been absent due to a major illness needs to be treated with sympathy and understanding. Communication is very important and needs to be balanced between checking up and ignoring. However, an assessment will be needed as to whether or not an individual will be returning to work and if so, when. Advice can be sought from the occupational health department and the individual's general practitioner, having regard to the requirements of the Access to Medical Records Act 1988.

If an individual is unlikely to return to his or her job, the manager should look at suitable alternative employment, although there is no obligation to create a special job. If there is no suitable employment, the individual may be eligible for ill-health retirement, otherwise the contract of employment will be terminated on the grounds of lack of capability to do the job.

It is important to seek advice from the personnel department on handling any termination of employment as the law requires an employee to be treated fairly and reasonably.

If an individual is likely to return, then contact is important and the return to work should be well-managed with, perhaps, the facility to come back on a part-time basis at first.

Short-term absences provide more of a problem to manage. If there is an underlying medical problem, as with long-term sickness, an assessment should be made as to whether or not the employee is capable to undertake the work, which will include medical information from the occupational health department and possibly the general practitioner. If the attendance is not likely to improve and is causing severe operational difficulties, the manager should look at the possibility of suitable alternative employment. If nothing can be found, the employer will be looking to terminate the employment on the grounds of lack of capability to do the job. As with long-term sickness, advice on the handling of these cases should be sought from the personnel department. If no single medical reason is behind the absence then the employee should be counselled to find out any underlying reason, such as domestic problems or dissatisfaction with work, which will need to be dealt with appropriately. Once these problems have been dealt with or if there is no particular reason, the employee will need to be advised that the absence level is unacceptable and targets should be set. If these are not met, the disciplinary procedure should be used.

Absence causes problems for all in a department and so should be dealt with promptly and fairly (Industrial Relations Legal Information Bulletin, 1989).

Discipline and grievance

The aim of any disciplinary procedure should be to correct performance. Rules set out the standards of conduct and make it clear what is required of employees, and they generally cover issues such as attendance, health and safety and misconduct. All units will have written disciplinary rules and procedures. A disciplinary procedure sets out what will happen when the rules are not observed and provides for fair and consistent treatment of employees. There are separate rules and procedures governing professional behaviour and professional misconduct.

Generally any breach of the rules should be dealt with fairly and promptly before memories fade. In many cases an informal counselling session is sufficient to resolve a problem without the need to invoke the disciplinary procedure. If not, a disciplinary interview is an opportunity to obtain all the facts and listen to the employee's story. The interview will normally be adjourned to decide whether or not to use the procedure.

A disciplinary procedure will normally have four stages:

1 Oral warning.
2 Written warning.
3 Final written warning.
4 Dismissal.

Usually the stages are progressed through until the employee improves or is dismissed. Most procedures, however, reserve the right to go in at any stage or skip a stage if the circumstances warrant such action. It is possible to dismiss an individual for a first offence such as gross misconduct and the local disciplinary rules may list the offences which will result in immediate dismissal. It is extremely important that the disciplinary procedure is followed correctly given recent legal developments.* Disciplinary procedures will have appeal rights built into them for individuals to invoke if they are dissatisfied.

A grievance procedure is a formal method by which an employee or employees can raise a complaint about an aspect of their employment. It usually comprises a number of levels which the employee can go to if not satisfied. The procedure enables dissatisfactions to be settled promptly and fairly.

Both discipline and grievance procedures are important to avoid industrial conflicts as they provide an open and systematic way of dealing with problems and breaches of rules.

Moving on

There are a number of reasons why an employee will be moving out of employment:

1 Dismissal.
2 Redundancy.
3 Retirement.
4 Ill-health retirement.
5 Death in service.
6 End of contract.

Dismissal

The final stage of any disciplinary procedure is dismissal. To dismiss someone fairly under the employment legislation, it must be on one of four grounds, or there must be some other substantial reason (Employment Protection (Consolidation) Act 1978 S.57):

1 Conduct.
2 Capability.
3 Qualification.
4 Redundancy.

An employee who has worked for 2 years (5 years for 8–16 hours per week) has recourse to an industrial tribunal to claim unfair dismissal. If the dismissal is found to be unfair, then the employer is liable for compensation and may be ordered to reinstate the employee.

Redundancy

Although technically a dismissal, redundancy is handled separately from conduct and capability issues. Redundancy occurs when the work is no longer needed and therefore the job no longer exists. Most organizations have agreed redundancy procedures which inform employees of potential redundancies as early as possible, and may allow for preferential interviews for other positions among other arrangements. There are statutory provisions covering handling redundancies which set out the rights of employees and minimum payments.

The key issue with redundancies is to keep employees well-informed of any developments and to select for redundancies clearly, in line with agreed procedures.

Retirement

Approaching retirement can be fairly traumatic. Many organizations offer preretirement courses which will offer helpful advice and may help an individual to adjust to retirement by offering a move to part-time work.

Ill-health retirement

Retirement on the grounds of ill health needs to be dealt with speedily and sympathetically. An

---

* The House of Lords' decision in the case of *Polkey* v *A E Daylon Services Ltd* [1987] IRLR 250HL re-emphasized the importance of procedure.

employee will need to be kept regularly informed of developments and may need counselling. The process should be smooth to avoid adding to anxieties and how these employees are handled is very important in demonstrating a caring attitude.

Death in service

This is always a distressing occurrence and managers will often need to be sensitive to the needs of friends and colleagues of the employee. It will be important to ensure that the relevant superannuation department is contacted to allow any benefits to be paid to the dependants as soon as possible.

End of contract

Some people move on because their temporary contract has ended or they have chosen to resign. Whatever the reason, when people leave they are often prepared to give useful and honest feedback about their work and the environment.

Handling the exit of an employee from the organization is as important as the induction process. A smooth and efficient process will minimize the disruption to the department. In the case of dismissal for misconduct, it can clearly demonstrate to staff the standards required by the organization. For those who move on for other reasons, how the exit is handled can demonstrate a caring attitude to staff by treating them well as they leave. It is important to remember that ex-employees can be useful ambassadors to potential recruits.

References

ACAS (1993) *ACAS Advisory Booklet No. 7: Induction of New Employees.*

ACAS (1990) *ACAS Employment Handbook.*

ACAS (1985) *ACAS Advisory Booklet No. 8: Workplace Communications.*

ACAS (1993) *ACAS Advisory Booklet No. 11: Employee Appraisal.*

ACAS (1990) *ACAS Advisory Handbook: Discipline at Work.*

ACAS (1992) *ACAS Advisory Booklet No. 12: Redundancy Handling.*

Armstrong, M. (1984) *A Handbook of Personnel Management Practice*, 2nd edn. Kogan Page, pp. 132, 152–153.

Audit Commission (1991) *The Virtue of Patients: Making Best Use of Ward Nursing Resources* NHS report no. 4. HMSO, London.

Barc, S. (1990) *Tolley's Drafting Contracts of Employment*, Tolley.

Brewster, C. and Connock, S. (1985) *Industrial Relations: Cost-effective Strategies.* Hutchinson.

British Psychological Society (1983) *Psychological Testing – A Guide.* British Psychological Society.

Department of Employment (1992) Employment Department Booklet No. 4 *Employment Rights for the Expectant Mother.*

Department of Health (1982) HC(82)10 Health Service Management. The Appointment of Consultants and Senior Registrars.

Department of Health (1977) HC(77)2 Health Service Management. Checks on Doctors' and Dentists' Registration.

Dyson, R. (1990) *Reshaping the Workforce – Breaking the Mould.* Mercia.

Health and Safety Executive (1974) *The Health and Safety at Work Act 1974 – The Act Outlined.* The Health and Safety Executive.

Industrial Relations Legal Information Bulletin (1990) The European Dimension. *Industrial Relations Review*, **404**, 2–9 and Report 467 Industrial Relations Services.

Industrial Relations Legal Information Bulletin (1989) Sickness Abroad. *Industrial Relations Review*, 386, 2–8 and Report 449 Industrial Relations Services.

Institute of Personnel Management (1980) *IPM Code on Occupational Testing.* Institute of Personnel Management.

Munro-Fraser, J. A. (1954) *A Handbook of Employment Interviewing.* Macdonald & Evans, London.

NHS Management Executive (1991) *A Management Development Strategy for the NHS.* NHS Training Directorate NHSME.

NHS Management Executive Value for Money Unit (1990) *The Role of Nurses and other Non-Medical Staff in Outpatient Departments.*

Phillips, A. and Winkless, T. (1991) Personnel identities. *The Health Service Journal*, 966–967.

Purseu, E. D., Champion, M. A. and Gaylord S. R. (1980) Structural interviewing: avoiding selection problems. *Personnel Journal*, November, 907–912.

Recruitment and Development Project (1990) 'Succession Planning' Recruitment and Development Report. *Industrial Relations Review and Report*, 20 February 1990.

Roger, A. (1952) *The Seven Point Plan*. National Institute of Industrial Psychology, London.

Statutory Instrument (1982) no. 276: The National Health Service (Appointment of Consultants) Regulations 1982 as amended by Statutory Instrument 1990 No. 1407: The National Health Service (Appointment of Consultants) Amendment Regulations 1990.

6.6 Decision-making in clinical teams

Roger Dyson

A study of decision-making has equal relevance for the everyday clinical work of the NHS as it does for relationships and behaviour in manufacturing industry. Its relevance to the NHS applies to the consultant leading a firm, to a nurse in charge of a ward, to the leading of a specialist clinical service, as well as to clinical directorates. The relevance of decision-making models will be demonstrated in this section by applying them to the issue of decision-making in clinical teams.

Clinical teams

The concept of the clinical team is central to the analysis in this chapter and requires a more precise definition. Initially the doctor – patient relationship was one-to-one; the doctor had no professional support team with the exception of voluntary carers, usually family. For the vast majority of people seeking treatment today, this one-to-one relationship between doctor and patient and doctor – patient – pharmacist remains the pattern. In today's hospital service, however, there exists a complex network of relationships between professional staff that centres on the treatment and care of the individual patient.

In the UK the tradition of specialization both within and beyond the medical profession has gone further than other countries in Europe. New professions are continually being formed as more highly specialized tasks lead to professional designations. In 1960 the establishment of the Council for the Professions Supplementary to Medicine provided the ultimate statutory recognition for many professions that had previously been regarded as simply medical auxiliaries. In more recent years art, drama, music and hearing therapists have all been added to the NHS list and in the current decade we can expect at least ambulance personnel and operating department practitioners to obtain professional or quasiprofessional status, despite the recent designation of both groups as NHS manual workers.

None of these groups has acquired professional status without the support of the relevant branch of the medical profession, and the increasing size and complexity of the clinical team or network that focuses upon the treatment and care of the individual hospital patient can be expected to continue to grow.

The distinction between team and network is important because any analysis of clinical activity demonstrates that team and network are in reality points on the spectrum. At one end of the spectrum a multiprofessional network involves many people in providing services to a given patient, but who may never meet and speak face-to-face about the patient, e.g. the registrar may never speak to the radiographer who takes the X-ray or to the medical laboratory scientific officer who performs the test. At the other end of the spectrum, a consultant psychiatrist may spend considerable time in team meetings with the clinical psychologist, nurse, physiotherapist, occupational therapist, social worker, etc., in considering the treatment and care of a particular patient. Between these points on the spectrum there are many variations and the most important and frequent is a dialogue between the doctor and just one other professional. The ward round may constitute a larger and more formal team meeting than this. In the context of this section clinical team refers to the group of professionals whose interaction involves some meetings and discussion, even though this may not occur for more than a proportion of the patients that they see.

Decision-making

Patients attend hospital for investigation, diagnosis and, where relevant, for treatment. If treatment is required the patient may require care during the treatment. The fact that there may be more than one diagnosis and that separate treatments may be conducted in parallel does not affect the basic relationship of investigation, diagnosis and treatment.

An important assumption in the analysis that follows is that after investigation patients have certain rights that they can expect to be honoured. They have the right to expect a single diagnosis, however complex or multifactorial that diagnosis has to be. They have a right to treatment that is timely with respect both to the diagnosis itself, and to their physical and mental condition. They have also the right to treatment and care that is both consistent with the diagnosis and that is also consistent between the different treatments and care regimes that are being administered by different members of the wider multidisciplinary clinical team. This right does not contradict the decision of a single consultant after investigation to pursue two avenues of treatment in an attempt to reach a firm decision about diagnosis.

The converse of these patient rights is that the patient also has the right *not* to be subject to wholly separate diagnoses by different professionals whose diagnosis may be mutually incompatible, or to receive treatment for a single diagnosis that is incompatible between one treatment and another. These assumptions about patients' rights will not be wholly acceptable. Indeed, in some quarters they have been hotly contested and this debate will be returned to at the end of the chapter. If the assumptions are valid, however, it follows that the multiprofessional clinical team that focuses upon the treatment and care of the individual patient requires some mechanism to ensure the various consistencies and timeliness that are the patient's right. This process can be described as management, leadership or coordination. The terms are not interchangeable and they imply differing degrees of authority to the person or persons whose role it is to exercise them, but in the analysis below leadership is accepted as the definition with which the majority of doctors (but not all) would feel most comfortable.

Models of decision-making in clinical teams

There are four basic models of decision-making relevant to clinical teams, although each model is capable of subdivision in a more substantial analysis.

Leadership

The leadership model is most frequently used to describe the traditional primacy of the doctor in the clinical team. The very first regional circular in the NHS (RHB48/1) referred to specialists (consultants) as having 'overall clinical responsibility' for hospital patients. This overall clinical responsibility was for patients referred by a general practitioner to a named consultant for investigation, diagnosis and possible treatment. It was this original framework that gave consultants their particular authority and responsibility for patients in the NHS and which has become called the medical primacy model. It was a model further enhanced by the Spens and Platt Reports of 1948 and 1961.

At its simplest, the leadership model ensures that the patient's entitlement to timeliness and consistency in treatment and care is achieved. This can be by ward rounds, by establishing clinical protocols, by requests and comments in patients' notes, and by the ordinary process of informal conversation in wards, corridors and on the telephone. What is crucial to the success of the leadership model is that the other parties in the team accept both the concept of the leadership role and the leader. Leadership does not mean autocracy, although autocracy is one type of leadership that has been and to some extent still is practised in the NHS and caricatured by the fictional character Sir Lancelott Spratt. Unreasoning autocracy can be deeply demotivating and distressing to other team members and can lead to outright revolts against medical authority, as revealed in the Normansfield Inquiry Report 1978.

The characteristics of a good leader include the willingness to defer to the specialist expertise of others and the ability to modify and change an initial judgement in the process of debate about clinical evidence. Charismatic leadership can be popular in a team of adoring acolytes, but not every consultant cast in the role of leader has dramatic charisma, and in many teams that function well, the leadership role is often only perceived as gentle coordination. The acid test of the existence and functioning of the leadership role, however, is the leader's ability to intervene to ensure timely treatment when it would otherwise not have occurred, and to ensure consistency of treatment on the occasion when clinical views differed and the patient's condition could permit no delay.

Consensus

A clear and strict definition of the consensus decision-making model is when all the members of the team have to agree before a decision can be taken and implemented. A subtly different but acceptable definition is that decisions can be taken when no member of the team objects.

Consensus entered the language of the NHS during the 10-year experiment with consensus decision-making management teams at area and district level between 1974 and 1984. It was replaced by the introduction of general management following the report by Sir Roy Griffiths. When historians of the NHS come to record that decade properly, the full extent of team breakdowns, regional interventions and early retirements will be revealed, but the lasting damage of consensus management was not in these more dramatic manifestations, but in the gradual drift away from firm and decisive management at hospital level as the desire to avoid difficulty and unpleasantness tempted many teams to back off from the hard management decisions that were required. The administrator, treasurer, nursing officer, consultant, community physician and general practitioner were too disparate a group for consensus to have had much chance, although in fairness there were some examples of conspicuous success.

The relevance of this to clinical decision-making is that the language of consensus traded within management teams drifted into clinical teams and encouraged, for example, a new view of the consultant – nurse relationship that was more a mirror image of the consultant and nursing officer relationship in the management team. It would be too simplistic to describe this drift as purely nursing-inspired. It involved many other professions in the clinical team and also had the support of some consultants, particularly those who worked at the judgemental end of the spectrum of medical specialties. In psychiatry and geriatrics systems were established in individual hospitals that recognized consensus teams of doctors, nurses and others to determine the admission of individual patients. This means that psychiatrists and geriatricians in these circumstances surrendered their right to make exclusive judgements about the suitability of a patient for admission. Some of these agreements provoked considerable local controversy, such as the Ashingdan case in 1981.

At the other end of the spectrum of medical specialties, it would be absurd to suggest consensus in an operating theatre. Between these extremes, however, and even with many consultants in the judgemental specialties, there exists a natural resistance to consensus as alien to the consultant's unique responsibility to the patient. The extent of consensus decision-making in clinical teams is hard to assess in detail because of the number of consultants who claim to operate by consensus but who would, in an emergency, still expect to step into a leadership role. Their claim to operate a consensus team is sometimes made deliberately to avoid possible conflicts between team members over issues of principle, and is sometimes simply a confusion of consensus and teamwork. Teamworking can be a style of leadership, just as it is a style of consensus.

Democracy

The idea of one person, one vote may seem strange in the context of the multidisciplinary clinical team, but it is included for completeness and it has been claimed to exist. In some of our run-down inner-city areas there are a number of walk-in clinics which attract patients/clients who have long since ceased to be effective members of a general practitioner's list, and who often belong to a homeless and vagrant population. For many, a single visit is all that will be made, irrespective of the need for regular support. These clinics are often staffed by some members of teams including psychiatrists, clinical psychologists, psychiatric and community nurses, social workers, etc. Decisions on diagnosis and treatment may have to be taken immediately without a second opportunity and in the absence of a doctor. Under such circumstances the majority view prevails and it is claimed that blank signed prescription forms are then used to implement the decision where medication is required.

Anarchy

The title of this decision-making model causes both controversy and hostility. It refers simply to a circumstance in which each person takes his or her own decision as he or she sees fit, with or without regard to the decisions of other people. In the clinical team this means that to some extent each member diagnoses, treats and cares for the patient in the way he or she thinks most appropriate, without necessarily having regard to the diagnosis and treatment of others in the team. Stated in such a stark way, it is often strongly rejected, particularly by doctors, but in reality anarchy defined in this way is growing in the NHS and may already dominate much of clinical care. It is growing because of the increasing rejection of teams (that almost inevitably require leaders) and their replacement with a model consisting of a series of unique and independent coequal professions. Within such a framework patients are cross-referred between professionals: a patient is referred to one person who alone takes the decision about diagnosis and treatment, until the patient is referred back or referred on to another member of the team who then exercises the same rights as the first.

People who support this view of the relationship between different clinical professions prefer to talk of cross-referral between teams of equals and reject the word anarchy. This is based upon the issue of 'with or without regard' to the decisions of other clinicians. If the nurse has regard to what has been done by the doctor and then takes his/her own professional decision, that is positive and responsible and not irresponsible, as the more common use of the word anarchy often implies. The problem with this euphemism is that it ignores the assumption about the patient's right to investigation, a single diagnosis and treatment that is timely and consistent with that diagnosis. If each professional is entirely independent of the other there can be no guarantee that the patient's right will be respected whenever there is a disagreement about either diagnosis or treatment.

There are strongly held and differing views about the relative value of chemical and behavioural therapies in the treatment of mental illness, to take just one example of how important such a difference of opinion could become for the patient. Across the main medical specialties even the concept of consent to treatment can be blurred where the patient is quite obviously willing to defer to whichever professional is giving advice. Cross-referral between teams of equals offers no mechanism for resolving differences of opinion, however honestly held, in the patient's interest and it is this possibility of inconsistent diagnoses and treatments that makes anarchy the more strictly correct definition of this particular decision-making model. In a political anarchy people are free to pursue their own ends irrespective of others, but they are also free, if they wish or if they are motivated, to behave responsibly and to respect the wishes of others as an *individual* act.

It is important to recognize that the models above are not alternatives with one being correct and the others wrong or rejected. In reality the model of decision-making may change between patients, and between diagnoses by the same consultant. The model of decision-making also changes imperceptibly over time, and the degree of drift from the traditional leadership model has been more pronounced in the south-east than in other parts of the country, although this is affected by variations between specialties and there is no simple geographical pattern. Nevertheless, there is evidence to suggest that decision-making in clinical teams is shifting away from the overt leadership model, and that the degree of anarchy is increasing as the non-medical professions seek a greater degree of equality with medicine.

Illustrations of the drift away from the leadership model

The doctor – nurse relationship is the most significant professional relationship in the majority of multidisciplinary clinical teams. Change can be considered on two levels. The first is simply the aggregation of minor changes that are seen by the doctor day-by-day and which are inevitably built up by hearsay and anecdote, given the lack of a properly researched study.

Changes in the doctor–nurse relationship occur in many tiny manifestations which, of themselves, taken out of context, would lead an individual consultant to be regarded as paranoid. There are many such small indicators of change: the diminution of the grand round to the round, and of the round to a sheepish attempt to catch the eye of a nursing auxiliary. How many doctors, when faced with the statement that nurses will no longer accompany them on ward rounds, have all too willingly accepted the arguments about nursing staffing levels in order to avoid a more difficult discussion about team responsibilities? Changing the bed names from Mrs Ferguson-Smythe to Mandy was met by most doctors with a superior lack of comment. The increasing difficulty of access to nursing staff at nights is a growing frustration to many junior doctors called to see a patient at night, but who then have to wait for the 'right' nurse to be available to speak to them in the absence of a nurse with overall nursing responsibility at nights. The inability to find appropriate clinical data about the patient within the voluminous nursing process reports is another indication of how effective clinical coordination can break down.

Considered at a more analytical level, these manifestations of change have more coherence: the infamous Salmon report of 1968 introduced an enormous nursing hierarchy which at one stage went from area nursing officer to ward sister by abolishing most matrons and introducing high turnover as an almost permanent condition of the staffing of many wards. The Salmon structure was eroded in the early 1980s and was dealt a quite savage death blow by the Griffiths Report. Today in a small number of hospitals the nursing officer at board level still retains managerial authority over nursing staff. But this model is now rapidly giving way to clinical directorates whose nurse manager is now the *final* level in the nursing management hierarchy.

The trauma of this change was considerable for nurse managers in post, and on the ashes of the old management structure the nursing profession has sought to build a safer and more permanent clinical hierarchy that would be free from the vagaries of management change. Clinical nursing specialists have appeared who have clinical authority over ward nurses by setting protocols and determining nursing practice, and they in turn are clinically accountable to a hospital director of nursing practice or some other title.

As the boundary between a clinical decision and a management decision can be unclear, nurses have drawn back some decision-making into the clinical arena in a way that is independent of management and doctors. Faced with disagreements with doctors at ward level, nurses can refer to a clinical nursing specialist, who in turn can refer to a director of nursing practice and this newer version of the old hierarchy can thus again exert control over the nurse in the immediate team.

Alongside this change has come the rejection on some wards of hierarchies based upon authority. These reject the managerial authority of ward sister in favour of independent nursing teams based upon qualified staff nurses. This does not contradict the establishment of clinical hierarchies referred to above, but is merely a further manifestation of the rejection of managerial authority within what is left of the nursing hierarchy in a few of the more radically disposed hospitals.

Taken in isolation, the development of stronger clinical leadership in nursing augurs well for the quality of patient care, as does the more recent development of primary care on the wards. A single nurse with continuous responsibility for planning, implementing and overseeing the nursing care of the patient from admission to discharge has to have many benefits. The implementation of primary nursing, on the other hand, is taking many different forms and in some sites appears to be the responsibility of people who have very different understandings of the role. In some sites it is used, as above, to reduce the managerial authority of ward sister. It occasionally leads to the separation of all ward staff into teams which can work, at a cost, in the day time, but which is almost impossible to work effectively with current night-time staffing levels.

It seems inevitable that primary nursing is here to stay but the method of its implementation is going to be quite crucial and its capacity for damaging the doctor–nurse relationship is very real. A strong case can be made for joint protocols before any practice or procedure is changed so that a cooperative environment is retained in the patient's interest. But when nurses try to insist on the unilateral right to change systems and protocols, the potential damage of the anarchy model is clear.

Nurses would protest that there is no reference here to doctors initiating unilateral change and this goes to the heart of the confusion about decision-making models. Doctors who see themselves holding the leadership role do not regard the introduction of change as beyond their clinical authority. Perhaps, however, it is time for the leadership role to be exercised more by consultation and with due regard to the interests of nurses.

The most negative element of these changes is seen when nurses refuse to medicate, refuse to take part in electroconvulsive therapy, refuse to proceed with the discharge of a patient, often on the grounds that they believe the medical request to be prejudicial to the interests of the patient and therefore prohibited by the UK Central Council Code of Nursing Conduct.

Advice to doctors in this position is often to avoid personalities and to focus upon the published clinical evidence for the treatment and its effects: testing nurses to put nursing research alongside medical research so that a fully informed decision may be reached. This does not always succeed in producing a mutually acceptable practice, but even when it does it marks a significant shift away from the basic leadership model of decision-making in which the adverse effects of anarchy are avoided, but only by substituting negotiation for real leadership.

Fortunately, the great majority of day-to-day working relationships are positive and patient-centred but the evidence of change is too great to avoid the conclusion of a drip-by-drip process of change that is continually eroding the traditional leadership model. Perhaps in future clinical directors should grasp the nettle and insist upon joint clinical protocols without the option of unilateral change within a single profession.

Exactly the same issues face the doctor in relationships with professional staff other than nurses: the obstetrician and midwife, the orthopaedic surgeons and rheumatologists with the physiotherapists, the physician and the speech therapist, the radiologist and the radiographer, the pathologists and the medical laboratory scientific officer, etc. Can an orthopaedic surgeon require physiotherapy? Can a physician terminate what he or she believes is unnecessary speech therapy for a stroke patient? Can an obstetrician insist that all pregnant women are seen by a doctor at least once during hospital-based antenatal care? Can an obstetrician walk the labour wards and intervene clinically at his or her own discretion? Can a pathologist establish in advance tolerances beyond which results must be referred to him or her before being reported? Can a psychiatrist require any clinical services of a clinical psychologist?

Each of these issues may be wide of the mark in many hospitals, but each has arisen as an apparently unresolvable dispute in one setting or another. The list could be far more extensive. It merely serves to illustrate the challenge to the traditional medical primacy leadership model and its replacement to a growing degree by the anarchy model of decision-making. Again, the same conclusions apply as for nursing, that the great majority of day-to-day working relationships are positive and patient-centred, but the same caveats also apply.

Analysing the change

The two previous sections have identified the decision-making models available to multidisciplinary clinical teams and have illustrated a drift away from the traditional leadership role of the consultant towards an environment in which those relationships can more justifiably be described as either anarchy or cross-referral between teams of equals according to one's view of the shift, and one's definition of terms. The degree of drift is highly complex. It is greater in some medical specialties than in others, there are definite geographical variations in the degree of change, the issues that have been the focus of change differ between and within particular professions and the change can be imperceptible, or on a few occasions it can be the result of traumatic interpersonal conflict. Often the isolated illustrations of change, given above, either seem to lack any logic or reason, or can seem to be based simply upon the inadequacy of particular individuals. Both assumptions would be wrong, for what they refer to are merely local manifestations of a broader trend that should be analysed at the macro level.

Changing clinical boundaries

Some of the changes are undoubtedly due to shifts in the clinical boundaries between professions, caused either for resource reasons or more usually because consultants in a specialty wish to focus more upon new and more exciting developments in their field, and less upon what is seen as routine and standard. Oxford's decision to employ a vein-stripper to relieve hard-pressed junior medical staff was logical given the resource pressure.

The much wider debate about the boundary between ward nursing staff and junior doctors and the extended role of the nurse is another classic illustration of the complexities of the personnel problem being resolved, subject to agreement, by expanding the clinical role of the nurse. There is much debate and research about the possibility of radiographers reading casualty film, or being trained to do so as clinical radiographers. This is not the policy of the Royal College of Radiologists, but the debate over the issue illustrates the direction and the same applies to the reporting of ultrasound, particularly obstetric ultrasound, by radiographers and midwives. These changes, as they occur, inevitably heighten the feeling of clinical independence and lead to perceived changes in the relationship between professions – a statement which is in no way meant to imply criticism.

Broader social and educational changes

In 1948 the academic distance between doctors and the rest was considerable and with it went considerable social distance and deference. The social changes of the last 40 years have led to a more egalitarian society, less deferential to social boundaries and to social hierarchies. At the same time the status of non-medical clinical qualifications has increased considerably at the formal level, whilst developments in medicine have concentrated upon acquiring and improving skills rather than extending formal qualifications.

Thus, clinical psychology, laboratory science, speech therapy and now radiography are all graduate professions, and nursing is rapidly extending towards graduate status for more and more of its members. In clinical laboratory science and elsewhere the requirement for formal qualifications at the postgraduate level certainly matches medical training. Against this background it is virtually impossible to argue that the nature of relationships between the professions within clinical teams could be expected to remain the same.

The Project 2000 proposals for changing the character of nurse training are now well under way and when their impact is fully felt on the wards and elsewhere it is hard to imagine that relationships between doctors and nurses will not change further in the direction outlined. A 3-year period of training that is much more academically based, and with a far smaller practical training element, will inevitably produce nurses more conscious of the 'proper' relationship between doctors and nurses, if less conscious of the implications of the practical duties that fall to nursing.

Professional ambition

The title 'professional ambition' is not used in a pejorative sense; it is quite appropriate for professions to seek to enhance their status within the NHS in which they work and within the broader society. It is a positive reflection on the skills of the non-medical professional leaders that in the last 20 years they have been able so dramatically to enhance their status relative to medicine. In doing so their interests have focused upon the patient and the quality of professional services to the patient. But it would be naive to assume that professional leaders have not been fully aware of the implication of their actions. Indeed, the proof of this lies in the claims made by single-profession trade unions, such as the Royal College of Nursing and the CSP, for higher remuneration to the pay review bodies. The increasing status and responsibilities of their professions *vis-à-vis* medicine and the use of the consultants' salary as a marker have demonstrated clearly their awareness of the significance of change. Indeed, those professional leaders with responsibilities for labour relations can be forgiven for feeling that if they increase the pressure on the change in status between doctor and nurse, they will inevitably assist their claims for improved terms and conditions for their members.

The Department of Health

The analysis of the role of the Department of Health in this period of change is extremely difficult. It is equally possible to outline a conspiracy model and a 'cock-up' model. Traditionally the Department of Health itself has always preferred the 'cock-up' model, which makes the conspiracy theorists even more certain that they are right. But the issues involved are serious and quite interesting.

The non-medical professions in the Department of Health are represented by professional heads or advisers who liaise with their own profession in the field. There is no doubt that these people have had some public visibility within their professions, as moderate advocates of the changes described in this chapter, and at the private level have often been far less moderate. By contrast, since Sir George Godber of blessed memory, the service has not *appeared* to have had a chief medical officer interested in these issues or concerned about their longer-term implications. The reality may be that chief medical officers subsequent to Godber have indeed sought to question, challenge and slow down the trends described, but if so they have managed to avoid news of it seeping out into the NHS. In fairness, ministers have been encouraged to seek chief medical officers with other interests.

The peculiar story about overall clinical responsibility is tailor-made for the conspiracy theorists. In 1985 the Department of Health issued a circular listing all the circulars that they intended to withdraw as part of a simplification exercise. These were sent out for consultation to all the relevant professions. After consultation, in 1986, a second and final list of circulars actually withdrawn was published and only one circular appeared on the second list that had not appeared on the first list. That was RHB (48)1, which included the reference to the 'overall clinical responsibility' of specialists and was the only formal instruction ever given to the NHS about the primacy of consultants. The matter was subsequently raised by the British Medical Association, who were referred to the sentence in the 1986 circular making clear that the withdrawal of circulars did not imply any change in policy. The failure to list RHB (48)1 in the 1985 circular for consultation was apparently due to the error of a very junior clerk in Epping, but for reasons too complex to go into it was not then possible to revoke the decision. The author can be forgiven slight hyperbole in the description of events, given that in essence they are correct.

The Nodder report on teams in mental health in 1980, recommending a formal transfer from the leadership model to the consensus model, was perhaps the first overt initiative of its kind, but more recent developments have sought to institutionalize changes in relationships in mental health. Following the Stanley Royd Hospital outbreak, a circular defining the duties and responsibilities of consultants in mental illness and mental handicap not only failed to refer to their 'overall clinical responsibility', but introduced the alternative of 'medical responsibility'. This satisfied many psychiatrists but circulars have since recognized the existence of nursing responsibility and clinical psychology responsibility without suggesting how or in what way these separate responsibilities should be exercised collectively within the team. As a formula it was as conclusive a shift from the concept of leadership to the concept of consensus as the earlier Nodder report.

This withdrawal of 'overall clinical responsibility' was also withheld in the circular concerned with the discharge of patients from hospitals, despite very strong medical pressure and the final version referred to the consultants, 'overall responsibility'. These events make one conclusion clear beyond controversy and that is that the withdrawal of the formula in 1985–1986 was quite clearly deliberate, and in private it is justified by civil servants as part of their duty to reflect changes in the NHS in the circulars and advice distributed from the Department of Health. If that is true, there must have been a serious debate and decision at the highest level of the Department of Health when the 1985–1986 changes were made, and one can only hope that the chief medical officer was at least aware of this. Whether the Department of Health is following or leads remains an open question.

Faced with these pressures and changes at the macro level, working consultants might ask why the medical view in this debate was not at least pressed hard by their own representative bodies. In the main, the Royal Colleges and Faculties have been the effective representative of academic medicine and of doctors in training, whose leaders were undoubtedly less exposed to these pressures than others. Also, in their dealings with non-medical professions, the Medical Colleges have almost invariably taken a benevolent, courteous and almost altruistic view of the aspirations of other NHS professions and have remained sympathetic to recognizable clinical language that has focused upon quality and the patient.

The position of the British Medical Association, as the consultants' principal trade union, has been harder to understand. Part of the answer may lie in the decision in the early 1970s to appoint a cadre of able but non-clinical industrial relations officers who have to some extent been impatient of interprofessional problems that might seem to undermine the common stand of the professional trade unions on matters of resourcing and of terms and conditions of employment. The investment of their major energy since 1988 in opposition to the NHS reforms has also inevitably directed attention away from this issue, despite its immediate day-to-day concern for many members.

Practical steps for managing clinical teams

For doctors who accept management responsibilities as clinical directors or otherwise, it is important to see the broader framework against which individual local changes can be measured. Section 6.1 outlined a framework for analysing and understanding the factors that influence behaviour at work and the way in which that behaviour is regulated. This section has sought to relate that broader framework to the NHS by examining the way in which clinical teams operate and take decisions, describing in the process the considerable change that has taken place in the last 20 years.

Curiously, whilst outside industry spent the 1980s restoring the significance of the leadership model and recognizing the legitimacy of trying to achieve a pattern of motivation that matched a necessary regulatory framework in the customer's interest, the experience of the NHS in the 1980s has been the reverse. Perhaps the NHS in the 1980s has simply been adjusting to and catching up with the trends of the 1960s and 1970s, with its movement away from the unitary to the pluralistic analysis of the NHS and in its downgrading of multiprofessional clinical leadership.

The lessons for the future are hard to tell, but for the clinical director there seem to be a number of strategic issues that need to be tackled and turned into policy if the process of change is to be orderly and controlled.

The interests of the patient

An early assumption in the section was the right of the patient to investigation, to a single diagnosis and to treatment that was timely and consistent with that diagnosis, irrespective of which professional staff were involved with the patient at any one time. *If* this describes the patient's right, then some framework has to exist for the management, leadership or coordination of the multidisciplinary clinical team to ensure that this is what the patient gets. If this is *not* the patient's right and if the patient is in effect to be moved about from professional to professional, each with his or her own independent right of action, the limits of that action within the directorate should be clearly understood as part of a coherent clinical philosophy.

It is not sufficient for doctors simply to argue their legal responsibility for the patient. Nurses are expected to follow a code of conduct and that code requires them never to do anything knowingly prejudicial to the interests of the patient. For breaking the code they can be struck off, as can a doctor from the medical register. What nobody has resolved is who decides what is in the patient's interest. When the issue is purely quantitative and relates to the accidental overprescribing of drugs, the issues are straightforward. When the nurse rejects the prescription because the doctor is wrong, in her or his opinion, the issues are complex and cannot be resolved simply by a restatement of the doctor's responsibility for the patient, or the nurse's responsibility to the patient under her or his code of conduct.

Joint clinical protocols

In the past, clinical protocols have changed within a profession unilaterally and without reference to the other clinicians in the team. These unilateral changes can often have a substantial financial impact, as well as an impact upon the way other clinicians are able to practise. Some clinical directors have now established that for patients treated in their directorate no clinical protocols will be changed (including medical protocols) unless and until they have been subjected to discussion and agreement against a background of knowledge that includes an assessment of the financial implications of the changed protocol. Individual consultants may be anxious about their clinical director exercising such authority, but without it the process of unmanaged drift, described in this section, cannot be brought to a halt.

Interprofessional disagreements

It is worth considering establishing a procedure for handling interprofessional disagreements within the directorate which allows for the safe and continuing treatment and care of patients whilst the disagreements are considered. One approach could be to establish that in the event of a disagreement the patient should continue to be subject to the traditional system of diagnosis, treatment and care until there has at least been an opportunity for the professional arguments to be considered away from the immediacy of the treatment of a particular patient.

Switching the debate away from personalities

In a clinical disagreement between professions, it is not likely to be possible to resolve a dispute on the basis that 'I am right because I am a doctor, and you are wrong because you are a nurse'. The best hope for the future lies in encouraging multiprofessional debate, based upon established research evidence, and the recognition of legitimate research developments. It should not be sufficient for any professional simply to say that clinical evidence and research are immaterial, because this is what my profession has told me to say and do.

Accountability

The perceived wisdom in the NHS at the present time is that management hierarchies should be as simple and as short as possible. Within this hierarchy accountability and responsibility should be clearly defined, with responsibility being exercised where responsibility lies. For most hospital clinical directorates the management of the ward is a crucial part of this framework, and the clarity of management accountability and responsibility should be matched by an equal precision and clarity of clinical accountability and responsibility. This does not just refer to the ward sister and above, but includes the key relationships within the ward where doctors and nurses interact to the benefit of patients.

It would be wrong to end this section by implying that a single illustration should be magnified into a major shift in behaviour. But in one hospital ward recently the nurses persuaded the consultants to conduct the round by discussion outside the ward because the presence of doctors and nurses around the bed was too daunting an experience for seriously ill patients. When a doctor needs to see a patient this is now done individually. In that ward a current suggestion is that patients should be brought to a private room at the end of a ward for medical consultation, so that doctors need never enter the ward proper. The author knows of only one case, but there may be others. This request highlights a classic dilemma for the doctor. A request couched in exclusively humanitarian terms and based solely upon saving seriously ill patients from unnecessary distress is one that is almost impossible to resist. Yet its consequence, if extended to all the wards that may contain seriously ill and dying patients, would be a power shift of significant proportions. Gradually the ward would become out of bounds to doctors and the nursing model of cross-referral between teams of equals would become more firmly entrenched as the ward becomes seen as a place where exclusively nursing care is given.

Before this goes too far there is still time to assert that doctors and nurses are part of a team and should work together in the interests of patients rather than as two divided professions meeting only at designated joint venues. The outcome is in the hands of the doctors and nurses themselves and how they conduct their practice hospital by hospital.

References

Department of Health: (1989) HC(89) 5 and LAC(89) 5 *Discharge of Patients From Hospital.*

DHSS (1980) *Organisational and Management Problems of Mental Illness Hospitals: Report of a Working Group*, (Chairman: T. E. Nodder).

HMSO (1948) *Report of the Inter-Departmental Committee on the Remuneration of Consultants and Specialists* (The Spens Report) Cmd. 7420.

HMSO (1978) *Report of the Committee of Inquiry into Normansfield Hospital*, (Chairman: Michael Sherrard, QC), Cmd. 7357.

Ministry of Health (1948) RHB (48) 1 *The Development of Consultant Services.*

Ministry of Health (1961) *Report of the Joint Working Party on the Medical Staffing Structure in the Hospital Service* (The Platt Report).

Ministry of Health (1966) *Report of the Committee on Senior Nursing*, (Chairman: Brain Salmon).

Section 7

Information and resource management

7.1 Measurement of health care

Alan Maynard

Introduction

It is surprising that health care systems everywhere have been managed for so long with so little information about so much of what they do. Until the 1980s politicians had allocated resources to the NHS and other health care systems on the basis of trust: they trusted clinicians and other professions to use funds effectively in the treatment of the sick. The traditions underlying the behaviour of doctors go back to the time of ancient Greeks when Hippocrates demanded that physicians adopted the individual ethic of doing the best possible for their patients, and not being diverted by self-interest and money.

It is remarkable that the professional ethic survived so long and it is as yet unclear whether its erosion by professional management will be cost-effective: professional codes of proper practice, if adhered to, may be cheaper than legions of expensive and ill-informed managers. However, be that as it may, politicians have become convinced that clinicians are unaccountable for their decisions and this deficiency must be removed by both *glasnost* and *perestroika*.

How has this decision been reached? This question will be addressed in the first part of this section. The information requirements of clinicians, purchasers and providers are addressed in the second part: what information do they need to manage their activities, and how can these needs be met? In the conclusion the issue of behaviour change is discussed: if it is possible to lead the clinical purchaser and provider horses to the water of better management information, how can they be persuaded to drink and adopt efficient patient care practices?

Existing management problems

Because of technological advance, the ageing of the population and new epidemics such as ac-

quired immunodeficiency syndrome, the demand for health care is expanding rapidly. However resources are finite and their rate of growth is usually slow, being determined in state-financed health care systems, such as the NHS, by the rate of growth of gross domestic product and the electoral cycle. Even in fragmented health care systems, like that of the USA, where expenditure growth rates are high and the spend is large (e.g. $800b or over 14% of gross domestic product in the USA) resources have to be rationed, as is proposed in Oregon (Klein, 1992; Maynard, 1992) and many citizens (37 million in the USA) have no health insurance.

In the early 1990s most health care managers have few data which are relevant to inform their choices about how to allocate resources between competing therapies and patient groups. The British government has introduced health care reforms and these changes require the purchaser to identify the health care needs of the local population and to buy those treatments which meet these needs in a cost-effective manner. Similar reforms have been introduced in the Netherlands, New Zealand, Sweden, Israel and Russia, and a variant of these market arrangements, managed care, dominates the USA health care system.

The data required for good clinical and non-clinical management can be divided into three categories: inputs, activities or processes and outcomes.

Input data

The NHS's measurement of inputs, especially expenditure and costs, is very crude. Finance managers until recently were required to stay within cash limits and their success was judged against this criterion and their finance systems were designed to ensure success. These managers wished to monitor and control nurse expenditure, catering costs, pharmaceutical outlays and other global budgets. They were not interested in the costs of a patient episode of care, let alone in using these data to fix prices for trading with purchasers or providers.

As a consequence the NHS, like all other health care systems, did not provide cost data. It was impossible to identify the cost of a procedure (e.g. a hernia repair), let alone the cost of a patient episode (e.g. the primary care, hospital, community care, patient and carer costs of repairing a hernia). To evaluate clinical practices, it is necessary to identify the opportunity cost of the procedure, that is the value of the foregone alternatives where a particular type of care is provided. Financial costs are not usually good measures of opportunity cost. Indeed, they are often the products of arcane book-keeping practices which mask opportunity costs.

To fix prices it is necessary to have information about cost flows for particular activities within the institution. Also it is necessary to be able to identify and apportion overhead costs (e.g. how much of the portering and electricity costs should be assigned to the price of a hernia repair?). In the evolving NHS market, finance managers are producing guesstimates of these costs, particularly for regional specialties (e.g. cancer and cardiology) and the elective surgical services bought by general practitioner fundholders. The range of prices offered by providers varies considerably (Table 7.1.1) and is probably a function of imperfections in financial data and practice, and variations in the length of stay.

The improvement of these price data, so that they reflect costs and act as efficient market signals to traders, will be costly and may involve the adoption of systems, such as diagnostic-related groups (DRGs), which have often covert incentives (fixed service prices induce hospital managers to reduce patient length of stay but require careful monitoring of outcomes and increased nursing inputs to care for a more dependent patient population).

Non-financial input data, for instance, patient throughput and labour utilization, are also imperfect. Many NHS hospitals continue to have inadequate patient information systems and, as a consequence, may be unclear about occupancy and utilization. Whilst all hospitals have payroll systems, these are usually inadequate sources of data about who is employed at what grade to do what task.

Process and activity data

Managers, be they providers or purchasers, have many demands for process and activity data. For instance, ward managers need to control nursing skill mix to produce good-quality patient care. What is the variation in nursing skill mix between different wards for similar patients and is it cost-effective for doctors or nursing assistants to be substituted for expensive, fully trained nurses? Some managers, for instance in the NHS management executive, have argued that resources can be saved by substituting less skilled for fully trained nurses with no adverse effects on patient care. Recent research, based on a limited but substantial sample, indicates that this counter initiative result may be invalid and that more skilled nurses produce better-quality care (Carr-Hill *et al.*, 1992).

The clinical skill mix is another area where there are disputes. Is the continued existence of the medical and surgical 'firm' efficient? With registrars and senior registrars being 'qualified doctors' in terms of European Commission regulations, there is a challenge to the continued

Table 7.1.1 Health care price (£): a selection from the early trading period

	Repair of inguinal hernia		Gastrectomy: partial or total	Total colectomy	Mastectomy
	Day	Inpatient			
Grimsby	303	1023	2041	2141	1347
York	477	737	2083	3413	1611
Kingston and Esher	250	644	2884	2884	1285
Clwyd	452	744	2715/3304	3957	1715
Winchester	333	658	2621	2621	1516
Kidderminster	293	926	2520	3263	1607
Wirral	278	658	2333	2443	1036
Bolton	179	739	2534	3168	1584

Sources: *Fundholding Magazine*, June 7, June 21, July 7 and July 21 1992.

existence of the firm. Have the consultants maintained the firm because it is efficient or because it reduces their involvement in work at unsocial hours and protects their private practice? The firm is unique to the UK health care market. Where is the evidence that it is efficient for patients and equitable to junior doctors? The institution appears to be the product of tradition rather than demonstrably efficient work practices.

Table 7.1.2 Geographical variations in surgical procedures in England: rate per 10 000 population (age- and sex-adjusted)

Procedure	District		Region	
	Low	High	Low	High
Hernias	10.0	20.0	8.5	14.5
Haemorrhoids	1.0	4.6	1.3	3.0
Prostatectomy	4.5	9.5	5.8	13.2
Cholecystectomy	7.0	11.0	5.7	9.7
Hysterectomy	7.5	15.0	18.1	28.7
Appendicectomy	14.0	21.0	12.9	19.4
Tonsillectomy with and without adenoidectomy	7.5	27.5	14.0	25.0

From Sanders *et al.* (1989).

Table 7.1.3 Plausible sources of variation at different levels of aggregation

Variation between	Morbidity	Supply	Clinical	Demand
General practitioners	S	0	L	S
Districts	M	M	L	S
Regions	L	L	S	M
Countries	L	L	L	L

L = Large; M = Medium; S = Small; 0 = no effect relative to others in row.
From McPherson (1984).

The independence of the clinicians and their firms has led to considerable variations in practices. Thus, general practitioners exhibit considerable variation in the level of use and type of antidepressants and non-steroidal anti-inflammatory drugs (NSAIDs; Keys *et al.*, 1992). These variations not only beg the question of the appropriate level of treatment but also of the effects of these practices on hospital utilization.

For instance, Fries *et al.* (1991), using US data, produced a toxicity index which showed that some NSAIDs were more toxic than others. There is evidence not only of varying NSAID toxicity but also of their excess use (Jones *et al.*, 1992). If general practitioners used less toxic and fewer NSAIDs, the number of stomach bleeds and subsequent deaths presenting in hospitals would be fewer.

The evidence about the variations in levels of surgical activity, even for so-called emergency procedures such as appendicectomy, is considerable. Some data reported by Sanders *et al.* (1989) are presented in Table 7.1.2. Priestman *et al.* (1989) have reported large variations in radiotherapy treatments offered to particular patient types with different forms of cancer. McPherson (1989) summarized the evidence about the causes of these variations (Table 7.1.3).

These results have been replicated in many countries, for example, Wennberg *et al.* (1987) found very large variations in medical practice in the USA. Such data beg the question: what is the appropriate level of care for particular patient groups?

Outcomes

There is a link in some cases between the level of activity and mortality outcomes: there is evidence of economies of scale whereby those surgeons with low levels of activity are more likely to kill their patients. There is some evidence for such relationships in vascular surgery and transplantation (Robinson and Luft, 1985; Maerki *et al.*, 1986). A relevant management question is: do such relationships exist elsewhere and do they exist also between clinical activity level and patient morbidity and speed of rehabilitation? Is the age of the general surgeon gone and should there be specialization rather than the perpetuation of the existence of this jack of all trades? Should specialization in general surgery be obligatory?

The exploration of such issues is incomplete. Most medical interventions are not supported by a body of good scientific evidence with regard to their outcome (Cochrane, 1972; Black, 1986). There is a lack of evidence not only about the duration of survival but also its quality. Survival information, such as it is, is for short episodes (e.g. data about mortality during inpatient stay can be acquired from the Körner information system) with little record linkage. There is no UK equivalent of the US Medical Outcome Study which consisted of a follow-up of a large group of patients from over two dozen hospitals for 5 years (Kravitz *et al.*, 1992).

The Medical Outcome Study measured not only hospital utilization and survival but also the quality of life of patients going through these hospitals. The quality of life (QoL) instrument used in this study was Short Form 36 (SF36). SF36 has been evolved over 15 years and has 36 questions about physical, psychological and social functioning. It has been used extensively in the USA (Stewart and Ware, 1992) and translated into several European languages, including English (Brazier *et al.* 1992).

This English form of the SF36 is being used increasingly, is very simple to use, and can be administered to patients in a few minutes. Its attributes, relative to the Nottingham Health Profile (NHP), have been demonstrated by Brazier *et al.*: the SF36 appears to be more sensitive and useful than the NHP. It has not been compared with another short generic QoL instrument, the EuroQol (EuroQol Group, 1990), which has not been used so widely.

Until survival data are linked and the quality of life of patients is routinely measured, clinicians and managers will continue to be ill-informed about the benefits of the treatments given to patients. They will continue to experiment on the job, with incomplete knowledge of outcome probabilities and little or no evaluation.

Inputs, activities and outcomes

NHS costs have been poorly measured and they and prices are poor measures of the opportunity cost (foregone value) of health care treatments. There are significant variations in medical and surgical practice; clinicians 'do their own thing', believing they offer the best treatment and produce good results. The evidence to support such assertions is absent: the outcomes of most treatments in widespread use today are unproven and have no scientific basis. The existing problems of clinical management are profound and being recognized by managers and patients who increasingly are questioning the clinical emperors with too few clothes!

Resolving the management problems

The resolution of the problems of ignorance about costs, variations (appropriateness of care) and outcomes requires careful measurement and continued questioning of medical practices. Can appropriate patterns of treatment be identified and agreed? How can the cost-effectiveness of competing therapies be measured? Can cost-effectiveness data and appropriateness consensuses be used to prioritize competing treatments – to decide who will be given treatment and who will be denied care, and left in pain and discomfort, perhaps to die?

Determining appropriateness

The general acceptance of wide variations in medical practice in all health care systems has led to efforts to reduce the dispersion by consensus conferences and other mechanisms to identify protocols for the appropriate treatment. This has been quite successful in some areas. For instance, the UK consensus conference on breast cancer treatment noted that there was little difference in survival after mastectomy and lumpectomy but much better quality of life with the latter (Consensus development conference – treatment of primary breast cancer, 1986). Morris *et al.* (1992) followed up the consensus statement and found that practices changed. However, they showed that there appeared to be geographical variations in the extent to which practice had changed: the preferred (conservative) practices had increased more in the south than in the north-west of England.

The setting of appropriate care standards is difficult. The empirical base to inform the process is, in most cases, seriously deficient. Not only have the authors of most clinical studies failed to measure the costs of the competing alternatives, they have also collected limited outcome data – usually narrow clinical measures rather than data on the duration and quality of survival. As a consequence there is a risk that appropriateness will be defined on the basis of publicly agreed expressions of consensus whose empirical basis is recognized as flawed and which are subsequently privately ignored by clinicians in their practices.

Alternatively, the consensus may be too influenced. In the USA and to some extent in the UK, lawyers adjudge negligence in terms of whether the clinicians followed best practice. Best practice can be defined as that which is professionally agreed as appropriate, particularly following a consensus conference. Consequently there is a risk that consensus statements, which may often be best guesses only, are taken as scientific pronouncements.

If the legal profession uses these guesses in this way, the medical profession may, when defining appropriateness, cover all eventualities and offer a wide and resource-intensive definition of appropriateness. These may be used to determine standards which minimize risk regardless of cost: perhaps this tendency can already be seen in anaesthesia standard-setting.

Not only may consensus agreements and standard-setting be inflationary, there is also the possibility that they will lead to conservative practices and impede medical innovation. As Mark Twain remarked, whenever you become a member of the majority it is time to pause and think about whether you are wrong. Feinstein (1988) has argued:

> The agreement of experts has been the traditional source of all the errors throughout medical history.

Unless the scientific basis for consensus conferences and the setting of appropriateness or treatment protocols is good, they will be double-edged swords. Their advantage is that they set standards by which practices can be judged. However, the standards may be wrong, difficult to change and inflationary. Such judgements can only be best guesses and it is essential that they are continually challenged and reviewed. To do this the volume of clinical trials which include cost and quality of life measurement, that is economic evaluation, must be increased significantly.

Economic evaluation

Types of economic evaluation

Economic evaluation involves the identification, measurement and valuation of all the relevant costs and outcomes of alternative treatments for a particular patient episode. Some cost minimization studies measure only the costs of the alternatives, assuming that the outcomes are identical. This assumption is often invalid in medicine and, as a consequence, cost minimization studies are of limited use.

Similarly, cost–benefit analysis is of limited utility in medicine. The objective of cost benefit analysis is to identify, measure and value all relevant costs and benefits in money terms. Not only are some of the costs (e.g. carer time) difficult to translate into money values, many benefits (such as reduced pain and increased mobility) are also difficult to value in these terms.

The most useful forms of economic evaluation in medicine are cost-effectiveness analysis and cost utility analysis. The use of the cost-effectiveness analysis technique facilitates the valuation of the costs of alternative treatments and their outcome, measured in terms of additional years of life (e.g. arising from renal dialysis) or reduction in blood pressure following cholesterol intervention. This approach, like all other forms of economic evaluation, is systematic and explicit. Its limitation is that the outcome measures across clinical specialties are not uniform. Thus, whilst cost-effectiveness analysis is useful in informing clinicians and managers about how best to invest scarce resources within a particular diagnostic category (such as what is the best way to treat renal failure), it does not inform choices between, for instance, chronic renal failure and investments in cholesterol reduction by exercise, diet or pharmaceutical interventions.

To remedy this deficiency, and inform choices between therapeutic categories, it is best to use another form of economic evaluation – cost utility analysis. This involves the identification, measurement and valuation of the relevant costs of the alternatives and the outcome, the latter being measured in some common unit across therapeutic categories, for instance quality adjusted life years (QALYs).

The uses of economic evaluation

These techniques, particularly cost-effectiveness analysis and cost utility analysis, are being used increasingly by purchasers to determine priorities. Thus in Australia from 1 January 1993 a pharmaceutical company can get a product licence to sell a new drug as it has done in the past. However, reimbursement of that new drug will be determined by new controls which require the company to carry out an economic evaluation to demonstrate that the drug is cost-effective. If the economic evaluation does not demonstrate cost-effectiveness, the company will be able to sell the drug (it is safe and efficacious and it has a product licence), but there will be no reimbursement from the public health care sector. Similar controls are being discussed in Canada and other countries.

The governments of New Zealand and the Netherlands are seeking to identify a core of demonstrably cost-effective health care services which will be provided by the state (Department of Health, 1992; Government Committee on Choices in Health Care, 1992).

These efforts are similar to those in Oregon (Klein, 1992; Maynard, 1992) and reflect a worldwide tendency by purchasers to use the techniques of economic evaluation to determine what treatments will, and what treatments will not, be reimbursed by public (e.g. UK-NHS and US Medicaid) and private (e.g. BUPA and US managed-care organizations) funding organizations. Such decisions will have obvious and profound effects on clinical practice.

Is economic evaluation sufficiently robust?

With public and private agencies worldwide using the techniques of economic evaluation increasingly, an obvious question is whether these techniques are sufficiently robust. Gradually criteria for the 'good' practice of economic evaluation are emerging: eight questions which should be used to interrogate the methods and results of all such studies are set out in Table 7.1.4. These are elaborated in standard texts such as Drummond *et al.* (1987) (see also Maynard, 1990).

There remain areas of economic evaluation (e.g. discounting to take account of time preference) where there are disputes (Cairns, 1992; Parsonage and Neuberger, 1992). However, despite this the virtue of economic evaluation is that it is explicit: previously implicit values and guesses are paraded for public inspection, challenge and improvement. Like medicine, economic evaluation is an art whose results should be evaluated and used with care!

The challenge of choice

Purchasers in the NHS and elsewhere all face the same problem – how to allocate scarce resource

amongst competing service demands? This economic problem is ubiquitous but in medicine it means that choices have to be made which determine who will die and who will live in what degree of pain and discomfort. The choices made by purchasers and clinicians need to be informed by data about costs and outcomes at the margin: that is, what health improvement is achieved by treatment when a little more or a little less resource is used?

If such efficiency questions cannot be answered, treatment may be unethical. If medical practice is inefficient, patients who could benefit from treatment will be denied it. Only efficient practice is ethical!

To pursue the goal of efficiency it is necessary to challenge existing practices and measure, clinically and economically, with care according to the principles of best practice in trial design. Purchasers anxious to synthesize the results of such work will demand 'league tables', such as that in Table 7.1.4, so that they can target their budgets on what apparently gives value for money. Such league tables have to be constructed and interpreted with care (Drummond *et al.*, 1992), and should be regarded as indicative rather than as definitive.

Overview

The use of the techniques of economic evaluation will facilitate the clearer definition of service treatment choices and provide data to inform decisions about resource allocation. Clinicians, economists and other health service researchers have a common interest in working together to improve methods and develop the knowledge base.

Conclusions: changing behaviour

The ignorance about inputs and outcomes is quite comprehensive. The literature on variations in medical practice is extensive. But how can clinical behaviour be changed? If the knowledge base is developed rapidly by economic evaluation being built into increased investment in clinical trials, better practices will be identified. But will clinicians change their behaviour?

There are examples of how well-designed and well-publicized trials have changed behaviour. Thus the results of the ISIS trial demonstrated

Table 7.1.4 Quality adjusted life year (QALY) of competing therapies: some tentative estimates

	Cost/QALY (£) August 1990
Cholesterol testing and diet therapy only (all adults, aged 40–69)[1]	220
Neurosurgical intervention for head injury[2]	240
General practitioner advice to stop smoking[3]	270
Neurosurgical intervention for subarachnoid haemorrhage[4]	490
Antihypertensive therapy to prevent stroke (ages 45–64)[3]	940
Pacemaker implantation[4]	1100
Hip replacement[4]	1180
Valve replacement for aortic stenosis[4]	1410
Cholesterol testing and treatment[1]	1480
Coronary artery bypass graft (left main vessel disease, severe angina)[4]	2090
Kidney transplant[4]	4710
Breast cancer screening[5]	5780
Heart transplantation[4]	7840
Cholesterol testing and treatment (incrementally) of all adults 25–39 years[1]	14 150
Home haemodialysis[4]	17 260
Coronary artery bypass graft (one-vessel disease, moderate angina)[4]	18 830
Continuous ambulatory peritoneal dialysis[6]	19 870
Hospital haemodialysis[6]	21 970
Erythropoietin treatment for anaemia in dialysis patients (assuming a 10% reduction in mortality)[6]	54 380
Neurosurgical intervention for malignant intracranial tumours[2]	107 780
Erythropoietin treatment for anaemia in dialysis patients (assuming no increase in survival)[6]	126 290

Sources: [1] Department of Health Standing Medical Advisory Committee (1990); [2] Pickard *et al.* (1990); [3] Teeling Smith (1990); [4] Williams (1985); [5] Department of Health and Social Security (1986); [6] Hutton *et al.* (1990).

that streptokinase was superior to tissue plasminogen activator used within 6 hours of a myocardial infarction. These results, sold vigorously by the Oxford researchers and groups such as the British Heart Foundation, changed practices very rapidly.

However, radiotherapists and surgeons appear to have been slow to change their behaviour in treating breast cancer in the light of Priestman's work and the publicity surrounding consensus statements. Perhaps too little effort is put into disseminating research results and funders have lessons to learn from the selling techniques of the pharmaceutical industry.

The case for augmenting information dissemination to change clinical behaviour should be determined by evidence about the cost-effectiveness of competing methods. The UK government has, in the period 1991–1993, spent over £100m on the introduction of medical audit. This expenditure has been complemented by time off, one half-day per month for all consultants, to discuss practices in the audit process. Unfortunately, and with some noble exceptions, this programme seems to have been poorly conceived and badly managed. There is evidence that it is very costly but there is no systematic evaluation of its cost-effectiveness.

An alternative strategy to change clinical behaviour is performance-related pay. At present consultants can get income from a variety of sources. Full-time employment in the NHS can generate an income of £49 000 per year. Private sector work, for the 12 000 consultants involved, produces an average income of £40 000 per year. Distinction awards, which are paid by hospitals to one in three consultants, can, at the A+ level, produce £45 000 per year. Domiciliary visits, insurance medicals and other activities also affect the pay packet of the clinician.

This payment package is a product of history and trade union (British Medical Association) bargaining. The managers of many NHS trusts as well as the doctors' pay review body are now examining the scope for reforming the payment package so that clinical behaviour is manipulated to achieve hospital and NHS goals (Bloor *et al.*, 1992). Whilst there is scope in principle to act in this way, there is difficulty in defining goals as well as uncertainty about whether alternative payment systems are cost-effective. Again, there is an urgent need to evaluate these issues rather than devise policy in an *ad hoc* fashion isolated from the knowledge base, as happened with the reform of the general practitioner contract (Scott and Maynard, 1991).

The recent reforms of the NHS may induce clinicians, purchasers and providers to measure performance more systematically and improve the efficiency with which scarce resources are used. There is, however, a risk that scarce resources will be sprayed at the measurement problem (and the related information technology policy), with little benefit to patient care. Clinicians and researchers always and everywhere should guard against the Marxist approach to management, which produces such waste!

The secret of life is honesty and fair play. If you can fake that, you've made it (Groucho Marx).

References

Black, A. D. (1986) *An Anthology of False Antitheses* Rock Carling 1984 Fellowship Nuffield Provincial Hospitals Trust, London.

Bloor, K., Maynard, A. and Street, A. (1992) *How Much is a Doctor Worth?* Discussion paper **98**. Centre for Health Economics, University of York.

Brazier, J. E., Harper, R., Jones, N. M. B. *et al.* (1992) Validating the SF-36 health survey questionnaire: new outcome measure for primary care. *British Medical Journal* **305**, 160–164.

Cairns, J. (1992) Discounting and health benefits: another perspective. *Health Economics* **1**, 76–79.

Carr-Hill, R., Dixon, P., Griffiths, M., *et al.* (1992) *Skill Mix and the Effectiveness of Nursing Care*. Centre for Health Economics, University of York.

Cochrane, A. L. (1972) *Effectiveness and Efficiency*. Nuffield Provincial Hospitals Trust, London.

Consensus development conference – treatment of primary breast cancer (1986) *British Medical Journal* **293**, 946–947.

Department of Health and Social Security (1986) *Forest Report. Breast Cancer Screening*. DHSS, London.

Department of Health Standing Medical Advisory Committee (1990) *Blood Cholesterol Testing: The Cost-effectiveness of Opportunistic Cholesterol Testing*. DOH, London.

Department of Health (1992) *The Core Debate: Stage One: How We Define the Core and a Review of Submissions* (prepared by the Bridgewater Group), Wellington, New Zealand. HMSO, London.

Drummond, M. F., Stoddart, G. L. and Torrance, G. W. (1987) *Methods for the Economic Evaluation of Health Care Programmes*. Oxford University Press, Oxford.

Drummond, M. F., Torrance, G. W. and Mason, J. M. (1992) Cost-effectiveness league tables: more harm than good? *Social Science and Medicine* **37**, 33–40.

EuroQol Group (1990) EuroQol – a new facility for the measurement of health related quality of life. *Health Policy* **16**, 199–208.

Feinstein, A. (1988) Fraud, distortion, delusion and consensus: the problems of human and natural deception in epidemiology studies. *American Journal of Medicine* **84**, 475–478.

Fries, J., Williams, C. and Bloch, D. (1991) The relative toxicity of nonsteroidal anti-inflammatory drugs. *Arthritis and Rheumatism* **34**, 1353–1360.

Government Committee on Choices in Health Care (the Dunning Report) (1992) *Choices in Health Care*. Ministry of Welfare, Health and Cultural Affairs, the Netherlands.

Hutton, J., Leese, B. and Maynard, A. (1990) *The Cost and Benefits of the Use of Erythro-*

poietin in the Treatment of Anaemia Arising from Chronic Renal Failure: A European Study. Occasional paper. Centre for Health Economics, University of York.

Jones, A. C., Berman, P. and Doherty, M. (1992) Nonsteroidal anti-inflammatory drug usage and requirement in elderly acute hospital admissions. *British Journal of Rheumatology* **31**, 45–48.

Keys, J., Beardon, P. M. G, *et al.* (1992) General practitioners' use of non-steroidal anti-inflammatory drugs in the Tayside and Fife reforms. *Journal of the Royal Society of Medicine* **85**, 442–445.

Klein, R. (1992) Warning signals from Oregon. *British Medical Journal* **304**, 1457–1458.

Kravitz, R. L., Greenfield, S., Rogers, W. *et al.* (1992) Differences in the mix of patients among medical specialties and systems of care: results from the medical outcomes study. *Journal of the American Medical Association* **267**, 1617–1623.

McPherson, K. (1989) Why do variations occur? In: Anderson, T. F. and Mooney, G. (eds) *The Challenge of Medical Practice Variations.* Macmillan, London.

Maerki, S. C., Luft, H.S. and Hunt, S. S. (1986) Selecting categories of patients for regionalization – implications of the relationship between volume and outcome. *Medical Care* **24**, 148–158.

Maynard, A. (1990) The design of future cost–benefit studies. *American Health Journal* **3**, 761–765.

Maynard, A. (1992) Priorities: follow the Oregon trail? *Medical Audit News* **2**, 20–22.

Morris, J. (1992) Regional variations in the surgical treatment for early T1/2 breast cancer. *British Journal of Surgery* **79**, 1312–1313.

Morris, J., Farmer, A. and Royle, G. (1992) Recent changes in the surgical management of T1/2 breast cancer in England. *European Journal of Cancer* **28a**, 1709–1712.

Parsonage, M. and Neuberger, H. (1992) Discounting and health benefits. *Health Economics* **1**, 71–76.

Pickard, J. D. *et al.* (1990) Step towards cost–benefit analysis of regional neurosurgical care. *British Medical Journal* **301**, 629–635.

Priestman, T. *et al.* (1989) The Royal College of Radiologists fractionation study. *Clinical Oncology* **1**, 63–66.

Robinson, J. C. and Luft, H. S. (1985) The impact of hospital market-structure on patient volume, average length of stay, and the cost of care, *Journal of Health Economics* **4**, 333–356.

Sanders, D., Coulter, A. and McPherson, K. (1989) *Variations in Hospital Admission Rates: A Review of the Literature.* Project paper 79. Kings Fund, London.

Scott, T. and Maynard A. (1991) *Will the New GP Contract Lead to Cost Effective Medical Practice?* Discussion paper 82. Centre for Health Economics, University of York.

Stewart, A. L. and Ware, J. E. (eds) (1992) *Measuring Functioning and Well Being: The Medical Outcomes Study Approach.* Duke University Press, Durham, NC.

Teeling Smith, G. (1990) The economics of hypertension and stroke. *American Heart Journal* **119**, 725–728.

Wennberg, J. E., Freeman, J. L. and Culp, W. J. (1987) Are hospital services rationed in New Haven or over-utilized in Boston. *Lancet* **1**, 1185–1189.

Williams, A. (1985) Economics of coronary artery bypass grafting. *British Medical Journal* **249**, 326–329.

7.2 Collection of patient-based data

Peter Jackson

Introduction

The primary function of any health care system must be to treat patients. This is a basic truth but one that needs to be constantly kept in mind when considering complex health care organizations. No matter what service they provide, all major organizations depend on good information systems in order to achieve good management. It follows therefore that any health care system must have good information about the way patients are treated. To provide a quality service, the patients' needs must be identified, treatment must be carried out efficiently and there should be a satisfactory outcome. The collection of data to measure these events must be patient-based and will require the commitment of medical staff if the information is to be accurate and meaningful. All doctors must accept that in addition to striving to provide good-quality medicine they have a responsibility to ensure that this process is monitored. The collection of good-quality data is therefore a fundamental requirement of any health service.

Historically within a hospital or similar unit there has been a division of managerial responsibility between general managers, who were responsible for the administration of the service, and clinicians, who were responsible for the treatment of patients. The general managers developed detailed information systems which provided data about the structure of the organization, for example staffing levels, and the activity levels, for example bed occupancy rates. This attempted to measure efficiency but with very little data on how effectively patients were treated. The clinicians' information systems on the other hand were poorly developed and sporadic, frequently confined to the occasional research study or a specific survey. Moreover there was no real incentive, from an organizational viewpoint, to collect routine data about treatment processes and outcomes. The clinicians were not regarded as being accountable to the general managers for the way they treated patients and therefore patient-based data were not considered important for the management of a health care organization.

Following the introduction of the Resource Management Initiative by the Department of Health and Social Security (1986) there was a major reappraisal of data collection within the NHS. This resulted in a drive to focus on the patient as a consumer, in much the same way that other service industries focus on their customers. Quality of service therefore became an issue not only for clinicians but also for general managers. The need for patient-based data has thus become an essential requirement for the whole organization. This type of information became even more important following the publication of the white paper, *Working for Patients*, by the Department of Health (1989). This established a requirement to perform medical audit and also laid the foundations for the establishment of an internal market with a separation of purchasers and providers of health care. Both these functions are dependent on having good patient-based data.

A further consequence of the Resource Management Initiative was the implementation of the recommendations made by Sir Roy Griffiths in the NHS *Management Inquiry* (Department of Health and Social Security, 1983) to bring doctors into the management structure. This was achieved by the creation of clinical directorates giving doctors a major role in the running of a health care unit. This has placed clinicians in a strong position to ensure that the development of information technology within the NHS provides appropriate clinical information. The primary reason for the introduction of computers must be to give clinicians, and other health care workers, the informational needs of the service they provide. The information requirements at a clinical or even a directorate level can then form the basis of that needed for more general management purposes. By aggregating data in this way – a bottom-up approach – the accuracy and credibility are maintained. Thus both clinicians and general managers will use a common database.

Data

What data to collect

National requirements

The NHS, from its outset in 1948, developed routines for collecting information about the hospital and community services for the purposes of management, planning and resource allocations. The most notable of these systems were the hospital activity analysis and the hospital inpatient inquiry. However as the organization grew in complexity, so did the data collecting systems, which ended up gathering a plethora of information, often duplicated, for different parts of the management structure. By the late 1970s it became apparent that much of the information being collected was not accurate, not relevant and not timely and as such was unsuitable for good management of the NHS. In order to correct the situation, a steering group on health service information was set up in 1980 under the chairmanship of Mrs Edith Körner. This steering group issued a series of six main reports, to which the name of the chairperson became attached. The first Körner report (Steering Group on Health Service Information, 1982) dealt with hospital-based services and the patients using them. It recommended the collection of a minimum data set about the characteristics of every individual patient. The information was to be collected on the basis of specific treatment events. These were defined as a consultant episode and a ward stay, which meant that when a patient changed to a different consultant or a different ward this could be identified. Data were also to be collected on the characteristics, availability and use of the service. It was also recommended that data collection should be standardized on the basis of the financial year and not the calendar year. The other Körner reports covered the informational requirements of patient transport services, staffing levels, paramedical services, community services and financial information. Taken together, the recommendations were intended to replace totally all the previous national information reporting systems.

The steering group was disbanded in 1984 after the proposals had been accepted. The challenge of trying to implement Körner has proved formidable and, although it has met with many problems, it has provided a major stimulus for the expansion of information technology within the NHS. There has been a rapid development of regional information systems and district information systems. At a hospital level the fundamental requirement has been to establish a master patient index containing data about every patient. This may then form the basis for a full patient administration system which will carry out many routine clerical functions such as the production of clinic appointment lists. Further developments can allow links with computers in other departments so that data can be passed easily around the unit. Whether a hospital has many systems networked together in this manner or develops a single hospital information support system will depend on local circumstances.

Local requirements

The main criticism of Körner has been that the information is not helpful for the management of an individual unit. The aggregated data are often perceived as being of value for producing statistics at a national level but with little relevance at a local level. Where this is the case the collection of data will be seen as a chore and given low priority. This means that it is invariably carried out at a site remote from the activity being recorded and with no feedback to the people performing the activity. This is a recipe for poor-quality data which will be incomplete and poorly validated. Much of the Körner data is of value at a local level if it is collected in an appropriate format. This means, on the clinical side, that all the information collected about patients is linked to the master patient index and can thus be related to an actual patient. When this is achieved the data items will be used locally, thus providing an incentive to ensure that they are of good quality.

An example of how the national requirements for activity data can be effectively used at a local level is shown in Figure 7.2.1. Aggregate information about average lengths of stay by specialty, or by consultant, is readily available but does nothing to help in identifying the reason for any variance. As a result the data usually do nothing to change or improve clinical practice.

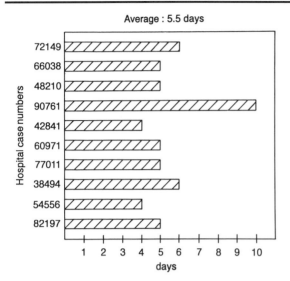

Fig. 7.2.1 Ectopic pregnancy: length of stay.

In the example depicted, the average length of stay for 10 cases of ectopic pregnancy is 5.5 days. At this level of detail the information is of limited usefulness. This length of stay would be accepted as being clinically reasonable and thus this fact would not stimulate any action. However, when the information on individual patients is looked at, there is an obvious outlier with a stay of 10 days, which is clearly abnormal. Because the information is presented in a format that includes the hospital case number the patient in question can be identified and the case studied in more detail. Lessons may then be learnt from this case that will help to improve the service for the future.

Clinical information

The collection of all clinical information must be done with the cooperation of clinicians if it is to be meaningful. This should not pose a problem as the information is required by doctors in order to audit their own work. They therefore have an incentive to ensure that the data collected are relevant and accurate. In view of the vast number of patients being treated within the NHS, it is essential to have a computerized clinical information system if a truly comprehensive database is to be achieved. The previous section has described how to ensure that activity data can be related to individual patients and clearly the more departmental systems that are linked through a master patient index, the more

information is potentially available. A fundamental requirement is to ensure that data entry is not duplicated and therefore all relevant patient-based information, from whatever source, should be available to the clinical information system.

The initial step for a doctor wishing to use a clinical information system is to identify what information is required from that which is already collected and then to consider carefully what additional information is needed. There is a temptation when first using a computerized data store to aim for the collection of a vast number of data items. This should be strongly resisted as the task of collecting, let alone analysing, the data will prove onerous. This will lead to delegation of responsibility, resulting in poor-quality data and the whole system will lose credibility. It is strongly recommended that to establish a system of data collection a small number of items is used initially. Before embarking on any data-collecting exercise the clinician should reflect on why each item is being collected. Information should be collected for a clearly defined purpose, not simply as a data-collecting exercise. In most cases the primary reason will be for audit purposes, either to monitor standards or to bring about a change in practice. This means that a basic amount of information is required about all patients. Any information system, however, should be flexible enough to allow more detailed studies, with extra data on specific groups being collected for limited periods of time.

For each data item to be collected there must be a satisfactory answer to each of the following:

1 For what purpose is the information required?
2 Is the data available from an existing source?
3 Is there a mechanism for collecting the data?
4 Is it possible to ensure the data collection is complete?
5 Is it possible to ensure the data is accurate?
6 Do the benefits from using the data justify the resources spent on collecting it?

All information systems should be allowed to mature with a periodic review of their function. Once confidence has been gained with the system then the use of the initial data items may well indicate where further information is required and these items can then be added. An equally important part of the review should be a reappraisal of all data items being collected and those that are not being used or do not fulfil the purpose for which they were intended should be either redefined or discontinued. Refinement of the quality of information must be a continuous process. For example, analysing the time spent by patients in the operating theatre may be a valid surgical audit measurement for a surgeon. If, however, the time is recorded from the patients' entry to departure from the theatre suite, this may not prove to be of use to the surgeon as the time taken for anaesthetic induction, recovery time, availability of porters and so on will influence the measurement. The time will then need to be redefined as the duration of the surgery, and the mechanism for recording the information will need to be reorganized.

Patient episode information

Because of the definitions laid down for the collection of Körner returns, most hospitals will record an inpatient episode as being an admission, subdivided only on the basis of a change of consultant or a change of ward. Outpatient events are generally recorded quite separately and there are arbitrary rules to distinguish an outpatient procedure from a day case. From the clinical viewpoint there is frequently an advantage in considering a consultant episode, that is, from the first contact with the patient until final discharge or death. This is particularly relevant to those specialties, such as the medical specialties, where a large proportion of the treatment is given on an outpatient basis. However, it would also be of help in grouping patients for comparative audit in surgical specialties where there may be an alternative between surgical or non-surgical treatment.

The minimum clinical information that should be available for the routine monitoring of each patient episode will include:

1 Initial diagnosis or presenting complaint.
2 Significant coexisting diseases.
3 Main diagnosis.
4 Type of treatment or operative procedure.
5 Complications of treatment.
6 Final outcome.

Although these items appear fairly basic, there can be considerable variation in how they are recorded. When the information is to be used by a group of clinicians then there has to be uniformity to allow sensible comparisons. A decision will be needed as to whether to record an initial diagnosis or the patient's presenting complaint. In general clinicians have been trained to think in terms of a definitive diagnosis but there are many occasions when a presenting symptom may be a more appropriate item. For example, in gynaecology there are many young women admitted to hospital with lower abdominal pain. Many of them have non-specific pain and are an interesting group to audit as there is a clear outcome, that is, freedom from pain. These may be more appropriately categorized by their presenting complaint as opposed to a presumptive diagnosis. There will then need to be agreement as to whether to include in this group those with a presumed diagnosis of constipation, pelvic congestion or irritable bowel syndrome and also those with a proven diagnosis such as pelvic inflammatory disease or endometriosis. It will depend very much on what use is to be made of the information as to how it should be recorded.

In terms of diagnosis the level of detail should be established at the outset. It may be sufficient to record a gynaecological diagnosis of infertility, but this could be divided into primary or secondary, and could be further subdivided into failure of ovulation or tubal factors, and so on. Clearly infertility subspecialists may well have a different requirement to the general gynaecologist but where data are to be used for combined audit, then a common denominator must be agreed. This of course will not prevent the individual clinician keeping more detailed information for his or her own use. In some cases there will also need to be agreed definitions for the use of a particular diagnosis and perhaps also an agreement on the terminology to be used.

The recording of coexisting disease and complications of treatment also need to be standardized within a unit. An obvious example arises with the recording of postoperative wound infections as different surgeons will have different definitions. Moreover, unless there is a mechanism for reporting the condition of all wounds, the surgeon who diligently records wound infections may appear to have a higher complication rate than a colleague who is less diligent about entries in the case notes. Human nature being what it is, there will always be a temptation to underreport complications when it is known that comparisons are going to be made. In fact, this might be an area where the effort taken to collect valid data is not justified and it may be more appropriate to look for an alternative measurement, such as a prolonged length of postoperative stay, to identify those patients with significant wound complications.

An area that has caused considerable difficulty has been the establishment of outcome measures. At its crudest, the discharge of a live patient is a good outcome, compared with the alternative. It used to be claimed that perinatal mortality was a reliable measure of the standard of obstetric care. However, whilst perinatal deaths are very important, their number – certainly those that could be classified as preventable – is now so small that they have little value for routine audit. Most specialties are similar and outcomes will be measured by the quality of life rather than mortality rates. In this respect surgical treatments are often easier to quantify than medical treatments. For example, a woman complaining of menorrhagia will be amenorrhoeic after a hysterectomy and a satisfactory outcome will depend upon the absence of any complications from her surgery. If she is treated by hormonal agents instead the outcome is not as easy to quantify and may well depend on an assessment of patient satisfaction.

Measurement of satisfaction can be fraught with complications and can be affected by other factors. For example, a woman may well be extremely satisfied with a sterilization procedure when questioned 6 weeks later but may express dissatisfaction at 6 months if she is having heavier than usual periods as a result of discontinuing her oral contraception at the time of the operation. Moreover the patient's assessment may conflict with the medical opinion. In a study of 75 individuals treated for hypertension, Jachuck *et al.* (1982) showed that the outcome was regarded as good in all 75 cases by the attending physician. This was based on the fact that the blood pressure was satisfactorily controlled. However, when the patients were questioned, only 36 felt that their quality of life had been improved and 7 felt that it was worse as a result of side-effects from the treatment. What was of particular interest was that when the patients' relatives were asked for an assessment, only one thought the treatment had improved the patient's quality of life. The other 74 stated that the patient was worse as a result of having treatment with a decline in energy and an undue preoccupation with illness.

In many cases the measurement of outcome will be complex and can best be resolved by a scoring system. The area where these have been used most widely is in rehabilitation medicine.

The patients' capabilities can be recorded by an activity of daily living assessment which will predict outcome and evaluate progress (Law and Letts, 1989). One of these scales, the Barthel index (Mahoney and Barthel, 1965), has been particularly useful in geriatric medicine and patients can be scored on admission, on discharge following treatment and can be followed up in the community by further scores. There is no reason why similar scoring systems should not be used in other specific areas. They could be used to cover patients' perceptions of their health and their satisfaction with treatment as well as their functional status.

How to collect data

With all data collection the aim should be to collect the information as soon as possible after the event and to have it recorded by the most appropriate person. The appropriate person is usually the one responsible for carrying out the particular task or making a particular decision. So, for example, the clerk will enter details for clinic appointments, the midwife will enter details of a normal delivery and the surgeon will record details of operative procedures. This will involve having computer terminals at appropriate sites throughout the unit and will involve a major educational and training exercise for the various staff involved. Attention must be paid to maximizing the benefits that can arise from using a computer in each area. Whenever possible, the very act of entering data should be an integral part of the routine operational task. This means that after entering data the clerk will be provided with the outpatient clinic list, the midwife will obtain the birth notification documents and the surgeon will have a letter for the general practitioner.

A decision has to be made at each level as to the most convenient way of entering the data. In most cases this will be by using a conventional keyboard with a user-friendly program. In certain circumstances the use of touch screens, light pens or bar code readers may be more appropriate. Where access to a terminal is difficult, handheld computers can be used and downloaded to the main database sometime later. The technology is available to suit most requirements and is still developing. For some clinical information it will be necessary to transfer the data from the hand-written case notes. It has been suggested that this task should be performed by the junior doctors as part of their contribution to the audit process (Ellis, 1989). However there is a time component attached to this and in many units it will be carried out more conveniently by either coding clerks or medical secretaries. There must be a clearly identifiable person responsible for the data entry and he or she will need to have appropriate training.

Complete data capture

The information about each patient must be as complete as possible. This will depend in a large part on the commitment of those using the system. Certain safeguards can be included in the computer program, for example a vital item such as a main diagnosis must always be recorded, whereas a complication of treatment can be an optional entry. This means that if a main diagnosis is not entered the program will not allow the person entering data to proceed until this section is completed. This will guarantee that the key items are always recorded. However if the data being recorded fulfil the criteria of being useful information then there will be sufficient incentive to have complete information on all items.

It is also important to ensure that data on all patients are captured on a clinical information system. When patients leave a hospital ward there may be a delay in entering the details or notes may need to be sent to another part of the hospital for coding. During this time a variety of things can interrupt the process, for example the patient may be readmitted, the notes may be called for by another department within the hospital or quite simply they may be lost. For hospital inpatient episodes a check can be made against all discharges and deaths recorded on the master patient index to confirm an entry of clinical information. For outpatient episodes the data capture can be compared with the lists of clinic attenders. This will ensure that any omissions can be identified and the data entry can then be completed.

Accuracy of data

Whether clinical information is being used for audit purposes or for the basis of management decisions, the medical staff must accept the responsibility for ensuring that it is accurate. The simplest procedure is for the main diagnosis and data from case notes to be recorded by hand at the time of the patient's discharge, or on completion of the outpatient attendance, by the doctor present at that time. The information on discharge can be collected as either a copy of the case summary or as a copy of the letter for the patient's family doctor. These sheets containing the clinical information can then be validated by the consultant or an appointed delegate before being passed on for entry into the clinical information system.

It is of considerable advantage if the person entering the data is actually present in the clinical area. This means either using a departmental coding clerk or the medical secretaries working in that specialty. Not only will they have easy access to case records but they will also have a close involvement with one department and will get to know how it functions and so will pick up residual errors. For example, the consultant's secretary will be familiar with most of the cases, having typed letters about them to the referring doctor, having put them on the waiting list, having prepared a theatre list and perhaps also having typed a case summary or discharge letter. Any variance with the coding sheet will then be spotted readily and, by being in the clinical area, can be easily queried.

The information system can also have validation checks built into the program. For example, a gynaecological diagnosis would not be accepted for a male patient and an obstetric entry would be queried if the patient was under 12 or over 45 years of age. These inbuilt checks can be taken to varying degrees of sophistication. The final stage of validation occurs, however, when the information is used. In carrying out medical audit and reviewing the clinical information, some of the inevitable human errors will be revealed. If one is looking at a group of patients with a main diagnosis of appendicitis and there is a case treated by herniorrhaphy, it will stand out as an error which can then be corrected.

Security of data

Clinical information must be respected as confidential and users of a clinical information system must be confident that it is secure. Unfortunately security must be regarded as relative and not absolute. The computerized data must therefore be at least as well-protected as hospital case notes. Each user of the system must accept responsibility for ownership of his or her particular section of information. Access to any data should be restricted by the use of a password or a series of passwords. This means that information at different levels can be obtained by using different passwords which can be allocated by the owner of the information. All users have a responsibility to ensure that their passwords are kept secret and it is a wise precaution to change them at regular intervals.

As patient-based information will be displayed on computer screens the positioning of the terminals is important so that information cannot be viewed by unauthorized personnel when the system is being used. When a terminal is left unattended it must be left in a safe mode needing a password to activate the system. There are also problems of security relating to the storage of disks containing patient data which should be treated in the same manner as hospital case notes. A final area of responsibility relates to the use of unauthorized disks on the system with the potential for introducing a computer virus. It is not unknown for the computer games enjoyed by the night staff to result in the introduction of a virus causing corruption of the system and the loss of a batch of records.

The problem of maintaining confidentiality becomes greater once various systems become networked across the hospital. There is an obvious need to share data so that duplicated data entry is eliminated but this has to be carefully regulated. It is preferable to establish ground rules for access at the outset. An individual clinician needs to be able to access all the information available on a named-patient basis. Groups of clinicians carrying out audit need to be able to see details of individual patients but at this level the information should be anonymous and should not contain the patient's name. Aggregate data on patients should be available for general managers but again the individual patients should not be capable of being identified, neither should the identities of individual doctors.

Coding

In order to use patient-based information effectively it is necessary to group cases into appropriate categories. This means that some form of classification must be undertaken which will then allow a code to be allocated to each condition. Medical diseases can be classified in a variety of ways, for example based on anatomical site or on the basis of aetiology. This can cause problems because a classification designed for national epidemiological statistics may not be appropriate for medical audit within a hospital department. It has also to be recognized that a classification is not the same as a nomenclature. A nomenclature consists of a list of all possible names whereas a classification usually lacks this detail and has a selected terminology. This means that the terms used in a classification may not always be those used in local practice.

The first steps towards a national classification of diseases were made after the introduction of the Act for the Registration of Births, Deaths and Marriages in 1836. Prior to this causes of deaths had been recorded at a local level in parish registers but with little uniformity. William Farr was the first medical statistician at the General Register Office of England and Wales, which was founded in 1837. He realized the need for a uniform nomenclature of diseases and a common classification in order to analyse causes of death. Although he introduced a classification of his own he also appreciated the value of having international agreement and did much to influence the International Statistical Congress (later to become the International Statistical Institute).

International classification of diseases

The present International Classification originates from the work carried out by Jacques Bertillon of Paris for the International Statistical Institute (Israel, 1990). This was based on the classification of causes of deaths in the city of Paris but was influenced by the work of William Farr in England. The Bertillon classification, which was adopted in 1893, was revised in 1900 when it became known as the International Classification of Causes of Death. Subsequent revisions occurred approximately every 10 years. The sixth revision in 1948 introduced the term diseases as well as causes of death and the classification was extended to cover non-fatal conditions. The World Health Organization took over responsibility for the classification with the sixth revision and promoted its use for the planning, monitoring and evaluation of health services in addition to its traditional epidemiological role. The current version is known as the *International Classification of Disease –*

Ninth Revision (*ICD-9*) and dates from 1975 (World Health Organization, 1977). In order to make it more appropriate for use in the UK the NHS management executive (1991) has produced a version of *ICD-9* with UK amendments and extensions. The tenth revision is due to be introduced in 1995.

The major problem with *ICD-9* is that it is a statistical classification and as such there are problems when trying to use it for clinical or audit purposes. Various adaptations have been produced, including an application for dentistry and stomatology, for oncology and for ophthalmology. In the USA a project was undertaken in 1977 by the Commission for Professional and Hospital Activity based in Ann Arbor, Michigan, to obtain codes that could describe the clinical picture of patients in more precise terms than those for statistical groupings and trend analysis. This resulted in the more detailed *Clinical Modification* (*ICD-9-CM*) published by the United States National Committee on Vital and Health Statistics (1980). This is widely used throughout the USA, Canada and Australia. Operative procedures can also be coded using *ICD-9-CM*.

Classification of operations

The standard system in the UK for coding operative procedures is the *Classification of Operations and Surgical Procedures* by the Office of Population Censuses and Surveys. This originates from the earliest British classification of surgical operations which was published by the Medical Research Council (1944). This was adopted in 1950 by the General Register Office which later became the Office of Population Censuses and Surveys. The third revision (*OPCS-3*) was produced in 1975 and was compatible with the World Health Organization International Classification of Procedures in Medicine, which coincided with publication of *ICD-9*. The currently used classification is the fourth revision (*OPCS-4*), which was implemented in 1987 (Office of Population Censuses and Surveys, 1987).

The main problem for coding surgical procedures is dealing with cases that have more than one operation performed. Frequently it can be difficult to decide which is the main procedure for coding. This is, once again, a reason why clinicians must have an involvement with the coding process. When multiple procedures have been performed there are problems when trying to group patients for audit purposes. For example, when a vaginal repair is performed with a vaginal hysterectomy in a patient with stress incontinence of urine, which is the main procedure? Moreover, it would be inappropriate to group this case with those where a vaginal hysterectomy, without a repair, is performed for menstrual problems. The analysis of data may therefore need to look for specified combinations of operative procedures.

Read codes

The Read Clinical Classification was devised by Dr James Read with the initial intention of providing a coding system for general practice (Read and Benson, 1986). In 1988 the Royal College of General Practitioners recommended that the Read codes should be the standard clinical way of recording medical data in general practice. This obviously had implications throughout the NHS and in 1990 the classification was purchased by the Department of Health (Chisholm, 1990) so that it now has crown copyright. Moreover an NHS centre for coding and classification has been established with the aim of maintaining and developing the Read codes.

The Read codes have been designed to be used by clinicians who want to record medical data on a computer system. They are intended to be comprehensive and cover symptoms, signs, diagnoses, procedures and medication, as well as other information such as occupation, diagnostic procedures such as laboratory and radiology, and preventive and other non-operative therapeutic procedures.

One of the main advantages of storing clinical data as a Read code is that the codes are structured in a hierarchical manner. This means that it is relatively easy to aggregate cases together, thus allowing analysis of the data at any level of the hierarchy. A further advantage is in the use of synonyms. The Read classification contains not only the official terminology, such as rubella, but also has a dictionary of synonyms which would include German measles. Because of this, patient data can be recorded in the format that is in common use. This makes the coding far simpler and more reliable as there is no guessing as to which code is the best fit.

The Read codes act as a superset to *ICD-9*, *ICD-9-CM* and *OPCS-4*, which means they can map on to these other classifications. This will be necessary for the provision of Körner returns which require this format and for the production of national and international statistics. The conversion of a Read code into one of the other classifications is achieved by a computer program and therefore no additional data entry is required. The objective of the Read codes is to bring together for the first time a classification and nomenclature that will cover the whole of medicine that meets the needs of both clinicians and managers.

Other classifications

There may be occasions when the general coding systems do not meet the requirements of a particular speciality and alternative classifications will be used. Probably the most widely used of these in the UK is the Systematized Nomenclature of Medicine (SNOMed), developed from the *Systematized Nomenclature of Pathology* by the College of American Pathologists (1977). Its use is confined mainly to pathology departments.

When any alternative method of clinical classification is considered it is important to ascertain if it will map unambiguously on to *ICD-9* and *OPCS-4*. If it does not do this, data entry will have to be duplicated because data are required in this format for national returns. This should provide a strong argument for using one of the standard classifications if at all possible.

Case mix

Collecting data at the level of the individual patient and ensuring that it is accurately coded provides the basic building brick for health care management. Information of such detail needs to be aggregated for both clinical audit and general management purposes. When each brick is of good quality the aggregate will be based on a firm foundation. The purpose of case mix is therefore to identify similar cases which can be meaningfully grouped together. It is important to recognize that there may be a discrepancy between the clinicians who desire case mix to provide groups of clinical similarity and the general manager who desires groups with a similar resource implication. In the light of what has

already been stated about focusing health care on the needs of the patient and of developing a common language between clinicians and managers, it should be the object of case mix to produce clinically meaningful groups which also have isoresource implications.

Diagnosis-related groups

The most widely used case mix grouping has been the diagnosis-related groups (DRGs) developed in the 1960s by Professor Bob Fetter at the Yale University School of Organization and Management (Fetter *et al.*, 1980). They were used by the US federal government as a way of trying to curtail the rapid rise in health care spending. Legislation was passed which meant that from 1983 a fixed price was paid by the Medicare programme funded by the Department of Health, Education and Welfare, depending on the patient's DRG (Bakken and Young, 1984). These payments cover about 40% of all hospital payments in the USA.

There are now almost 500 DRGs which fit into 23 major diagnostic categories based on body systems (Jenkins *et al.*, 1990). Each DRG comprises a group of patients with similar characteristics. The grouping is based on six key items – the principal diagnosis, operative procedure, comorbidities and complications, age, sex and discharge disposition. The DRG was originally based on *ICD-9-CM* data but the version used in the UK takes groups from *ICD-9* and *OPCS-4*. DRGs are generated by a grouper program using the data in the clinical information system.

Modification of the DRGs has been necessary for child health and also for psychiatry. The DRGs only cover inpatient episodes and, in an attempt to put costs on outpatients, the ambulatory visit groups have been developed.

Health care resource groups

With the implementation of resource management by the Department of Health there was a drive for the case mix analysis to be based on DRGs. There were however problems in that they are relatively crude groupings which frequently have little clinical relevance. Their biggest problem is that they are based on US case mix and clinical practice and their relevance to British costings is not proven. DRGs also do not take into account measures of severity of disease or quality of care.

Health care resource groups (HRGs) were introduced by the Department of Health in 1992 primarily to provide a British alternative to DRGs (Sanderson, 1992). HRGs for each specialty were developed by separate working parties, although at present not all specialties are covered. The requirements were that the groups would be suitable for local resource management, would be clinically acceptable and could be defined using routinely available data. This means that clinical coding must be in *ICD-9*, *OPCS-4*, Read codes or compatible systems. Other data items that might be required, such as the patient's age, are generally available from the Körner data set. The HRGs are based on clinical practice within the UK and are therefore more homogeneous in resource use than DRGs.

Severity of disease

The measurement of the severity of a disease can be important for many aspects of health care management. From the clinical aspect the severity of a disease may determine whether treatment is given on an outpatient basis, or as an inpatient, or even on an intensive care unit. There can be a correlation between severity and outcome, making this a valid factor to consider for clinical audit. Certainly it is standard practice to allocate malignant disease a staging which not only determines the type of treatment given but which acts as a prognostic indicator of survival rates. It is also true that severity of a disease will have an implication on the resources used for its management.

Most of the work on recording severity of disease has come from the USA and most of this has been motivated by financial requirements. Reimbursement of hospitals based on a standard payment for each DRG assumes that the hospital average matches that for the country as a whole. If for any reason the hospital has a bias towards the more complex range of any DRG, perhaps because it is a special referral centre, then it will be underfunded. For this reason attempts have been made to make DRGs more specific by adding some measure of severity. These have included the severity of illness index (Horn *et al.*, 1983) and the patient management categories (Young *et al.*, 1982), both of which have depended on a clinical judgement and have

therefore been hard to standardize. More recently, staging of disease (Gonnella *et al.*, 1984) has been introduced in which all disease categories have been divided into four main stages by a panel of specialists. To date these classifications have had little value in the UK but they may have a part to play in the future with the development of contracts between purchasers and providers of health care.

Severity of disease scoring systems have been devised for clinical purposes. Probably the most widely used is APACHE, an acute physiology and chronic health evaluation (Knaus *et al.*, 1985), which can be applied to all critically ill patients. In APACHE II 12 different observations are scored from 0 to 4 and extra points are added depending on the patient's age. The total count correlates closely with mortality and its principal use is in intensive care units. For example, surgical patients with an APACHE score less than 5 have a 1% mortality rate, whereas when the score is over 35 the mortality rate is 86%.

Use of data

The value of clinical-based data has already been stressed and indications have been given about how it can be useful. Certainly there is no value in collecting data unless they are going to be of value. This section will look at just two specific areas of data usage. The first is concerned with measuring the efficiency of a health care unit and the second with the efficiency and effectiveness of each patient episode.

Performance indicators

Performance indicators were developed in 1981 as a means of providing information for general managers within the NHS. An initial set of about 145 was produced by the Department of Health and Social Security; this was then supplemented by a set from the interauthority comparisons consultancy at the Health Services management centre at Birmingham University. In 1983 a joint group on performance indicators was established with eight working groups covering acute services, children's services, the elderly, mental illness, mental handicap, support services, estate management and personnel.

Performance indicators were intended to ensure quality in the provision of health care. There are now about 425 indicators, based on data already collected at a regional level, which will allow comparison between hospitals in England and Wales. They measure efficiency but do not measure quality of care and for this reason are more correctly named health service indicators (Department of Health, 1990). The results are supplied on floppy disks and provide graphic displays as well as commentaries (Lowry, 1988). Examples of first-line performance indicators include:

1 Actual length of stay – based on bed occupancy at midnight.
2 Turnover interval – the time a bed remains empty.
3 Actual throughput – number of patients per bed per year.
4 Notional days to clear the waiting list.

The greatest danger of using health service indicators is that they rely purely on a statistical average for activity and do not reflect the quality of care (Kirk, 1988). There is in fact a danger of creating a situation of diminishing averages. This means that whoever has the worst indicator, for example length of stay, will be pressurized to discharge patients earlier. This of course will lower the average and put someone else on top. It can be seen how this system can drive towards cheaper health care but without any real safeguards to prevent the quality of care being reduced.

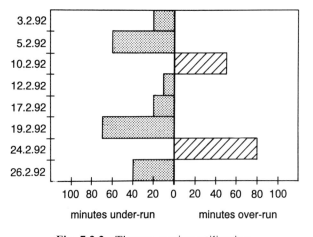

Time allocated : 24 hrs 00 mins

Time used : 22 hrs 20 mins

Fig. 7.2.2   Theatre session utilization.

In many instances more valid indicators of performance can be obtained from data being collected by the various departments. For example, a surgeon may find it helpful to see data relating to the usage of theatre, as displayed in Figure 7.2.2. This will enable him or her to identify occasions on which there was a significant over-run or under-run. This type of information is likely to help the individual surgeon monitor his or her efficient use of resources, whereas the health service indicators will be of value at a unit management level.

Profiles of care

A profile of care is a description of the standard treatment for any given condition. The profile may be set by an individual consultant for his or her own use or it may be a collaborative venture by a department. The complexity of the profile will depend on the amount of data being recorded at patient level. It will include the expected length of stay, diagnostic investigations carried out in pathology and radiology, drug therapy and operative procedures performed. It could also include complication rates and outcome measures where these are recorded. The profile should be as comprehensive as possible to give a complete clinical picture and also, because each item can have a value attached, a realistic costing.

Profiles of care are a convenient way of carrying out audit using a large amount of computerized patient-based data. In fact the original profile can be obtained by using the computer to give an average for the patients already treated in the group that is being studied. This can then be modified by the clinicians and future treatment can be monitored by comparison with this profile. The groups may be based on a diagnostic category, a surgical procedure or a case mix group such as a DRG or HRG. They are most appropriate for conditions that are relatively high-volume or that are high-cost, though clearly they can be applied to any grouping. A general surgical department in one district general hospital found that 67 diagnoses covered 80% of the inpatient workload and that 49 procedure codes covered 80% of the operations performed. Some specialties had smaller numbers, for example in gynaecology 28 diagnostic groups covered 80% of the workload and 10 groups covered 80% of the operations. In general medicine the numbers are more daunting, with 146 diagnostic groups needed to cover 80% of the work; however the top 15 diagnoses will cover 40% of the case load.

Profiles of care can be used at any level of detail depending on the type of review being undertaken. A department could undertake a regular monthly review of the commonest groupings looking at only a few key parameters in order to carry out a form of occurrence screening. At a slightly more detailed level, several parameters may be considered for a periodic assessment of a particular topic. With ectopic pregnancy, for example, the following could be identified:

1 Any admission more than 1 day preoperatively.
2 Any stay greater than 6 days postoperatively.
3 Any previous admission up to 3 months before diagnosis.
4 Any readmission within 3 months of treatment.
5 Any deaths.

This would then highlight those cases where a more detailed review of their case records was required. By doing this, cases would be identified where treatment was less than ideal, with delay in performing surgery, previous admission when the diagnosis was missed, significant complications of treatment and so on. The remaining cases – hopefully the large majority – could be accepted as having been treated appropriately as they lie within the profile.

The use of profiles should be multidisciplinary and therefore they will form the basis of collaborative care plans. Once profiles have been established, they can be used for setting standards and monitoring performance throughout a unit. There is, however, a much wider use: with uniform case mix it will be possible to carry out meaningful comparisons of different units across the country. An established profile for a given condition is also of value as an educational tool and can be a reference source for junior doctors, nurses and other health care workers. Because the financial information is linked through the clinical information system, the profile of care will also reveal the cost of treating each patient, facilitating an audit of efficiency. Profiles of care will therefore have an increasingly important role to play in the negotiation of contracts between the providers and the purchasers of health care.

References

Bakken, C. L. and Young, D. S. (1984) Changing American medicine. *British Medical Journal* **288**, 956–957.

Chisholm, J. (1990) The Read classification. *British Medical Journal* **300**, 1092.

College of American Pathologists (1977) *SNOMed: Systematized Nomenclature of Medicine*, CAP, Chicago, IL.

Department of Health (1989) *Working for Patients*. HMSO, London.

Department of Health (1990) *Health Service Indicators Guidance Dictionary*. HMSO, London.

Department of Health and Social Security (1983) *NHS Management Inquiry*. HMSO, London.

Department of Health and Social Security (1986) *Health Service Management – Resource Management (Management Budgeting) in Health Authorities*, Health notice HN(86)34. HMSO, London.

Ellis, B. W. (1989) How to set up an audit. *British Medical Journal* **298**, 1635–1637.

Fetter, R. B., Shin, Y., Freeman, J. L., Averill, R. F. and Thompson, J. D. (1980) Case mix definition by diagnosis related groups. *Medical Care* **18**, 1–53.

Gonnella, J. S., Hornbrook, M. C. and Louis, D. Z. (1984) Staging of disease. A case-mix measurement. *Journal of American Medical Association* **251**, 637–644.

Horn, S., Sharkey, P., Bertram, D. *et al.* (1983) Measuring severity of illness: homogeneous case mix groups. *Medical Care* **21**, 14–25.

Israel, R. A. (1990) The history of the International Classification of Diseases. *Health Trends* **22**, 43–44.

Jachuck, S. J., Brierley, H., Jachuck, S. and Willcox, P. M. (1982) The effect of hypotensive drugs on the quality of life. *Journal of the Royal College of General Practitioners* **32**, 103–105.

Jenkins, L., McKee, M. and Sanderson, H. (1990) *DRGs: A Guide to Grouping and Interprtation.* CASPE, London.

Kirk, R. M. (1988) Personal view. *British Medical Journal* **296**, 999.

Knaus, W. A., Draper, E.A., Wagner, D. P. and Zimmerman, J. E. (1985) APACHE II: a severity of disease classification system. *Critical Care Medicine* **13**, 818–829.

Law, M. and Letts, L. (1989) A critical review of scales of activities of daily living. *American Journal of Occupational Therapy* **43**, 522–528.

Lowry, S. (1988) Focus on performance indicators. *British Medical Journal* **296**, 992–994.

Mahoney, F. I. and Barthel, D. W. (1965) Functional evaluation: the Barthel index. *Maryland State Medical Journal* **14**, 61–65.

Medical Research Council (1944) *A Provisional Classification of Diseases and Injuries for Use in Compiling Morbidity Statistics*, Special report series no 248. HMSO, London.

NHS management executive (1991) *International Classification of Diseases, 9th revision, with UK amendments and extensions*. St Anthony, Alexandria, VA.

Office of Population Censuses and Surveys (1987) *Classification of Surgical Operations and Procedures* 4th revision. OPCS, London.

Read, J. D. and Benson, T. J. R. (1986) Comprehensive coding. *British Journal of Healthcare Computing* **3**, 22–25.

Sanderson, H. (1992) Measuring case mix. *British Medical Journal* **304**. 1067–1068.

Steering Group on Health Service Information (1982) *First Report to the Secretary of State – Hospital Facilities and the Patients Using Them*. HMSO, London.

United States National Committee on Vital and Health Statistics (1980) *International Classification of Diseases, 9th revision. Clinical Modification*, 2nd edn. US Government Publishing Office, Washington, DC.

World Health Organization (1977) *International Classification of Diseases: Manual of the International Statistical Classification of Diseases, Injuries and Causes of Death, 9th Revision 1975*. WHO, Geneva.

Young, W., Swinkola, R., Zorn, D. *et al.* (1982) The measurement of hospital case mix. *Medical Care* **20**, 501–512.

7.3 Fundamental aspects of computers

Patrick Cryne

Introduction

In the world of computing there is no such thing as future-proofing. Over the past 10 years the rate of change would have confounded even the most far-sighted industry expert seeking to make predictions in the early 1980s. For those making buying decisions about computers, whether involved in selecting a machine for playing amusement games or for high-performance business transaction processing, the choice is by no means clear if the key criterion is to avoid early obsolescence.

Why is the future such a short-term prospect in buying computers? Just as the rate of change in medical equipment is accelerating, the dynamics of computing are no less rapid. Indeed, the increasingly sophisticated microchips that constitute the building blocks of computers have the same evolutionary origins as those components that drive forward the technical innovations that take place in medicine.

In writing about computers the risk is that the text shares the same rate of obsolescence as the technology it describes. Nevertheless, this section seeks to describe developments in computing that clinicians increasingly need to know in general, and specifically, some of the applications and benefits that will change working practices in patient management.

Computer evolution – from valves to chips

The growth of the computer industry is without parallel in the world economy. In the late 1960s there were less than 100 business computers operating in the UK. By the end of the 1980s there were in excess of four million. Of course the development and staggering success of the personal business computer account for a considerable amount of this growth. However, it is true to say that the processing power of the present generation of personal computers would significantly outperform the giant machines that dominated computing even 10 years ago. What has given rise to the explosive growth in computing over the last 30 years, and what does it mean for today's computer user?

To look at the reason for growth involves looking at computers at the component level. Very simply the accelerating rate of change coincides with the development of the key components that contain the base instructions for computers. The original computers contained vacuum tube valves which were more mechanical than electronic in their construction. By the early 1960s the transistor had taken over as the key logic component of the computer and was 300 times smaller than the vacuum valve. However, perhaps the most significant development in the history of computing emerged in the early 1960s with the development of microchip technology. The intervening period has seen the rapid exploitation of this technology. In its computing context a microchip can be defined as miniaturized electronic circuits mass-produced on a tiny chip or wafer of silicon. Silicon has been used as the most common medium for microchip technology because of its conductive properties and cost. Inevitably, microchip technological advances will introduce other conductive materials as computer developers strive to put more and more complex circuits into smaller and smaller spaces. At present, chip technology has advanced to the extent that in mass production, a single miniature silicon chip can contain the circuitry equivalent to 100 000 transistors in earlier generations of computing.

The two main uses ascribed to silicon chips in common parlance are memory chips and microprocessors, although they are used for other functions within computers, for example controlling disk drives, printers and video displays. Economies arising from silicon chip mass production, a process which is largely automated (with computers making their own components), mean that costs of the essential circuitry of computing are a fraction of those incurred 10 years ago and set on an ever-downward path. It is this development that has made possible the diffusion of computer technology throughout society with the consequent economic and social impact.

Mainframes, minicomputers and microcomputers

There was probably never a time when one could define the difference between these three classifications of computers by reference to the technology used because by the time the microcomputer arrived, the basis of its circuitry was already in use in mainframes and minicomputers. And yet the terms have stuck in common usage. The extent to which they have any real meaning is determined more by processing power and organizational use than by reference to the inherent technology.

The mainframe computer was originally named because of the metal cabinet that housed the central processing unit of computers in the late 1950s, when there were no minicomputers or microcomputers. If it has any real meaning now, it refers to large central computers meeting the corporate needs of a major organization. Such machines typically will run hundreds of terminals and manage many gigabytes (billions of characters) of data storage.

The expression minicomputer emerged in the early 1960s with the development and mass production of the PDP range of machines from Digital Equipment Corporation. Other companies followed this lead and the minicomputer industry was born. Initially, minicomputers were directed towards engineering and scientific applications; however, their use has been extended into commercial areas as software suppliers recognized the demands from the market for relatively low-cost business systems. The arrival of the minicomputer has had a significant impact on the computing industry as they grow in power to occupy the roles formerly discharged by small and medium-sized mainframes. The latest generations of mainframes and minicomputers share common technological architectures, so how does one distinguish between them? Again, the best classification is by reference to use rather than by technology. Minicomputers can best be defined as multiuser machines

designed to meet the needs of a small company or a department. A typical user population for a minicomputer-based system might be between 10 and 100.

The mid 1970s saw the origins of the microcomputer as engineers and scientists began to exploit the diverse uses of silicon chip microprocessors. The earliest microcomputers appeared in the USA as do-it-yourself kits, with Commodore, Tandy and Apple emerging as early manufacturers of personal computers. The embryonic applications for the microcomputer were basic word processors and spreadsheets which lacked the credibility and viability for anything other than personal use. The biggest boost to the emerging microcomputer industry came when IBM launched its personal computer in 1981. Suddenly, the microcomputer gained respectability in the business world which IBM dominated through its mainframe and minicomputer products. IBM's entry into the microcomputer market also gave a major fillip to the software systems industry as companies began to recognize the huge growth potential of personal computers.

Just as the distinction between the mainframe and the minicomputer has become blurred with the convergence of technology, the distinction between the minicomputer and the microcomputer has lost its clarity. When personal computers first arrived, they were designed as single-user machines comprising one integrated circuit. Today's microcomputer is considerably more powerful than even the mainframe of 10 years ago. Microcomputers can be made to run remote terminals and to link with other computers over communications networks. The concept of the microcomputer as a purely personal machine is no longer an acceptable definition.

Having established the case that the distinction between the mainframe, the minicomputer and the microcomputer is difficult to define in terms of basic technology and is more a matter of power and purpose, what does this mean for the evolution of computing within organizations? At present each classification of computer has its domain. In a hospital, the mainframe still has a role in processing high-volume, extremely dynamic patient transactions, for example in patient administration systems. The minicomputer, initially targeted at the departmental level to meet the needs of laboratories, is encroaching on this domain as power and performance increase with technological advances. The microcomputer is now challenging the departmental role of the minicomputer as the advent of local area communications networks provides the means for personal computers to be linked to share large amounts of data storage, printers and business functions.

In the foreseeable future it is probable that the distinction between mainframes, minicomputers and microcomputers will disappear altogether and the buyer of computer resource will be left with the decision on how much computing power is needed to support the systems to be operated. Already, many computer suppliers spearhead their marketing message with claims for the upgradability of their computers in terms of the amount of additional processing power, memory or storage that can be added to an initial configuration. Unfortunately, many naive buyers of computer systems will be only too aware that the upgradability has limits which are soon absorbed by business growth, development of new computing functions and the hunger of new software packages that seek to exploit the latest technological innovations.

Despite this cautionary message on the limits to upgradability, the trend has been established that will see increasing convergence in computing technology. Although the current generation of computers will not deliver it, the computing industry is within sight of being able to deliver a mainframe computer on a microchip, thereby completing the convergent process. The implications of this development will have a revolutionary impact on society in general and business organizations in particular. The cost of providing computer power to individuals within organizations will tumble and machines will replace people at an increasing rate in those functions that are purely task-related. The imperative for the individual will be to understand and exploit the capabilities of computers on an increasing scale, not at the technology level necessarily, but as an aid to managing their own activities and those of the organization as a whole.

The computer software industry

Just as the component technology of computing has been through an evolutionary process, the same can be said of the industry that has grown up by supplying the application systems that run on computers. The first service companies to follow on from the development of mainframe

computers were the bureau organizations that could provide cost-effective transaction processing in a period when the cost of entry into computing was extremely high. Typical services offered by bureaux were accounting and payroll processing.

The emergence of the minicomputer and the realization that they could be used as business machines led to the founding of software companies that specialized in the supply of programming services. As customers looked to reduce the costs of their systems and software companies looked to control the cost, quality and serviceability of their offerings, computer application packages started to emerge in the common business areas. This trend has continued to the extent that most organizations will look to adopt package solutions to their business systems requirements rather than incur the costs and delay of developing bespoke software. It is now very rare for business organizations to develop bespoke software to meet their business computing needs except in highly specialized areas. In the hospitals, most computer-based operational systems running on mainframe and minicomputers are based on package software, for example patient administration systems, radiology and pathology systems and the newer applications dealing with ward ordering and resource management.

However, it is in the microcomputer field that the computer software package has made the most significant gains. The cost of developing software varies little, whether it is intended for a mainframe, minicomputer or microcomputer. Development costs are more a function of the scope of the application than the machine which hosts it. Given the low relative costs of microcomputers, it is often seen as incongruous to incur heavy development costs for bespoke software to run on them. As such, the microcomputer has become the host to a wide range of software packages across the range from games to sophisticated business systems.

The proliferation of microcomputers that has occurred since the mid 1980s has encouraged a considerable growth in the package software market. That growth has also been accompanied by a recent market rationalization in which there have been a few major winners gaining significant market share, but also a very high number of losers who have left the market. In some sectors of the software market the fall-out rate has been 90% over the past 5 years as suppliers fail to retain their customer base as the rate of change in microcomputer technology compels continuing new investment in software products. The microcomputer software market has recently become less volatile, but it cannot be assumed that the market shake-out has been completed and, inevitably, there will be further casualties as companies fail to respond to the needs of their customers to improve their products whilst also suffering reduced profit margins to maintain competitiveness. Like all maturing markets, the situation in any software application will inevitably resolve into a few dominant suppliers with others seeking to establish profitable niche areas. For those selecting computer software, the safest guide will be to choose from those suppliers which have the strongest customer base for their product portfolio. The barriers to entry in the mainstream software market are now very high because of the cost of following technological change and competitive pressures. Even in niche areas, new suppliers will need to be confident of their market analysis and cost control before they can enter the market with confidence of a long-term future.

The terminology of computing

So far we have been looking at the evolutionary developments. However, to maintain a dialogue on computing today and to form a view about strategies for the future, it is necessary to understand some of the current terminology of computing. Just as the language of medicine is foreign to laypeople except at the most basic level so too is the language of computing. As with medical terms, it is impossible to transmit a full and detailed understanding of the true meaning of the jargon which prevails in computing in a few words. Nevertheless, in order that the layperson may be able to ask the questions that will enhance understanding of computing issues, it is worth looking at some of the currently used terms and exploring their meaning.

Open systems

In the development of computing throughout the 1960s and 1970s individual manufacturers built machines in accordance with their own specifications and without any regard for the approach taken by others. The result was that each manufacturer's computers could only work with specific printers, terminals and other peripheral equipment designed specifically for them. Similarly, software had to be developed specifically for each manufacturer's computers. This had the effect of 'locking in' customers to a particular computer supplier and, as a 'hostage', the customer had little control over the expansion costs as computing needs grew. As a consequence of this unsatisfactory situation (from the point of view of the customer at least), the late 1970s and 1980s have seen a burgeoning interest in the development of standards that will allow greater connectivity between computers and peripherals, and indeed, between computers from different suppliers.

In general terms, open systems has a wide meaning. Not only is it used to define the connectivity options described above, but it is also used to describe the capability to transfer business systems from one supplier's machine to another without modification of the software. In this general sense, computer systems sales staff will promote very strongly the 'openness' of their offerings. However, the term open system can have a more precise meaning as determined by the International Standards Organization, which is currently working on several hundred standards covering information processing. The most important area of work has been in the field of open systems interconnection (OSI), which sets standards for computer systems suppliers which are intended to allow different computers to exchange information, irrespective of the make, operating system or other characteristics.

Increasingly, the health sector is insisting that suppliers of computer systems conform to OSI standards in order that connectivity can be assured and that investments in equipment can be protected. The UK government's Central Computer and Telecommunications Agency advises the public sector and suppliers on standards that are recommended through its Government Open Systems Interconnection Profile (GOSIP).

Fourth-generation languages

The existence of a fourth generation of computer languages points to the existence of earlier generations of programming tools. It is not worth dwelling on the contributions made by the first and second generations of computer programming languages, even if they could be defined precisely. However it is relevant to consider, not the past contribution, but the present role of third-generation languages in the development of computer systems. Most computer systems that have been developed for business applications and have been in use for a number of years will have been written using a third-generation programming language. This is particularly true of mainframe and minicomputers-based systems. These types of systems will have been developed using traditional analysis and programming techniques and will probably have been written using the COBOL or FORTRAN programming languages or later derivatives. These languages are for use by programming specialists and, whilst using English-like statements, are largely unintelligible to the layperson. Languages like COBOL, although offering many short-cut commands to the programmer, still require the definition in detail of all the procedures that the computer must perform in order to complete the processing task. Because of this COBOL programming is extremely verbose and requires proper structuring in order to ensure that the program runs efficiently and can be easily maintained.

The advent of fourth-generation programming languages offers those developing programs a measure of freedom from the highly structured approaches needed previously. Simplified, English-like commands typify fourth-generation programming languages, which have been designed for on-line use, often by the end-users of computer systems. The development and use of fourth-generation languages have been constrained to date by the cost of the processing power required to run programs which, although easier to develop and understand, may sacrifice some of the efficiency of more structured programming languages. Despite this constraint, fourth-generation languages are gaining ground as computer processing power becomes cheaper in relative terms.

Perhaps the fastest rising star in the fourth generation of computing languages is structured query language (SQL). Originally developed by IBM, SQL can be used to access a growing range of databases on mainframes, minicomputers and microcomputers. SQL is an elegant and concise query language with only 30 commands which can be used to create statements which are close to simple English natural language statements. Typically queries will be typed into computer terminals and the results will be displayed on screen. As more and more database products provide support for SQL, the use of this fourth-generation language will grow rapidly and microcomputer users, in particular, will develop skills in this language.

Relational databases

Almost in parallel with the emergence of the fourth generation of computing languages has been the development of relational databases for use in computer systems.

Originally, computer databases followed a hierarchical structure, much like an inverted tree diagram or an organization chart. In order to progress through the data in the database the user was required to specify the path to be taken. This type of database tends to lack flexibility to the extent that it is difficult to extend the scope of data capture or define new paths through the data without a major reorganization of the database. Hierarchical databases have their strengths in application areas in which the required paths through the data are predictable and stable. Basic accounting applications are often based on hierarchical database models since many of the functions to be performed are repetitive and the outputs required are often in standard formats. Hierarchical databases are still used extensively in business applications because they offer high performance in accessing and organizing data, particularly in support of routine and repetitive tasks.

Relational databases follow a fundamentally different approach. The basic principles followed by relational databases were defined originally by Edgar Codd of IBM in a paper published in 1970. However, it is only since the late 1980s, with the arrival of fourth-generation computing languages and the growth of computing power that the relational database has gained its hold on information-processing and retrieval. In a relational database the data are not organized in prescribed paths. Instead, the data is stored in simple two-dimensional tables. A query on a relational database may be satisfied from a single table but, if necessary, tables may be linked together using data items that are common between tables. The results of the query will also take the form of a table. Suppose, for example, a database lists patients, their age and diagnoses in a table, as shown in Table 7.3.1

Table 7.3.1

Patient number	Name	Age	Diagnosis
12698445	Cryne, Jean	39	Fractured femur
14563890	Armstrong, Kate	12	Appendicitis
16456798	Thompson, Anna	14	Tonsillitis
23354368	Fenton, Beryl	65	Fractured cheek bone
89786566	Wood, Peter	60	Fractured pelvis

Another table might contain a list of doctors and their patients (Table 7.3.2).

Table 7.3.2

Doctor	Patient
Dr Allison	14563890
Dr Calvert	89786566
Dr Gibbons	12698445
Dr Gibbons	16456798
Dr Taylor	23354368

A query may ask: 'List in alphabetical order the names of all patients of 60 years of age or greater who have suffered from a fractured bone, together with their age and the name of their doctor'. Such a query would result in Table 7.3.3.

Table 7.3.3

Patient	Age	Doctor
Fenton, Beryl	65	Dr Taylor
Wood, Peter	60	Dr Calvert

This simple illustration does little to convey the immense potential power of the relational database. A complex query on a relational database might involve joining many large tables just to service a request for information which may never be repeated. It is the capability of the relational database to service queries on an *ad hoc* and flexible basis which creates the superiority over traditional hierarchical databases. Given this flexibility, why are relational databases not used exclusively to store all forms of data, irrespective of the application area? The answer is quite simple. Relational databases are slower in performance than precisely defined hierarchical systems for most predictable queries and functions. Nevertheless, relational databases are gaining ground quickly and it is likely that they will dominate data storage and retrieval for

management information systems in the remainder of this decade.

Initially, IBM was seen as the major player in the relational database but the growth prospects in this market have drawn in new players. The most notable of these in the health sector in mainframe and minicomputing are Oracle and Relational Technology with its Ingres product. At the microcomputer level Ashton Tate with its dBase range of database products is probably the best-known seller.

Perhaps the most exciting development opened up by the arrival of relational databases is the possibility of distributing databases across several computers. Under this model, computers located in the office environment can run systems that manage local data, but can also communicate with other remote computers to share and exchange data. Clearly, this capability can be achieved with hierarchical databases and third-generation programming languages. However, the prospect offered by relational technology and the new generation of computing languages is the potential for the non-specialist to be able to query databases spread over a number of geographically dispersed computers without needing to understand where the information resides or how it is structured.

Operating systems – MS-DOS, OS/2, Unix and all that

In the early development of computers the master control programs that manage the computer's internal functions were based on the proprietary software of the manufacturers. In recent years the computer industry has moved towards the use of a limited number of operating systems that are able to exploit the advancements in microchip technology.

In the microcomputer field the dominant operating system over the past decade has been MS-DOS, developed by Microsoft. Without a doubt the market position of MS-DOS owes much to its adoption by IBM as the operating system (with minimal variations) for its range of personal computers. The IBM variant is marketed and sold under the name PC-DOS. The combination of IBM and MS-DOS has done much to advance the cause of microcomputing by setting a direction that the rest of the market could not ignore and was obliged to accept as a *de facto* standard. The phrases **IBM-compatible**,

IBM clone and IBM-alike have entered the terminology of computing as suppliers seek to combine MS-DOS and equivalent microcomputer architecture to those adopted by IBM, but with a more competitive cost structure. Only Apple has sought to buck the trend towards MS-DOS with any measure of success, although more recently even they have moved towards greater compatibility with the *de facto* standard.

However, nothing is forever in computing, so what price the future of MS-DOS? In the short term the hold that MS-DOS has established will endure because of the investment that application system developers and microcomputer users have made and will wish to protect. In addition, Microsoft has continued to update MS-DOS through new releases (currently Version 5.0) that allow the operating system to grow its functionality and performance in line with developments in microchip technology. However, MS-DOS does have a major drawback in that there are limits to the amount of internal memory with which the operating system can work. Ten years ago these memory limits were thought to be so high that they would not constrain application system developers or deny users the performance they needed. Today, the memory constraint is limiting the capabilities of many microcomputer-based packages as new features are introduced to improve usability, functional capabilities and performance in handling large volumes of data. Packages such as Lotus 1-2-3, Excel and Windows are straining the capacity of MS-DOS to support them.

To break the current memory limits inherent in MS-DOS, Microsoft has developed a new operating system called OS/2. Additionally, OS/2 provides the capability to run more than one program simultaneously and incorporates a presentation manager which gives microcomputer users screen displays based on graphical icons that make the skills needed to exploit the technology easier to assimilate and use. Once again, IBM has endorsed Microsoft's new operating system as the choice for its latest range of microcomputers. Whether this development will result in wholesale defections from MS-DOS to OS/2 is by no means certain. A major determinant will be the willingness of application system developers to reinvest in making their products run under OS/2. In turn, their decision will be forced by the demands of users for new and better application systems. For the time being MS-DOS remains the leader, with millions of microcomputer users working with the operating system daily as an integral part of conducting business processes.

At the mainframe and microcomputer levels, standardization of operating systems has not emerged as smoothly as in the microcomputer area. Operating systems proprietary to computer suppliers have been the norm until recently. For IBM, ICL and Digital Equipment Corporation the main operating systems used in the health sector have been VM, VME and VMS respectively. There is no doubt that proprietary operating systems, whether intentionally or fortuitously, have had the effect of locking users into a particular computer vendor, since application software does not easily transfer from one operating system environment to another. The overall effect of this has been to protect the pricing of mainframe and minicomputer equipment for the benefit of the vendors and to restrict the choice of application software for the buyer to those systems that will run in the selected operating system environment.

Clearly, the health sector, with its paucity of investment resources in the information technology area, has been poorly placed to make extensive commitments to proprietary operating systems. When it has needed to commit to a major investment in an application area that involves proprietary approaches, the health sector has centralized expenditure through regional health authority computer departments, bureaux and consortia arrangements to gain economies of scale. Patient administration systems, general ledger, payroll and personnel systems are examples of application areas where these types of arrangements have been used to finance mainframe and minicomputer-based packages, often running under proprietary operating systems.

With the health service reforms that have followed the White Paper *Working for Patients* published in 1989 the move has been towards greater autonomy for hospitals and other health care delivery organizations. The opportunity for hospitals to come together and share computing resources has diminished with the reforms as the management of the organizations seek to exercise greater control and ownership over their data and the information that it can generate. Information is being seen increasingly as a valuable corporate resource that contains potential competitive advantage in any internal market for health care services. Seizing that competitive advantage depends on having the depth and accuracy of data and being able to convert it to information which has the right content, presentation and timeliness for the business purpose in hand. In order to allow hospital managers to develop their own in-house information departments, major changes are needed in the costs of computing over those involved in the historic approach. Fundamental to a change in the cost base of computing has been the need for the emergence of a more open approach in which different vendors offer mainframe and minicomputers which run the same operating system, thereby allowing software to be transferred between different computers, thus giving equipment choice to the buyer. Inherent in this choice is the opportunity to switch suppliers in order to get the best possible buying terms.

In pursuit of the portable operating system, the health sector experienced something of a false dawn with the early promise of the Pick operating system. Named after its designer, Richard Pick, this operating system is targeted mainly at the minicomputer range of machines and is built around its own relational database and query language. It has established a reasonably strong presence in the health sector in niche application areas, largely because of its ease of use. In particular, McDonnell Douglas and General Automation have promoted Pick as their main operating system for their mid-range computers. Despite this initial success, Pick has lost ground in the last few years with the emergence of Unix as the preferred portable operating system of some of the major minicomputer vendors. IBM, ICL, Digital Equipment Corporation, Hewlett Packard and Bull have all developed ranges of Unix-based minicomputers in order to follow the growing market demand for portable software solutions, not just within the health sector, but within the computer market place in general.

Unix is an operating system for a wide variety of computers throughout the range from mainframe to microcomputers. It is written in a highly portable software language called C. It was developed originally at AT&T Bell Laboratories during the early 1970s for sophisticated work in computer science and research. Unix consists of a central part, known as the kernel, which controls the computer's operations, and an outer part known as the shell. The shell is directly accessed by users and interprets their instructions for the kernel.

For much of its early years Unix was largely confined to academic communities where its technical sophistication could be exploited and its complexity could be handled. Throughout the 1970s and early 1980s, the antitrust regulations in the USA prevented AT&T from commercially developing Unix and it entered the public domain where different variants started to emerge. As a result of these separate lines of development, many incompatible versions of Unix have appeared in the market place, thereby threatening the potential of the operating system to support system portability. With AT&T gaining the right to market Unix in the early 1980s, the process of conversion towards a common standard commenced. By the end of the decade leading computer manufacturers and software suppliers were already collaborating closely to define standards for Unix. Most major procurements of Unix-based systems in the health sector now require conformance to a standard called POSIX, which has been drafted by the US Institute of Electrical and Electronic Engineers and has been taken up by the International Standards Organization.

The growth in the number of installed Unix systems over the past few years has been remarkable. Most leading computer suppliers, including AT&T, IBM, Digital Equipment Corporation, ICL, Hewlett Packard and Bull, now have a range of dedicated Unix machines. There are in excess of one million Unix-based systems installed worldwide, compared with approximately 30 000 Pick-based installations. In the health sector many of the software applications used in hospitals are being converted or rewritten to run under the Unix operating system and it is now mandated in many new computer system procurements.

Expert systems

Perhaps one of the areas subject to the most hype in computing currently is that of expert systems. Many sales representatives wishing to sell computer systems which use structures of rules to optimize problem solutions will describe them as expert systems, but do these applications genuinely make equivalent or superior assessments of situations and derive answers better than a human professional? Certainly some computers can solve complex problems using a rules-based approach, but are they really capable of holding a knowledge base and making inferences from it as part of the problem-solving process? The answer in the foreseeable future of computing is a resolute no!

One of the areas in which expert systems have been used in the research field has been that of medical diagnosis. In this type of system a patient's symptoms are requested and these are compared with the information supplied by doctors and the computer offers an 'opinion' on what might be wrong. The results from these systems to date have been less than perfect and doctors' careers are safe, even into the long term.

So what is an expert system, and why has progress been limited to experimental projects or the most simple applications? An expert system holds the knowledge of an expert in the form of a table of rules that assist non-experts as they attempt to solve problems. The knowledge base consists of a series of if . . . then rules, together with programming logic that allows inferences to be drawn from the knowledge base. Typically, these systems engage the user in a dialogue, prompting for the supply of information needed to assess the problem. Special languages have been developed with an inference capability, for example PROLOG and LISP.

However, creating an expert language is more difficult than it appears. This is because a surprisingly large proportion of expertise is based not on rules, but on guesses, hunches and intuition. In addition, an expert system relies on vast amounts of information being gathered to build up the knowledge base. If one considers the number of rules that would need to be established within an expert system to allow a medical diagnostic conclusion to be drawn with a high degree of confidence then it would soon reach thousands. An expert system based on several thousand if . . . then rules also has to manage the interrelationships between those rules. As the rules grow, the performance of the system declines rapidly and becomes erratic and unstable. When one considers that most fields of human expertise involve far more than 10 000 rules, it is hardly surprising that expert systems are unlikely to displace human professionals such as doctors, lawyers and accountants. Nevertheless, research will proceed in this area of computing directed towards improving computer languages, more efficient capture of knowledge and exploiting the growth of computing power.

Networking – LANs, WANs and all that

Initially, microcomputers were developed as stand-alone machines for running personal systems. The linkage of microcomputers within a local area by high-performance cables so that users can share data and expensive peripherals such as disk storage and printers is commonplace. A recent survey showed that over 50% of microcomputers used in business today are linked by means of a local area network (LAN). This is likely to grow considerably over the next few years as networking technologies improve and database systems grow in their capability to manage data distributed over many computers, whether mainframe, minicomputer or microcomputer. The current generation of LANs ranges tremendously in size and complexity. Some LANs may be confined to linking a few microcomputers to a printer, whilst others may connect several hundred microcomputers to large data storage devices (file servers) and electronic mailing systems. Because connectivity is the core issue involved in networking computers from potentially different suppliers, standards have been defined which govern the flow of data over networks. The most common standard network protocols are EtherNet and Token Ring, which share the market virtually equally.

Whereas LAN technology operates over short distances, typically within an office or building, a wide-area network (WAN) is concerned with long-distance communication over cables or even satellite links to connect computers. LANs and WANs can be linked together via gateways to allow computer users to access both local data storage devices and printers, and to link to a remote location to use the computer resources at that site. The growing capabilities of networks offer to revolutionize the work place and working practices. The prospect of the end of the office as the place of work is looming for many types of occupation. In future, employees will be able to stay at home and still have access to all the information and communication channels necessary to conduct business effectively. This development will have a major impact on the cost structure of business and those able to exploit this opportunity presented by networking developments and advances in related technology will gain a considerable competitive advantage.

The language of microcomputing

The terminology used to describe mainframe and minicomputer technology will, for the large part, remain in the province of the computer professional. However, the ubiquitous nature of the microcomputer means that the terminology used to describe the features and functions of these machines will become an integral part of the language needed to conduct business in the modern economy. Those unable to hold a basic dialogue in microcomputer-speak will be at a disadvantage in the office community of the future. The remaining paragraphs of this section are devoted to giving the reader an elementary understanding of some of the most common terms in current parlance.

One of the companies that has had a considerable impact on the growth and direction of microcomputing throughout the world has been Intel. Intel designs and manufactures microprocessors. Intel was selected to provide the microprocessors for the first IBM microcomputer and has maintained that relationship. As the industry in general has accepted the IBM microcomputer as the *de facto* standard, so Intel's position has been strengthened as arguably the leading microprocessor design organization. Of the leading microcomputer companies, only Apple, with its MacIntosh range, has bucked the trend by using Motorola as its supplier of microprocessor technology. The growth in the power and capabilities of microprocessors over the past decade has been phenomenal. Those who make their living from marketing microcomputers have been quick to realize that the microprocessor used in the microcomputer epitomizes its performance. They have also realized that the consumer, whether an individual or a corporation, is growing in sophistication and marketing needs to reflect a growing technological awareness of the consumer. As a consequence, much of the marketing of microcomputers has moved away from emphasis on the functions that can be performed, since these are conditioned by application packages that have portability between different suppliers of microcomputers. Instead, the current thrust of marketing is focused on the power of the microprocessor at the heart of the system and its cost. Originally, the most commonly used microcomputers used the Intel 8086 or 8088 microprocessor. Although many of these machines may still have a useful life running old applications, the current generation of microcomputers has moved on.

The microprocessors that have dominated microcomputing over the last few years are the Intel 80286 and 80386 and the immediate future involves the Intel 80486. These processors, which tend to be known as the '286, '386 and '486, have become key marketing differentiators between generations of microcomputers from different suppliers. So what's in a number, and does it really matter which microprocessor lies at the heart of a microcomputer? The '286, '386 and '486, as the numbering sequence suggests, have an ascending order of power and capability, which is material as microcomputer software and packages grow in their sophistication and performance requirements. The '286 was introduced in 1984 to give a performance boost to those microcomputers running the MS-DOS operating system. It offered the additional advantage of being able to work with faster printer technology than previously available. Since it was designed principally to work with MS-DOS, it suffered in performance terms when the new IBM OS/2 operating system emerged and Microsoft started to release new generations of easier-to-use, but immensely more sophisticated, software. These developments in software are destined to relegate the '286 to the annals of microcomputing history.

The Intel '386 processor represents a major advance over the earlier '286. It was introduced in 1986 with a capability to work with up to four times as much memory as the '286. However, the radical advance that the '386 brought was the capability to run several different software applications concurrently. For example, a microcomputer user could run a spreadsheet package and a word processor package at the same time through the capability of the '386 microprocessor to separate its memory into discrete blocks. To be able to operate in this mode does, however, require special software which manages the process of switching between different applications that may be running simultaneously. One of the software products which manages concurrent processing on microcomputers is Microsoft Windows, which is considered further below.

Whereas the '386 microprocessor represented a major technological advance over the earlier '286, the '486 provides only an incremental step over the '386. The Intel '486 microprocessor provides the potential for the microcomputer to use even more memory, with a 16-fold increase over the '386. Furthermore, the '486 has extended transistor circuitry that incorporates the mathematical capabilities that previously had to be provided on separate microprocessor chips. The power of the '486 microprocessor is astounding when compared with the capabilities of even mainframe computers of 10 years ago. At present, the challenge is for software suppliers to provide the applications and functionality to utilize this processing capability. However, the immediate past suggests that this gap will be closed very quickly through innovations in software in response to business needs. In fact, all the evidence supports the view that the rate of obsolescence of microcomputers, through the capability of applications to absorb the growing power of microprocessors, will accelerate. In response to this, many companies will no longer capitalize expenditure on microcomputers, recognizing that the potential life of machines is very short, not through wear and tear, but through technological obsolescence.

Having examined the role of the microprocessor in current advances in the capabilities of microprocessors, and having raised the issue of the vast amount of memory that the '386 and '486 processors can manage, it is worth a brief explanation of the role of memory and its relationship with the microprocessor. Memory is the microcomputer's primary storage (sometimes known as random access memory or RAM). It is not to be confused with secondary storage, for example diskettes, disk drives or tapes. Memory is effectively the microcomputer's work space which it uses to store data, to which the microprocessor needs direct access when performing computations or prior to printing or storing data on disks. Application software packages will also need to have access to part of the microcomputer's memory, again as work space for direct use. The microcomputer's memory is comprised of microchips with the necessary circuitry to hold data values as long as constant electrical power is available. Once the microcomputer is switched off the memory is cleared of its contents.

The amount of memory that a microcomputer has available is measured in terms of bytes. For the layperson, a byte is equivalent to a single character. So to record this chapter of the book in microcomputer memory would require approximately 10 000 bytes. When microcomputers were initially introduced the memory capacity was limited to little more than 8000 bytes (or 8 kilobytes, shortened to 8 kbytes or even 8K) and therefore they had no use in the business sphere and were confined to hobbyist and educational use. The first microcomputer introduced by IBM in 1981 was released with 16K of memory and

was termed a personal computer, which did not suggest any serious commercial use. In 1983, IBM's PC-2 was introduced: this offered 64K of memory, expandable to 256K. Initially the cost of manufacturing memory chips was so high and the future of microcomputing so uncertain that MS-DOS was designed with a capability to manage a maximum of 640K of memory. Such has been the success of microcomputing and the growth of the applications that are performed on them that with hindsight this is now seen as a major mistake and a threat to the future of MS-DOS as the *de facto* microcomputer operating system.

The cost of memory with advances in the manufacturing processes is now very low and microcomputers can now be supplied with direct storage capabilities that could not be dreamt of, even in mainframe computing, less than a decade ago. Whereas expressing memory size in the form of kilobytes was an effective shorthand a few years ago, this scale is no longer appropriate as microcomputers grow in power. Now it is necessary to describe memory in terms of megabytes (approximately 1 million bytes or 1000 kilobytes). Secondary storage in the form of disk drives is now being supplied with the capability to store data in terms of gigabytes (approximately 1000 megabytes or 1 million kilobytes or 1000 million bytes). One can forecast without danger that soon the direct memory of microcomputers will be expressed in the form of gigabytes and the capacity of the microcomputer to invade all aspects of business life will have truly arrived. To turn a capability into a practicality will require microcomputers to become easy to use, even by those with the least technical aptitude.

Ease of use in microcomputing has been elevated to the status of a science and given the terms human–machine interface, end-user interface or computer ergonomics. Different types of interface have been tried and tested in the market place. The traditional method of communicating with the microcomputer has been the keyboard which, although highly efficient for those with typing skills and manual dexterity, represents a barrier to the majority of potential users. Touch-sensitive display technology has been tried as a potentially easier interface for computer users. This involves designing computer screens with a pressure-sensitive panel which allows the user to select computer options by pressing the screen at the appropriate place. The limitation with this type of technology is that the complexity of the dialogue that can be conducted with the computer must be limited. Typically, touch screens are used to provide basic information to users from a limited range of options. Applications using the technology are mainly in the public information area or for initiating simple transactions. For example, banks sometimes use the technology to allow customers to order cheque books or request information on services. Non-critical applications are best suited to this technology.

Another technology tried in the field is voice recognition. Of course, the ideal solution to the end-user interface would be through the medium of voice. To be able to speak to the computer and initiate even the most complex transaction is commonplace in science fiction. The practical limitations of current technology are well short of this aspiration. The reality is that, even in the most advanced systems, computers can recognize fewer than 500 words of human speech. Even in these systems the error rate in voice recognition is relatively high and care has to be taken to ensure that the computer is synchronized to the specific voice pattern of the user. This constraint in the use of voice recognition means that its application is limited to specialist areas. One of the more socially useful applications areas for voice recognition is in providing computer support for blind users, particularly when combined with voice synthesis in which the output from the computer is in the form of synthesized speech. Voice synthesis is also an emerging technology for other areas of disability where the user has lost the capacity to speak clearly. Perhaps one of the most famous users of a voice synthesizer is Professor Stephen Hawking, who had to look to the USA to provide the technology to meet his needs. It is unlikely that voice recognition or synthesis will provide a means of controlling input to, and output from, computers in a mass market sense in the medium term. However, it remains the optimum solution to the end-user interface problem.

Having looked at interfaces that have limited application or have failed to win support, it remains to consider the technologies that have grabbed and held the imagination of computer users. Initially, microcomputer users had to memorize commands and type them in order to run application programs. Those with strong technical knowledge may still prefer this mode of dialogue with the microcomputer. Menu-driven applications then emerged to allow computer users to run programs without the need to know any commands. In the most complex systems hierarchies of menus may be involved in which the user refines his or her choice by being offered increasingly specific menu options. Some systems will combine a menu-driven approach with a 'fast path' capability in which commands can be entered to eliminate steps in the menu hierarchy. This development allows both the advanced users with detailed computer training as well as those with minimal technical understanding but sound application knowledge to use the same system in the way each prefers. Menu-driven systems have been virtually perfected in business systems and it is unlikely that any significant further innovation is possible in this area.

The innovation that is replacing the menu-driven user interface, particularly in microcomputing, is based on three components. Firstly, it is based on the use of graphics to provide on-screen symbols or icons which, if selected, cause a computer function to be performed. The icons are usually drawn to allow the user to make a reasonable inference of the process that will arise from its selection. For example, a graphical representation of a printer might reasonably infer that print options will be offered if that icon is selected.

Secondly, this type of approach, often described as an iconic or a graphical user interface (or GUI), offers the option of selecting the icon by keyboard, but is more often accompanied by a mouse device that directs an on-screen pointer to the desired icon. The mouse is usually equipped with one or more buttons that are clicked when the pointer has identified the icon to be selected. Most commonly, the pointer is directed to the preferred icon by rolling a ball housed within the mouse. All leading microcomputers will be equipped with a connection into which a mouse device can be plugged.

The third component to accompany the GUI and mouse device in securing a new generation of microcomputer users is windowing technology. Known in technical circles as an applications program interface (API), windowing allows two or more applications to be run simultaneously, each of which can be viewed through its own window. Windows can be overlaid on the screen with the current application occupying a window in the foreground while the others reside in the background. The windowing environment

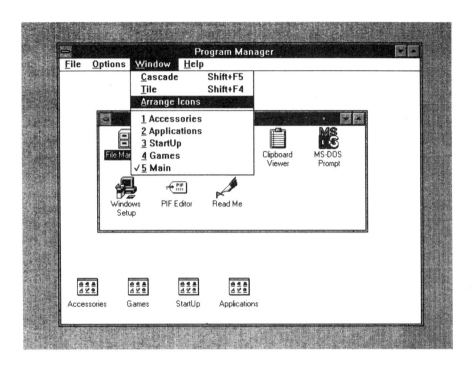

Fig. 7.3.1 Example of Microsoft Window screen presentation.

has other features associated with it, such as pull-down menus, scroll bars, multiple type fonts, facilities to move data between applications in different windows and many other capabilities unique to this type of interface.

The combination of these three components to allow users to use applications to a high degree of sophistication without technical knowledge and minimal keyboard expertise is usually attributed as an innovation to Xerox, with Apple introducing it to the microcomputer mass market. Later Microsoft adopted a similar approach with its Microsoft Windows product, which creates an environment in which multiple MS-DOS applications can be run concurrently. Windowing technology has also been adopted by IBM to provide the program management functions for its latest range of OS/2-based microcomputers.

Such has been the success of windowing technology that many application package suppliers are producing versions of their systems specifically designed to work in conjunction with

Microsoft Windows and allow users to use icons and mouse technology consistently between applications. Figure 7.3.1 above shows an example of a Microsoft Windows screen presentation. The collective power of Microsoft, IBM and Apple in the microcomputer industry is more than sufficient to ensure that icons, the mouse and windows will be the basis of the end-user interface to microcomputing until the technical constraints on the exploitation of voice as a medium of communication with computers can be overcome.

Personal systems for the clinicians

Having looked at the development path for computers in general and microcomputers in particular, it is now appropriate to consider the type of systems that is likely to be of most value to the clinician for personal or office use. Of course no two individuals are the same and the need for

Table 7.3.4

Basic personal systems	Shared systems	Specialist applications
Word processing	Electronic mail	Desk top publishing
Computer spreadsheet	Facsimile	Statistical package
Personal database	Diary management	Expert systems
Graphics	Compact disk drives	Computer imaging

systems will vary with the role, functions and interests of the person concerned. However, Table 7.3.4 suggests a classification of micro-computer-based systems for clinicians, although over time those systems once considered specialist will tend to become commonplace as office system packages integrate more functions and information needs increase in sophistication.

Basic personal systems will operate on a microcomputer which will have its own second-ary disk storage and local printing capability. With the falling costs of printer devices, event-ually even personal system users will be working with laser printers as the norm, whereas impact and inkjet printers have been the norm in the past.

Of all the potential microcomputer applications to gain the widest use, word processing is the most common. Word processors have grown rapidly in capabilities from basic text editors to comprehensive applications capable of not only formatting text automatically, but also integrat-ing graphics within documents. There is no bet-ter example of how word processing has altered an industry so fundamentally as that of the newspaper sector. Word processing has altered the method of manufacture of the finished pro-duct and also changed the skills set of those still engaged in the industry. Its impact is less dra-matic in other industries, but none the less signi-ficant. As everyone gains computer literacy through current education programmes, the in-clination for those who need to produce textual material to use a computer directly rather than have a secretarial intermediary will grow. The link between documents and mailing systems that can disseminate them quickly to the in-tended recipients will encourage this trend further. The word-processing packages that dominate the microcomputing world at present are Micro-soft Word and WordPerfect, although there are others such as WordStar and Display Write. This area of the software market is extremely dynamic and versions change rapidly, incorpor-

ating new functions and capabilities. Market positioning will inevitably change in this environ-ment.

Closely behind the word process application in its market success has been the spreadsheet ap-plications, which had their origins in the ac-countant's columnar worksheet. In its early form this type of application presented the microcom-puter user with a matrix of rows and columns into which text, labels, numbers and formulae could be entered. The benefit of this type of application was concerned with automating many of the arithmetic tasks involved in prepar-ing this type of worksheet and avoiding the need to recalculate manually when one or more of the figures or formulae being used were changed subsequently. Spreadsheets became very popular with those involved in budgeting or planning and were used as modelling tools for exploring the implications of different scenarios. The ap-plications of spreadsheets have been extended out of the accountant's domain into other man-agement areas that have a requirement to model, plan or account for activities. Spreadsheet appli-cations have acquired many new features since the early packages such as VisiCalc were intro-duced. Microcomputer software developers have sought to extend the spreadsheet concept to pro-vide a three-dimensional modelling tool. Further-more, the applications have been developed to integrate other functions, for example, graphics and database management capabilities. For the accountant this type of application will continue to be a considerable boon. However, this type of application could also assist the clinician not just in a planning and modelling context, but also in relation to providing easy-to-use analyti-cal tools to support research activities. Some of the market-leading suppliers in this application area are:

1 Microsoft (with its Excel application).
2 Lotus (with Lotus 1-2-3).
3 Computer Associates (SuperCalc versions).

Whilst spreadsheet software is increasingly including basic database capabilities, these functions are limited by the boundaries and format of the worksheet concept. Consequently there remains a strong market for specialist microcomputer databases which allow data to be captured easily and flexibly, yet also possess powerful *ad hoc* reporting capabilities to control the content, ordering, formatting and general presentation of the information that can be retrieved. There are a large number of commercially successful applications of this type in the market which include:

1 dBase IV (Ashton Tate).
2 Paradox (Borland).
3 FoxBASE+ (Fox Software).

Again, spreadsheet applications have incorporated a graphics capability in many of the present market offerings. However, the quality and flexibility of the graphics, as with the database capabilities, may not be sufficiently functional or flexible for some requirements. Where the graphics must be of a standard close to, or equivalent to, those required for desk top publishing it may be necessary to consider a dedicated graphical reporting package. Some of the most commonly used graphics packages in the market currently are:

1 Harvard Graphics (SPC Software Publishing).
2 Freelance (Lotus).
3 Micrografx Designer (Micrografx).

Care must be exercised when using graphics packages for high-quality publishing purposes, since low-cost microcomputer packages may have limitations which affect the resolution of the images that can be produced.

Some of the benefits that organizations expect to receive from investment in microcomputers can only be achieved through better communication and sharing of corporate information. The growth in the installation and use of microcomputer networks is making it possible for individuals to share high-cost storage and printer devices and to share software rather than to hold individual copies of computer packages. Some computer packages have been developed for use with local area communications networks and support the concept of sharing software and data files. Increasingly, the microcomputer will become the window through which the individual will obtain access to corporate resources and

be able to disseminate information to colleagues. Shared systems to support better communications will include high-performance printers, electronic mailing and messaging facilities, diary and meeting scheduling capabilities and corporate educational and training material stored on compact disks (CD-ROM). Only now are shared systems being offered in anything like an integrated fashion. Over the next few years clinicians will need to be prepared for major changes in working practices as office support services and communications arrangements become increasingly automated. The potential benefits to the patient in terms of increased efficiency and effectiveness are considerable, but the organizational change processes will exact a high cost.

Although individuals or groups may have requirements outside the normal range of systems used by the majority, it is becoming increasingly possible to meet those specific needs within the same technical architectures used to run more general applications. Already, any microcomputer package must for its medium- and long-term future deal with the *de facto* standards set by IBM, Microsoft and Intel. In addition, packages need to be able to operate within communications networks which conform to open systems interconnection standards. Thus clinicians looking to use specialist applications like statistical packages or dedicated desk top publishing are strongly advised to select only those packages that can run in the systems environment that is being used for more general computing needs. In those areas where computer applications are dependent on emerging technologies, for example capturing pictures and text in digitized form, or expert systems that require specialist languages and high-performance processing, it is more difficult to be prescriptive. Any investment in these areas will need to recognize that entering the market early may have a high cost and low integration capabilities. Only a realistic cost-and-benefit analysis can give guidance on whether the investment is justified.

Corporate systems for hospitals

Although the level of investment in information technology in most hospitals compares unfavourably with commercial organizations of the same size, most hospitals will have computerized their patient management systems. Past investment has typically addressed the functional needs in the various operational areas of the hospital. Many investment decisions will have been taken on local operational need, rather than in the context of an overall information technology strategy. Because of this, many hospitals will have a diverse array of systems with duplication in the data entry taking place. The Department of Health has undertaken two significant exercises over the last few years that have sought to change this position. Firstly, the resource management initiative gave rise to what has been termed case mix management systems which, as well as meeting a range of management information needs, were also charged with providing a patient-based database of clinical and financial activity by drawing data from existing hospital operational systems. This approach was both pragmatic in terms of interfacing existing sources of data with the latest in database management technology, and also innovative in that it led to a detailed analysis of the technical issues involved in linking existing systems.

The second initiative was the hospital information support system (HISS) project, where the issue of finding a fully integrated approach to a hospital's operational and management information needs could be met with an avoidance of the need for any duplication in data capture. A number of pilot sites have implemented systems consistent with the HISS initiative, but it is too early to determine the full benefits that will be made in terms of the quality and costs of the patient care process. The very least that they can be expected to achieve is a much-needed stimulus to the computer industry to identify better the functional requirements of hospitals in the UK and to deliver that function within the context of a systems approach that offers the following features:

1 A standard operating system portable across different suppliers' computers.
2 A portable database management system based on relational technology.
3 Open communication standards for allowing the transfer of data and documents across local and wide area networks and between different manufacturers' computers.
4 Cooperative processing between microcomputers, with their high end-user functionality, and traditional mainframe and minicomputer technology with its high-volume data-processing strengths.
5 Standard end-user interfaces to allow easier access and exploitation of the capabilities of computer systems.

6 An opportunity for the individual to meet local personal computing needs through microcomputer-based software solutions delivered through the same terminal that also allows access to corporate systems and information.

There is a strong basis for assuming that this vision will be capable of being met within the medium term since many of the technologies are available now. The impetus to turn the technological capability into an integrated systems approach specifically for the hospital operating as a business and service entity will come, not from suppliers pushing their products at the market, but from end-user demand for better information to improve the lot of patients and pressures to contain the costs of service provision.

Future trends in computing

The section started with the premiss that it is difficult to predict the rate of growth in computing technology, with the particular risk that it will be underestimated. However, whilst the rate may be difficult to judge, there is more clarity about the direction, although new innovations could potentially disrupt any predictions. With this caveat, it would be reasonable to assume the following:

1 Consolidation of the position of Unix as the standard operating system for general business purposes will continue, and its use for microcomputers as well as mainframe and minicomputers presents a major threat to MS-DOS and OS/2. The portability of operating systems will be accompanied by the capability to have the same opportunity with databases and application functions.
2 Microchip technology will continue to advance at a pace and the prospects of ultimately arriving at the position where a mainframe can be delivered on a single piece of silicon or similar semiconductor medium seem certain within the medium term.
3 Computer memory capabilities will continue to expand in line with the growing capabilities of software applications. The availability of low-cost memory for computers will allow better end-user interfaces to be developed that will encourage more computer users, which will in turn create more demands for technical innovation.
4 The speed of communication between systems will be increasingly based on optic fibre technology, with conventional cabling being ultimately replaced as the preferred medium. The demand for higher performance, coupled with lower costs, will drive this development.

These trends will take computing into virtually all aspects of personal and business life. The opportunity, for those prepared for the change and who have an understanding of the benefits to be obtained and knowledge of how they might be delivered, is enormous. For those unable to assimilate the skills and resistant to the trends the future is bleak.

Reference

Department of Health (1989) *Working for Patients*. HMSO, London.

7.4 Choosing the right computer system

Sheila Bullas

This section is written in the context of choosing the right computer system to support general and clinical management.

Background

Until recently systems have often been chosen at a regional level and implemented in hospitals. This was at a time when there was little information technology in hospitals, few information technology skills locally, systems were complex to implement and the cost was a great deal more than it is today. However, one aspect made the choosing of the computer system easier than it is today. That is, each computer system had a distinct function. Systems would be purchased to meet the needs of, say, the pathology department or to provide for patient administration. There was little need for individual systems to exchange data or talk to each other.

Many of the individual departmental systems that have been procured and many systems being purchased now are required to exchange data or to integrate in such a way that information does not have to be entered into each of the different systems. In particular, a system that is to support resource management or audit will receive data from operational systems, that is systems used for the day-to-day activities of the hospital. The time-consuming and expensive task of keying in data again will thus be avoided.

New operational systems, such as order communications and results reporting, need to exchange data with systems such as the patient administration system if the patient's basic details are not to be keyed into each individual system. It is quite common at present for different systems to hold their own basic patient details or index. Apart from the duplicated effort, a change in one system is not reflected in others. For example, if one department finds that a patient has changed his or her address, they may change it on their own system but the change will not necessarily be communicated to other systems where the address is used. A key development is therefore to ensure that a common master patient index is available to all systems – not a trivial technical issue in many cases.

Figure 7.4.1 shows an advanced technical configuration of systems having access to common patient basic details and obtaining management information as a byproduct of the operational systems.

This shows how much communication between systems there is likely to be in the future. This should be done in such a way that it is obvious to the user which system is being accessed; users should be able to go to their terminal, switch it on, identify themselves and then have access to all the systems they need to use. With the diverse nature of information systems in most hospitals, it will be some time before this is a reality. It has been known for users to require four different terminals on their desk to access four different systems, each with a completely different command structure, requiring much training and perhaps stress counselling. Careful choice of future systems can, at least, stop the situation getting any worse.

Increased experience of the use of computer systems means that people are making more informed choices but the choice itself is in many ways more complex now because of the variety of systems available, the need for systems to communicate with each other, and the difficulty of preventing gaps or overlaps in what the different systems do, particularly when they come from different suppliers.

User involvement

Throughout the NHS one can find systems that have been imposed without sufficient consultation with the people who are expected to use those systems. The system may not be liked, not perceived to be suitable for the local circumstances and therefore not providing the benefits that

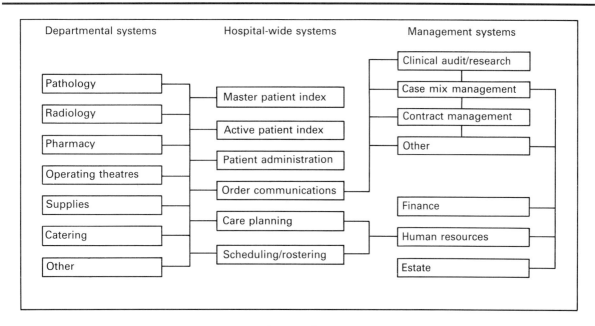

Fig. 7.4.1 Technical configuration of systems.

may be expected from it. Elsewhere the same system may be liked, used enthusiastically and provides the benefits. It is certainly true that there are horses for courses; while the system was appropriate in one situation, it was not in another. But in many cases the only difference is the degree of user involvement in the selection of the system. It is now accepted that those who will be using the system must be very much involved in its selection from the earliest stage. If users are not involved in the selection of a system, it will not be as successful as it could be, however good the system itself is.

This is particularly important where the system is to support clinical or general management where the benefits are derived from the use of the information to make decisions to change what is done or how it is done. For operational systems, use of the system may be the only way for staff to carry out their day-to-day tasks. For example, recording patient details on a system may be the only routine way to register them, order a pathology test or obtain a meal. For systems that support resource management and audit, there is no operational reason for them to be used. User involvement in selection of the system is one of the most effective ways to ensure commitment and enthusiastic use.

The range of systems available is extensive, with all suppliers keen to extol the virtues of

their own offering. At the last count there were 12 systems available that could support resource management, some of which would also support audit, budgeting and contracting (NHS Management Executive, 1991a). There were at least 22 personal-computer-based medical audit systems (Anderson Consulting, 1990). The range of personal computer hardware and software for word processing, spreadsheets, desk top publishing and other personal applications is endless. How can you choose the right system?

Information and information technology (IT) strategy

All hospitals need to develop a broad understanding of their overall approach to IT – a strategy. The aim of the strategy is to ensure that systems are planned and used properly (Central Computing and Telecommunications Agency, 1989). The strategy helps at all stages of planning, purchasing and implementing systems and not only makes the choice of system easier, but improves its chances of successful use. If systems are not properly planned, they can limit effectiveness and constrain options for the future. This is particularly true now that systems need to communicate with each other and where systems are used by many different people throughout the organization and not just a single department.

The strategy aims to answer three questions relating to information and information systems:

1 Where are we now?
2 Where do we want to be?
3 How do we get there?

If no existing systems were implemented and there were no constraints of time scale, available money or political imperatives, the development of a strategy and the selection of systems would be easy. This is, however, a luxury not often found. There will be existing systems which may be doing a good job and fit into a development path for the future. There may be systems which are coming to the end of their useful life or do not do a useful job and need to be replaced. The effectiveness of existing systems provides opportunities and constraints in choice of systems for the future.

In determining where we want to be, it is important to identify opportunities and the role that information systems might have in exploiting these opportunities. Central initiatives with associated monies for the introduction of systems, such as resource management and audit, present opportunities which may determine priorities for particular systems if the opportunity is to be exploited. If selection is made, taking into consideration the overall strategy of 'where we want to be' and 'how we get there', the strategy will help in selection, rather than if particular choice is allowed to drive the strategy.

For example, if the strategy were to specify a preferred supplier of systems to be company A in order to ease communication between different systems, then the choice of a system to support resource management or audit would give preference to systems from this supplier and only if a suitable system were not available from this supplier would consideration be given to other suppliers. If, on the other hand, the strategy was to specify an open-systems policy, whereby systems running on a range of suppliers' hardware but conforming to a common open systems standard were given preference, the choice of systems would be widened, the risks associated with a single supplier reduced but the difficulty of communication between different systems, different command structures and gaps and overlaps in functionality increased.

Changes in structures, policies and processes within the organization need to be taken into consideration, as will the interdependence of systems and any particular problem areas.

There is no single way to meet the information systems needs. 'How we get there' needs to consider a range of options which will take into account constraints and opportunities in finance, staff numbers and skills. These will need to consider any imperatives requiring a short-term solution which will be fitted in to longer-term plans and it will need to consider what is technically feasible.

Choosing systems in the light of an information and IT strategy reduces the risk of chaos, expensive mistakes and difficulties of integration of systems in the future.

The strategy can help to indicate preferred options for hardware and systems software that the system is based on. It can help to indicate preferred options for suppliers of applications. It can help determine what functions should be sought in individual systems and which systems need to communicate with which. For example, a basic case mix system, as described in the core specification (NHS Management Board, 1989), will support resource management, whereas one of the more sophisticated systems will also support audit, budget reporting and contracting. Alternatively, these different aspects may be supported by different systems that communicate with each other.

General

Whatever type of system you require, you need to be sure you know what you want it to do. For larger systems, a detailed statement of need will be written. The aim of this is to define the problem, not the solution. You will describe what you want the system to do and how you want it to be done, if you want to use particular methods or have standards to which it must conform. For example, you may want to specify what coding systems are used for diagnosis and operative procedures or what hardware standards are specific for your hospital. The statement of need is not intended to describe the technical solutions – it is for the suppliers to describe how they will tackle it. It will describe those things that the system must do and those which may be desirable. It is tempting to try to put everything you want a computer to do in the same specification but it may not be sensible for a single system to do everything.

For smaller systems, it is equally important and useful to write this down. This provides a checklist against which you can judge suppliers' offerings. For larger systems, the statement of need and a summary have a major role in the formal procurement process. A model document for case mix management systems is available as a guide (NHS Management Executive, 1990a). This document includes:

1 A description of elements of the organization affected by the system.
2 A functional specification (description) of the system you are seeking to procure.
3 An analysis of the required data.
4 Any specific systems requirements, including hardware, software, communications, security.
5 Performance requirements, including assumptions on sizing and use of the system.
6 Reliability requirements, including acceptable time before repair or replacement in the event of a system failure.
7 Support requirements, which may cover training, project management, implementation, physical environment, engineering, maintenance and software support.
8 Details of the procurement process and time scales.

The statement of need is a formal document against which suppliers submit a proposal stating what their system can and what it can't do. This proposal forms the basis of assessment of the individual offerings and is also used to determine whether the chosen supplier delivers what has been agreed in a subsequent contract. Unless you are procuring a general package such as a word-processing package, it is useful to seek a formal response from the supplier, whatever size the system.

You will want to see several systems demonstrated by different suppliers and make sure that they can demonstrate all the features you require in the system. Without the checklist, it is easy for suppliers to demonstrate all the good features of their system and gloss over some features that you consider essential but are not provided by their system. The principle of *caveat emptor* applies.

You should also ask to see the system working in at least one other hospital and talk to the people using it. There is a great difference between seeing a demonstration from a supplier and seeing how the system actually performs in the operational situation. Be careful, however:

the system appropriate for one hospital may not be appropriate for you; organization and standards may be different and the success may be due more to the people using the system rather than the system itself. A supplier, if still in business, can always demonstrate one successful site. Ask for a full list and call several sites at random to check general satisfaction with the system. The random check also offers the opportunity to ask about the support services the supplier offers.

It doesn't matter how good the system itself is if the supplier is not going to be around in a year's time to provide support and maintenance and to provide updates to the system. In this respect, promises and a contract mean nothing. Check out the financial status of the company. Your local supplies department or the NHS computer procurement centre can help you with this. You can never be sure – companies come and go, even large ones, but at least you can reduce the risk you are taking.

You will want to understand what support is required, what is available and how much of this is included in the purchase price and what additional costs you will incur. If you have a formal operational requirement, your requirements for support will be included in this and a formal response will be obtained from the suppliers. In any case, there are a number of questions you may wish to ask, depending on the nature of the system:

1 What training is required and what is available?
2 Is this provided on the user's site or supplier's site?
3 For a larger system, who is going to provide project management?
4 Will the supplier install the software and get it up and running?
5 Who will set up any necessary data files?
6 For a larger system, are there any special environmental conditions required?
7 If you operate in an unusual physical environment in terms of, say, local electricity supply, will the equipment function correctly?
8 When you get a fault with the hardware, how will it be repaired and how quickly?
9 When you have some difficulty with the software, is there someone you can call who can help?

Large systems

For any system expected to cost over 100 000 ecus or about £80 000 European Community rules for procurement apply. Systems such as

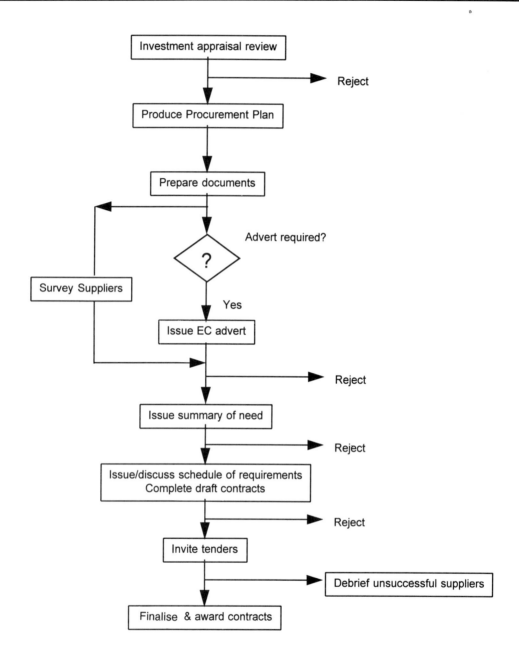

Fig. 7.4.2   Procurement process.

case mix management and order communications and results reporting come in this category. These regulations are quite complex but are more simply described in a guide published as part of a case mix procurement pack produced by the resource management unit of the NHS management executive (1991b).

The formal process for the procurement of a large system is shown in Figure 7.4.2 and described in *POISE, a Guide for Managers* also from the NHS management executive (1993). This full process can take a minimum of 43 weeks to complete.

The choice of system will involve a team of people with different skills and responsibilities.

For case mix management, for example, the range of skills that need to be brought to the team include project management, general management, medical, nursing, information, and finance. The team will, hopefully use a recognized methodology for project management, such as PRINCE (NHS Management Executive, 1990b), to ensure that the specification, selection and implementation of the system are properly planned and managed and take into consideration everyone's views, particularly those of the people who will be using the system.

In a simplified form, the same methodology can be used for smaller systems; at least the same principles apply.

The whole project is split up into a number of stages which might be, for example:

1 Specification.
2 Procurement.
3 Installation.
4 Implementation.

A project board takes overall control of the project and comprises an executive who provides overall project guidance and assessment throughout the project; a senior user who represents users of the system; and a senior technical representative with responsibility for technical implementation. In this way the business, user and technical aspects of the system are considered at the highest level.

A project manager is appointed who has day-to-day responsibility for management of the project from beginning to end. Each stage of the project will have its own stage manager, who may also be the project manager in a small or simple project. This person is responsible for ensuring that the products of the stage are produced on schedule, within budget and to high-quality standards. The stage manager is supported by a business assurance coordinator who maintains the schedule and budget; a technical assurance coordinator who monitors technical integrity; and a user assurance coordinator who represents users' interests.

Technical guides are available to ensure that all the relevant questions are considered at each stage of the project. These have been developed over many years using the experience of people who have been through the process of selecting systems. No one needs to start with a blank sheet of paper to define what needs to be done, whether this is in questions that need to be answered when specifying the system, preparing an operational requirement or drawing up a contract for supply.

Personal computer systems

Selecting large expensive systems is time-consuming if expensive mistakes are not to be made. The process of public sector procurement is subject to all manner of regulations to ensure open competition both nationally and defined by the European Community. It can be frustrating when, for a sum within your own budget, you may be able to purchase a personal computer system which will be able to deliver some benefits immediately while you wait for the greater benefits that can be obtained from the larger systems. You may want to purchase a personal computer system which can deliver more personal rather than corporate benefits.

You should ensure that whatever is purchased will not become useless within a short time and that the system you purchased can be used to access any of the existing or future systems you will need to access, for example, patient administration or order communications. You will not want to have two or more computer screens on your desk to give you the full range of access to the information you require.

Your hospital may well have a policy on hardware or software or both. Buying hardware or software which is in general use throughout the hospital has all manner of advantages. There may well be advantageous discounts because of the number of systems purchased. There may be support and maintenance available for any difficulties that are experienced in use. If you have a fault on your machine, provided you have copies of your data available, you may be able to swap to another computer while yours is being repaired. Training programmes may be readily available or trained staff who understand the system may be available to cover holidays and sickness for use of the system by secretarial staff. This is particularly important for such facilities as word processing. Most of the leading word-processing packages are much the same these days; you may as well get the advantages of using the one that others throughout the hospital are using.

The small system to support audit has certain advantages. It can certainly provide benefits in a much shorter time scale than a large system designed to support the whole hospital. It does, however, have certain disadvantages. The most important of these is that, unless the system is linked to the operational systems of patient administration, pathology, etc. the data will have to be keyed into the system separately – a time-consuming, expensive task which can lead to the introduction of inaccuracies.

Another disadvantage of the small system, unless integrated with other systems of the hospital, is that the information is presented differently in the different systems because definitions are different or inaccuracies are not identified and corrected. It helps if everybody is 'singing from the same hymn sheet' so that discussion can move away from 'my information is accurate', 'no, mine is right' to 'what does it mean?'

References

Anderson Consulting (1990) *Computers in Medical Audit. A Guide for Hospital Consultants to Personal Computer (PC) Based Medical Audit Systems*. West Midlands RHA.

Central Computing and Telecommunications Agency (1989) *Strategic Planning for Information Systems. The Information Systems Guides*. Wiley, Chichester.

NHS Management Board (1989) *Case Mix Management System, Core Specification*. Resource Management Directorate.

NHS Management Executive (1990a) *Model Operational Requirement for a Case Mix Management System*. Resource Management Unit.

NHS Management Executive (1990b) *PRINCE Methodology*. Central Computing and Telecommunications Agency.

NHS Management Executive (1991a) *Casemix Systems Survey, version 3*. Resource Management Unit.

NHS Management Executive (1991b) *Casemix Procurement*.

NHS Management Executive (1993) *POISE, a Guide for Managers*.

7.5 Data protection and security

Barry Barber

Introduction

The importance of data protection is that it seeks to put in place a set of well-known basic rules which provide an environment within which computer-based personal information can be processed. There are, obviously, many difficult situations encountered by health professionals in the course of their work where there are considerable pressures to maintain confidentiality of certain information coexisting with pressures to make disclosures of that same information on the grounds of public interest. These problems are usually best settled by experienced health professionals who are conversant with the relevant legislation and who have weighed the consequences of alternative courses of action within the context of the basic professional, ethical and data protection guidelines. They can be called upon to justify their decisions to a court or to a disciplinary body of their peers. This long-established process has provided the foundation for the practice of medicine and its associated health professions and it ensures that difficult situations that were not envisaged by those devising regulations can be sensibly addressed.

Information systems security is a wider term than simply that of data protection and confidentiality. It includes all aspects of:

1 *confidentiality* of all information held within the information system, whether the information is personally identified or not;
2 *integrity* of the system and its information in the sense that it is all functioning correctly and the information has not been altered either accidentally or maliciously;
3 *availability* of the system and its information whenever it is needed.

This approach takes the modern view of information system security and is consistent with the best UK and European Community (EC) practice. There are circumstances when the issues of integrity and availability may require even more

attention in health care systems than may be required in respect of the issue of confidentiality. Data protection covers most of these issues in respect of information that can be personally identified but it gives an additional general right to the individual to obtain a copy of the record held about him or her (subject access). In health care, confidentiality is usually concerned with personally identified information where the amount of information passed to an individual in the health care environment is restricted to what the individual needs to know to deliver appropriate health care to the patient.

For convenient reference, the material presented in this section is arranged in the conventional fashion, starting from a data protection standpoint which is then developed to cover access to non-computer health records and the changing European environment in data protection. The subject is finally explored from the standpoint of information systems security.

Medical ethics and the duty of care

The Hippocratic oath is usually regarded as the first attempt to outline some of the basic requirements for the satisfactory practice of the profession of medicine. It included the concepts of working for the benefit of the sick, refraining from the misuse of drugs, not seducing patients and maintaining confidentiality. Medical ethics and the duty of care are major topics which require whole books for an adequate discussion. The fundamental issue is one of the individual acceptance of professional responsibility for the processes of care and of accountability for the safety of these processes.

The importance of data protection

Data protection has come to mean the various issues raised in the Data Protection Act 1984 or in the Council of Europe Convention 108 for the

Protection of Individuals with regard to Automatic Processing of Personal Data (1981) in respect of information that is personally identified. The issue of confidentiality is part of data protection and it has always been a significant issue in health care because it provides the basis on which patients tell their physicians details of their ailments, disabilities, private life and confidential circumstances so that their situation may be fully understood and their problems addressed. Without this degree of trust between the patient and the health professional, significant issues would be missed and treatable problems would remain untreated. The Council's recommendations on automated medical data banks was published in 1981.

The need for security

The three concepts of security – confidentiality, integrity and availability – were outlined above. However, the reasons for the present concern about information systems security arise from the developing arrangements for care within the NHS, the developing technology available for handling information systems, both large and small, and the use of those systems. The key issues arise in the following ways:

1 The number of systems, terminals and terminal users has increased enormously and the chances of things going wrong have likewise increased.
2 The systems now hold more sensitive information and breaches of confidentiality can be more serious.
3 The systems are now used to hold information required for treating patients and errors in the information may lead to errors in the treatment of patients.
4 More staff who are inexperienced in the use of computer systems are using the systems and hence they are less likely to notice errors.
5 More staff are reliant on computer systems to handle their work.
6 Technically the information systems are much more reliable than they were previously and the information they provide is accepted more uncritically than would previously have been the case.
7 The NHS management executive's strategy is reliant on the use of information systems to achieve national NHS objectives of providing integrated, continuous health care.
8 More information systems are networked together to provide wider access or data linkage, resulting in potentially greater opportunities for unauthorized access.

9 Information systems are beginning to edge into the area of safety critical systems where patients may die as a result of errors in system design, system implementation, data input, routine operations or system maintenance.
10 The UK Data Protection Act 1984 requires personal information to be kept secure.
11 The Council of Europe Convention 108, which has been ratified by the UK, states that 'Appropriate security measures shall be taken'. This is interpreted in the explanatory memorandum as 'adapted to the specific function of the file and the risks involved' and 'based on the current state of the art of data security methods and techniques in the field of data processing'.
12 The draft EC directive concerning the protection of individuals in relation to the processing of personal data is currently being revised but it is likely to require greater security in the harmonized European information systems environment and it proposed 'dissuasive sanctions in order to ensure compliance'.

The introduction of computers in health care

From the point of view of the utilization of computers in health care, the health professionals have to advise the computer specialists of their security requirements. The issue of the confidentiality of the information to be held within the computer systems is normally addressed; which individuals can see what information and in what circumstances and which individuals can change what information? Most of the systems developed to date have addressed these confidentiality issues in the sense required by the specific clinicians at the institutions concerned in implementing the computer system. The current challenge is to translate these specific requirements into generic concepts which will be satisfactory in a UK and European context. In addition, it is necessary to educate clinicians so that they can specify their requirements for the other components of information systems security, namely integrity and availability as these issues may be even more important than the issues of confidentiality.

Confidentiality of personal health information

Good clinical practice requires the sharing of information about a particular patient between those concerned with the care of that patient, including those concerned with facilitating that care by processing information. In each case the individual requires information on a 'need to know' basis for the activities with which they are concerned. This engenders a dynamic tension between sharing information that may not be needed and withholding information which appeared to be irrelevant but yet which would have altered the processes of delivering care. Health professionals recognize the conflicting requirements inherent in this 'need to know' approach with the practice of modern health care delivery within the multidisciplinary, multisite context stretching from tertiary hospital care to community care with the involvement of the local authority services and informal carers. Everyone concerned with the NHS needs to be aware of the professional requirements for confidentiality in handling information about patients and they should be subject to clauses in their contracts of employment in respect of these issues if they are not already subject to professional disciplinary procedures. Appropriate training should be given where necessary, with follow-up reminders from time to time. This approach helps to develop a caring community within which information can be shared without risk of damage to patients.

The approach to the Data Protection Act 1984

A history of the development of the concepts of data protection is an interesting one that is outlined in the *Encyclopaedia of Data Protection* (Chalton *et al.*, 1988). In the early 1980s, within the context of the developing EC, it became clear that the UK would be in danger of being excluded from important information systems business if it did not put a suitable data protection regime in place. The minimum requirement was to enact domestic legislation corresponding to that required by the minimum safeguards of Convention 108, which could then be ratified. This awareness resulted in the Data Protection Act 1984.

Report from the confidentiality working group (1984)

One of the reports of Edith Körner's health services information steering group, from the confidentiality working group, which was chaired by David Kenny, provides a much needed description of current best practice (Department of Health, 1984). It describes the confidentiality requirements of the NHS in some detail and with some clarity.

Survey and issues

The working group carried out a month-long survey in the medical records departments of six health authorities of the number of requests made for the release of patient information. The 1273 requests represented about 53 requests per week for each health authority and it was discovered that: 'Staff guidance on the maintenance of confidentiality was often little more than a brief talk about its importance during professional training or as part of an induction course'. The working group concluded that:

> There is very little legal protection of a patient's claim to confidentiality . . . If information is disclosed without his consent and without legal sanction, he can sue for breach of contract or breach of confidence although the cost of bringing civil proceedings is often prohibitive. In practice, however, he relies primarily for protection on the ethical codes of the professional bodies, on the administrative procedures and on staff recognising that confidentiality must be maintained if a relationship of trust between the patient and those caring for him is to be retained . . .
>
> A breach of confidentiality occurs if anyone, deliberately or by accident, gives information gained through his work to a third party without the patient's consent. Consent may, however, be implied, e.g. for information to be used for the continuing care of the patient, and there are certain, limited, circumstances when confidentiality has to be breached, e.g. to meet statutory requirements or because other public interest is considered more important than the patient's right to confidentiality. What is important is that a patient's data be disclosed only in specified circumstances and subject to approved procedures.

The theme of all the guidance in the report is that identifiable patient information must not be disclosed unless:

1 It is required for the care of the patient.
2 The patient has given consent for disclosure.
3 There is a legal requirement to disclose.
4 It is in the interests of the patient or of the general public that the information be disclosed and these interests are considered to override the duty to maintain confidentiality.

Handling the disclosure of personal health data

The handling of disclosure has five components.

1 The health authority must not disclose information to third parties without the patient's express or implied consent.
2 The health professionals have a duty to keep personal health information confidential and to disclose data only to those who need the information for the care of the patient.
3 These health professionals obtain the personal health data from patients and they entrust these data to the safe-keeping of health authorities on the understanding that their professional obligations will be respected.
4 The authority has a responsibility to ensure that internal disclosures to staff and authority members are not made for any other purposes than the health care of the patient concerned.
5 Personal health information relating to a person other than the patient must not be disclosed to third parties or staff, even with the consent of the patient, for any purpose other than the health care of that patient.

The only exceptions were the following categories of disclosure:

1 Required by law.
2 Required by court order.
3 Required for the investigation of a complaint or some essential management function.
4 Authorized by an ethical committee.
5 Required for the prevention, detection or prosecution of a serious crime.
6 Required to safeguard national security.
7 Required to prevent a serious risk to public health.

All exceptional disclosures were to be logged and monitored.

Recommendations

The fundamental recommendations of the working group were that each health authority should develop a policy for protecting and keeping confidential patient information. This policy should be publicized in patients' leaflets, in staff training, handbooks and contracts. This policy was to be supported by establishing management arrangements to ensure that it was implemented and audited. Finally, the health authority should be publicly accountable for its performance in this area by monitoring its policy and publishing statistics, 'at least annually', of 'the number and nature of the exceptional disclosures of patient data'.

Council of Europe

The Council of Europe is active in a wide variety of activities such as human rights, data protection, bioethics and its reputation is justifiably high. A number of the relevant recommendations are listed in the bibliography including those related to personal data used for scientific research and statistics (Council of Europe, 1983a), social security purposes (Council of Europe, 1983b), police sector purposes (Council of Europe, 1987), direct marketing (Council of Europe, 1986) and computerization of medical data in hospital services including university hospitals (Council of Europe, 1988). In respect of data protection and information systems security the following matters stand out. The Council of Europe Convention 108 for the Protection of Individuals with Regard to Automatic Processing of Personal Data is the current world data protection standard. The Council's *Regulations for Automated Medical Data Banks* (Council of Europe, 1981) are currently being revised. It has also developed recommendations on computer-related crime (Council of Europe, 1989).

Other international organizations

International Medical Informatics Association (IMIA)

IMIA grew out of Technical Committee 4 of the International Federation for Information Processing as a special interest group of national societies concerned with the development of health informatics in all its aspects. Within the UK the British Computer Society provides the representation from the various health informatics specialist groups. The objective is to provide the most effective representation from the health care informatics community, including all types of practising clinicians computer specialists concerned with health care systems and health care managers. A world congress, MEDINFO, is held every 3 years. IMIA working group 4 has produced two monographs entitled *Data Protection in Health Information Systems; Considerations and Guidelines* (Griesser *et al.*, 1980) and *Data Protection in Health Information Systems – Where do we Stand?* (Griesser *et al.*, 1983).

European Federation for Medical Informatics

The European Regional group of IMIA, the European Federation for Medical Informatics holds European congresses and has a working group which addresses data protection and security in health information systems.

European Commission

The EC is funding a programme of advanced informatics in medicine during the period 1992 to 1994. This includes the secure environment for information systems in medicine project which aims to provide public deliverables in respect of a harmonized approach to data protection and security in health information systems across Europe. This initiative has produced a useful monograph *Health Informatics: Handling Health Data in Europe in the Future* (European Commission, 1991). It provides a valuable successor to the monographs of IMIA working group 4.

European standards bodies

The main European standards body is the Comité Européen de Normalization (CEN) and it established a technical committee to address the issues of medical informatics standards. This committee secured representation from all the member bodies of CEN, which extends beyond the limits of the EC and published a *Directory of the European Standardization Requirements for Healthcare Informatics* (Comité Européen de Normalization, 1993). It has a working group dealing with health care security and privacy, quality and safety. In addition, the European workshop on open systems has established an expert group on health information systems as well as a security coordinating group. The UK has set up a corresponding pattern of bodies to feed information into the European groups and to receive the results of their work.

UK Data Protection Act 1984

The key definitions established by the Data Protection Act 1984 are listed below but they leave open a wide variety of issues which may be addressed by other legislation. The boundary between these areas will change with changes in the fundamental data protection legislation, such as may happen following the expected promulgation of a revised EC directive on data protection, and with the interpretation by the courts of the meaning of various aspects of the legislation. It should be noted that the UK Data Protection Act 1984 does not define the terms computer, privacy or ownership of data. The issue of the ownership of data is a particularly contentious issue and computer specialists have usually tried to focus attention on the much more specific matters of who requires access to a system in order to:

1 create a computer record;
2 read that record, or specific parts of it;
3 update that record, or specific parts of it;
4 amend that record, or specific parts of it;
5 delete that record, or specific parts of it.

Ownership is a very broad term and it tends to evoke concepts that may either not be applicable or may not yet have been defined in UK law. It is usually better to be more specific as to exactly what is intended rather than to face the ambiguities of an ill-defined concept which tends to generate expectations that cannot yet be fulfilled.

UK Data Protection definitions

The Data Protection Registrar has developed a series of eight guidelines to assist in the understanding of the act which form a convenient starting point for any examination of these issues (Data Protection Registrar's Office, 1989 a–h). The following definitions arise from the Data Protection Act 1984, together with the associated health order:

Data

Data means 'information recorded in a form in which it can be processed by equipment operating automatically in response to instructions for that purpose'.

Personal data

Personal data means 'data consisting of information which relates to a living individual who can be identified from that information (or from that and other information in the possession of the data user), including any expression of opinion about the individual but not any indication of the intentions of the data user in respect of that individual'. It is worth noting that Convention 108 comments that 'identifiable persons' means a person who can be easily identified: it does not cover the identification of persons by very sophisticated methods.

Living individuals

The UK Data Protection Act 1984 is not concerned with anything other than the automatic processing of the personal data of 'living individuals'. Information about dead individuals or 'legal persons' is not covered, nor is information which cannot be processed automatically and hence most manual records are excluded.

Exclusion of manual records

It is, however, clear that there are some areas of overlap where, for instance, material has been gathered with the intention of processing but which has as yet not been processed. Furthermore, information which has been obtained as a result of processing, such as a computer print-out, is subject to the law regarding disclosure even when the original computer records have been erased but is not accessible to a subject access request. Thus, a typical medical record which has laboratory test results from a laboratory computer included is additionally covered by the data protection rules on disclosure where disclosure from the rest of the record may only be covered by the professional rules of confidentiality.

Personal health data

Personal health data is defined in the health order as 'Personal Data consisting of information as to the physical or mental health of a data subject if:

1 the data are held by a health professional;
2 the data are held by a person other than a health professional but the information constituting the data was first recorded by or on behalf of a health professional'.

Health professionals

Health professionals are listed in the health order and comprise the following categories:

1 Registered medical practitioner.
2 Registered dental practitioner.
3 Registered optician.
4 Registered pharmaceutical chemist or druggist.

5 Registered nurse, midwife or health visitor.
6 Registered chiropodist, dietician, occupational therapist.
7 Registered orthoptist, physiotherapist.
8 Clinical psychologist, child psychotherapist, speech, art or music therapist employed by a health authority or equivalent.
9 Scientist employed by such an authority as a head of a department.

Processing

Processing means 'amending, augmenting, deleting or re-arranging the data or extracting the information constituting the data'. Any operation 'that is performed only for the purposes of preparing the text of documents' is excluded from the definition of processing. This distinction can be a very fine one and many activities that might be carried out for convenience on a computer go beyond this word processing exemption. References usually do not qualify because it would be normal to provide a reference and update it when subsequent references were requested. Bibliographies would need to be registered unless all the authors are no longer alive. In general, the best approach is to register some data usage if there is the least doubt that the activity is exempt either by definition or because it comes clearly within some exemption.

Processing personal data

Personal data is processed if any of these processing operations take place 'by reference to the data subject'. Virtually any computer system using standard software can be used to set up some data usage that requires registration and this need only take a very short time. For instance, a standard contact list would have name, address, telephone and fax numbers but even this is only exempt if it can be held that the telephone number is required 'for the purposes of distributing information'. However, if additional information is included as to the particular interests of the individuals in order to target this information distribution, then it must be registered. Certainly, if the record includes details of the nature of these contacts or notes about any discussions then these would also have to be registered. Again, it is usually easier to register in doubtful cases rather than expend the energy in ensuring that the staff keep within some rather complex exemption.

Data subject

Data subject is 'an individual who is the subject of Personal Data'.

Data user

Data user means a person who holds data and the person may be either a living individual or a 'legal person'. Within the NHS it is likely to be a health authority or a NHS trust or a general practitioner. The General Medical Services Committee of the BMA has issued a code of practice for general medical practitioners with a forward by the data protection registrar.

Holding personal data

Data is defined as being 'held by a person' if:

1 'the data form part of a collection of data processed or intended to be processed by or on behalf of that person'; and
2 'that person (either alone or jointly or in common with other persons) controls the contents and use of the data comprised in that collection'; and
3 'the data are in the form in which they have been or are intended to be processed' 'or (though not for the time being in that form) in a form into which they have been converted after being so processed and with a view to being further so processed on a subsequent occasion'.

Computer bureau

A computer bureau is operated by a person if:

1 'as agent for another person he causes data held by them to be processed'; or
2 'he allows other persons the use of equipment in his possession for the processing of data held by them'.

This definition is much wider than the colloquial understanding of a commercial computer bureau in that it includes any one person or organization who causes personal data to be processed for a data user or who allows a data user to process data on his or her equipment. It is, therefore, desirable for most organizations to register as both a data user and a computer bureau to cover situations where processing is undertaken for others or equipment made available to them.

Disclosing

Disclosing has a special meaning within the act as follows:

'Disclosing', in relation to data, 'includes disclosing information extracted from the data'. Where the 'identification of the individual who is the subject of Personal Data depends partly on the information constituting the data and partly on other information in the possession of the Data User, the data shall not be regarded as disclosed or transferred unless the other information is also disclosed or transferred'.

The following general exemptions to the non-disclosure provisions are included within the act:

1 Disclosure to a data subject or a person acting on his or her behalf.
2 The data subject or any such person has requested or consented to the particular disclosure.
3 The disclosure is by a data user or a person carrying on a computer bureau to his or her servant or agent for the purpose of enabling the servant or agent to perform his or her functions.
4 The person making the disclosure has reasonable grounds for believing that the disclosure falls within any of the foregoing paragraphs of this subsection.

There are a number of non-disclosure exemptions that will be noted later but these exemptions essentially form part of the definition of what is meant by disclosure.

Powers of the Data Protection Registrar

The first mechanism for enforcement of the Data Protection Act is the appointment of the registrar and staff. He or she has three specific major powers under the act to enable him or her to carry out these duties effectively. 'If the Registrar is satisfied that a registered person has contravened or is contravening any of the Data Protection principles' he or she may serve that person with an enforcement notice or a deregistration notice as a means of securing compliance with the act. He or she may serve a transfer prohibition notice where he or she is satisfied that the transfer is likely to lead to the contravention of any of the data protection principles. The data protection tribunal provides a mechanism for data users and computer bureaux to appeal against a refusal of registration or against any of these notices issued by the registrar.

It is clear from these requirements that a breach of the data protection principles is not, in itself, a criminal offence but non-registration or failure to comply with a notice requiring compliance with one or more of the principles is an offence. The cumulative effect of these powers can, in any specific situation, ensure that a data user does comply but the volume of data usage that the data protection registrar has to oversee is so extensive that it is believed that a cultural change will be required before compliance will become general. The current perception of much of NHS management is that data protection died when it became clear that the volume of subject access requests was low. However this perception is slowly changing as NHS trusts have to register as data users. It is believed that management will be more receptive to the security implications as they understand the issues more clearly and that the process of implementing the security within the NHS will bring the additional data protection activities along in its train.

Offences under the Data Protection Act 1984

The second major mechanism for the enforcement of the act is the courts. The act creates 10 new offences as follows:

1 Holding personal data without being registered or without having applied for registration.
2 Knowingly or recklessly holding data, using data, obtaining or disclosing data or transferring data other than as described in the register entry.
3 Knowingly or recklessly operating as a computer bureau in respect of personal data without being registered as such.
4 Not keeping a registered address up to date.
5 Knowingly or recklessly supplying the registrar with false or misleading information on application for registration or change of particulars.
6 Failure to comply with an enforcement notice.
7 Failure to comply with a transfer prohibition notice.
8 Knowingly or recklessly disclosing personal data without the data user's authority.
9 Intentional obstruction of a person executing a warrant.
10 Failure, without reasonable excuse, to give reasonable assistance in the execution of a warrant.

The act contains an exemption from prosecution clause which the registrar believes will apply to health authorities. However, it should be noted that authorities and their servants and agents will be guilty of an offence in law if they contravene the requirements of the act. This exemption does not in any way exempt health authorities from the need to register their data-holding and usage or the need for them fully to comply with the act. Their servants and agents can certainly be prosecuted even if the authority itself cannot, and of course the authority is open to claims for compensation for damage and associated distress.

Rights of data subjects to sue for damage and distress

The third major means of securing compliance with the act is the rights of the data subject to sue through the courts for compensation for damage and associated distress arising from:

1 Loss of data.
2 Destruction of data without the authority of the data user.
3 Disclosure of, or access to, the data without the authority of the data user.
4 Inaccurate data – data which are incorrect or misleading as to any matter of fact.

In addition, the courts may order a data user to comply with a subject access request or to rectify or erase incorrect data.

Warrants for entry and inspection

The powers of the registrar are very substantial in certain circumstances, bearing in mind that many organizations cannot function without their associated information systems. Warrants for entry and inspection can be issued on the application of the registrar if he or she has reasonable grounds for suspecting:

1 that a criminal offence under this act has been or is being committed;
2 that any of the data protection principles are being contravened by a registered person.

Such a warrant may allow the registrar 'to enter those premises, to search them, to inspect, examine, operate and test any data equipment found there and to inspect and seize any documents or other material found there'. Normally, adequate written notice will be given of the request for access but 'the foregoing provisions shall not apply if the judge is satisfied that the case is one of urgency or that compliance with those provisions would defeat the object of the entry'. Obstructing someone executing a warrant is an offence.

In an extreme case it would be possible to arrive one day to find that a warrant had been executed and documents removed to such an extent that the systems could no longer be safely operated. The minimum action of an individual facing the execution of a certified warrant is to request copies of anything that is seized.

The eight data protection principles

Although all eight data protection principles seem eminently reasonable, it is surprising how powerful they are as a body for assessing the way in which personal data has been handled. All eight principles apply to all personal data held by data users. The eighth principle, which requires that personal information is kept secure, is the only principle which has to be observed by computer bureaux. The data protection principles are described in part I of schedule I of the Data Protection Act 1984 and part II contains specific interpretations of these principles and they are discussed in the registrar's *Guideline 4* (Data Protection Registrar's Office, 1989d). However, the interpretation of these principles will develop as experience grows of their application in various circumstances and as decisions of the registrar, the data protection tribunal and the courts accumulate.

1 'The information to be contained in Personal Data shall be obtained, and Personal Data shall be processed, fairly and lawfully'.
2 'Personal Data shall be held only for one or more specified and lawful purposes'.
3 'Personal Data held for any purpose or purposes shall not be used or disclosed in any manner incompatible with that purpose or those purposes'.
4 'Personal Data held for any purpose or purposes shall be adequate, relevant and not excessive in relation to that purpose or those purposes'.
5 'Personal Data shall be accurate and, where necessary, kept up to date'.
6 'Personal Data held for any purpose or purposes shall not be kept for longer than is necessary for that purpose or those purposes'.
7 'An individual shall be entitled at reasonable intervals and without undue delay or expense to be informed by any Data User whether he holds Personal Data of which that individual is the subject; and to access to any such data held by the Data User; and where appropriate, to have such data corrected or erased'.

8 'Appropriate security measures shall be taken against unauthorised access to, or alteration, disclosure or destruction of, Personal Data and against accidental loss or destruction of Personal Data'.

Data protection within the NHS

The approach to handling the various aspects of data protection within the NHS is described in some detail in the *NHS Data Protection Handbook* (NHS management executive, 1988). There is no need to repeat the requirements at this level of detail but the key issues as seen in retrospect are indicated below.

NHS Data Protection Handbook

The key chapters in this handbook addressed the key issues as follows:

1 The Data Protection Act 1984.
2 Administration and implementation within the NHS.
3 Ensuring compliance within the NHS.
4 Subject access: the provision of copies of personal information for individuals.
5 Handling disclosure: the provision of personal information without consent.
6 A model NHS code of practice for complying with the Data Protection Act 1984.
7 Particular issues relating to specific application areas: child health systems.
8 Data protection requirements for computer systems.

The handbook also contains appendices which outline the functions that needed to be discharged to establish an appropriate data protection regime, a checklist for testing the adequacy of the data protection arrangements in NHS organizations and a series of relevant references to appropriate reading material and training videos.

The act allows the Secretary of State, the Home Secretary, to make orders relating to a variety of issues and these were duly embodied in the health order and the social work order. Following these orders the Department of Health issued a series of guidance circulars covering the interpretation of various aspects of these orders. These were:

1 *Data Protection Act 1984: Modified Access to Personal Health Information* (Department of Health, 1987a).

2 *Data Protection Act 1984: Social Work Orders etc: Individual's Right of Access to Information* (Department of Health, 1987b).
3 *Data Protection Act 1984: Modified Access to Personal Health Information* (Department of Health, 1987c).
4 *Data Protection Act 1984: Modified Access to Personal Health Information* (Department of Health, 1989).

The Data Protection Act 1984 has been discussed extensively in many other places but one specific issue that is important in health care is the extra provision in the health order that requires a health authority or NHS trust holding personal health information to seek the professional opinion of an 'appropriate health professional' before giving subject access in respect of whether there is any need to withhold any information in the record because it 'would be likely to cause serious harm to the physical or mental health of the Data Subject' or because it would be likely to disclose to the data subject the identity of another individual.

The *NHS Data Protection Handbook* is being updated to reflect the NHS reforms and NHS information systems security requirements.

Registration of data usage

As each NHS trust is launched it is necessary for it to arrange for its own data protection registration, thus finding itself in a similar position to that of health authorities when the Data Protection Act was first implemented during the period 1985/86. It is essential that all organizations processing personal data should register, as processing without being registered is an absolute offence under the 1984 Act. Clearly, the new NHS trusts are in a better position than the health authorities were originally when they first registered because their activities will already have been registered under its former authority and there is now some considerable experience of the working of the act since it came into force. The work of registration can best be handled in the following way:-

1 Carry out a rapid census of computing equipment and data usage.
2 Discuss the use of the computing equipment with relevant departmental heads or responsible specialists.
3 Obtain the parts of the health authority's previous registration relevant to the new trust.

4 Ensure that staff receive training in handling data protection.
5 Appoint an individual to handle the initial registration.
6 List draft registrations for each department. Once the basic data have been accumulated, it is possible to begin drafting the registrations to cover the work of each department, including:
   (a) Purposes of data usage.
   (b) Data subjects.
   (c) Data classes.
   (d) Data sources.
   (e) Data disclosures.
7 Cluster groups of similar draft registrations. Registrations with the same purpose and similar data subjects, classes, sources and disclosures from different departments can be included under one form in order to reduce the administrative effort of registration.
8 Categorize the registrations for the registrar. When the expected volume of subject access requests was fairly high it was considered useful to group registrations concerning:
   (a) Patient purposes.
   (b) Staff purposes.
   (c) Contractor and supplier purposes.
   (d) Word-processing facilities.
9 Prepare the forms for transmission to the data protection registrar.
10 Copy the forms and get them signed by the chief executive.
11 Post them by recorded delivery.

The Health and Social Work Orders and Department of Health guidance

In order to assist health authorities in the process of implementing the Data Protection Act 1984, the Department of Health issued a series of four health circulars outlining specific issues of which authorities needed to be aware (Department of Health, 1987a–c, 1989). The Health Order (HMSO, 1987a) defines personal health data, as indicated previously, as personal data consisting of information as to the physical or mental health of the data subject if:

1 the data are held by a health professional; or
2 the data are held by a person other than a health professional but the information constituting the data was first recorded by or on behalf of a health professional.

The order contains a list of health professionals. The purpose of defining personal health data was to allow certain limited exclusions to the general subject access arrangements of the Data

Protection Act 1984. These exclusions relate to information that:

1 'would be likely to cause serious harm to the physical or mental health of the Data Subject or any other person';
2 'would be likely to disclose to the Data Subject the identity of another individual (who has not consented to the disclosure of the information) either as a person to whom the information or part of it relates or as the source of the information or enable that identity to be deduced by the Data Subject either from the information itself or from a combination of that information and other information which the Data Subject has or is likely to have'.

It should be noted that personal health information as defined in the Health Order is still subject to the arrangements of the Health Order even when it is held, for instance, by a social services department. The Social Work Order (HMSO, 1987b) specifically excludes personal health data and it is necessary for them to obtain advice from an 'appropriate Health Professional' in respect of the issues of serious harm and the disclosure of identity.

Appoint a data protection coordinator to ensure compliance with the Data Protection Act 1984

The process of registration is only the initial step in complying with the Data Protection Act. It sets the scene and initiates a continuing process which requires human resources to make effective. The volume of human resources is not yet clear but the situation where many health authorities put in staff to handle their registration when the act came into force and then withdrew these staff when it became clear that there would not be a large volume of subject access requests has left them vulnerable to idiosyncratic complaints which the data protection registrar will have to investigate and which may reveal glaring gaps in their compliance with the act.

The approach of the NHS management executive's information management group was to initiate a programme from the Information Management Centre in Birmingham to link together all the issues of data protection and information systems security as a coherent whole, thus approaching the matter from the slightly different standpoint of security. However, in order to ensure that things happen it is necessary to assign someone the function of carrying out the work

required and they must be given a significant time and resources to carry out the necessary work. In addition, they must report to a sufficiently senior level of management to command the attention of other busy individuals within the organization. It is simply not sufficient to add the functions on to an already overcrowded job description with no prospect of the individual ever having time to carry out the necessary functions.

Non-disclosure exemptions

The Data Protection Act lists a series of non-disclosure exemptions in addition to those already noted in the definition of disclosure. They include the following items:

1 *Disclosures required by law.* These must be restricted to the specific items required by the law if this exemption is to apply. It does not cover general disclosures of other material but it is restricted to the items specified in the relevant law.
2 *Disclosure for national security.* This is not likely to apply frequently within the NHS but a certificate from a minister of the crown would indicate that this exemption was being invoked.
3 *Crime and taxation.* There is an exemption for the prevention or detection of crime, the apprehension or prosecution of offenders or the assessment or collection of any tax or duty. The Association of Chief Police Officers devised a code of practice which includes a form requesting personal information within this category. No NHS disclosure should take place in reply to a police request without a proper written request on such a form. The form does not constitute evidence that the request falls within the exemption but it should be taken into account by those needing to make a decision on such a request. Equivalent information and declarations should be sought from any taxation authorities with requests in this category.
4 *Urgently required for the prevention of injury or other damage to health of any person or persons.* The issue concerning disclosure in this case would be the reasonable belief that there was danger of injury or damage to someone's health. This concerns the normal operation of the NHS and relevant staff would be able to form professional judgements on this issue directly.

'Fair obtaining' of personal information

The registrar in *Guideline 4*, when discussing the implications of the data protection principles, outlines a number of issues that he would wish to examine when considering whether information contained in personal data has been 'obtained fairly' as required by the first principle:

1 Could the person supplying the information reasonably be expected to appreciate, without explanation, the identity of the data user and the purposes for which the information would be used or disclosed? If not, why did the data user not explain them to the person?
2 Did the data user explain why the information was required and why it might be used or disclosed? If so, was the explanation complete and accurate?
3 Did the person ask about the uses and disclosures of the information, and if so, what reply was made?
4 Was he or she under the impression that the information would be kept confidential by the data user? If so, was that impression justified by the circumstances and did the data user intend to preserve that confidence?
5 Was any unfair pressure used to obtain the information? Were any unjustified threats or inducements made or offered?
6 Was he or she improperly led to believe that he or she must supply the information, or that failure to supply it might disadvantage him or her?
7 Did the data user have any particular knowledge about the person from whom he or she obtained the information either because the person was one of a specific group, for example young people, or because he or she had a personal relationship with the person? If he or she had no such knowledge, would the explanation he or she gave concerning the collection and intended uses be understood by the ordinary person in the street?

If the Data User requests information about individuals either from themselves or from others, either orally or by filling in a form, the user should try to make sure that no-one is misled as to who the information is for, why the information is required or why it will be used or disclosed. If the identity of the Data Users and all the intended uses and disclosures are clear from the context in which the information is being supplied, no further explanation should be necessary. In some cases however, there may be additional uses and disclosures which the person supplying the information could not reasonably be expected to know about. Then the duty to obtain information fairly requires steps to be taken to make him aware of the true position. This will usually be done by briefly explaining the intended uses, disclosures and users. A general description will usually be sufficient. ·

The Data User must always be fair to the person from whom he obtains the information. The information might be about an individual different from the person from whom it was obtained. In some circumstances the concept of fairness may require him to give some thought to the individual to whom the information relates as well as to the person from whom it was obtained. The fairness has to be judged in each case in relation to a particular piece of information. If different pieces of information are obtained separately, each must be fairly obtained.

Guidance from the registrar regarding 'open postcards'

The age-old practice of some parts of the Health Service of sending out postcards inviting the attendance at hospitals or clinics for purposes which may or may not be indicated should be discontinued as it involves the disclosure of personal health information to anyone who happens to pass by.

Key issues in the implementation within the NHS

After the organization's data usage has been assessed and registered it is necessary to manage the whole data protection activity. The issues of establishing and maintaining compliance with the act are addressed in detail in the *NHS Data Protection Handbook*. It includes the basis for a code of practice together with job functions and checklists for compliance. The following brief outline indicates the approach to the main issues:

1 Establish a senior committee to oversee data protection and security issues.
2 Training and awareness of staff.
3 Establishing the arrangements for handling subject access requests.
4 Monitoring changes in data usage and equipment.
5 Maintenance of registration.
6 Compliance with data protection principles.
7 Establishing a secure environment for processing.

The implication of the reforms and what needs to be done

The NHS reforms, as set out in the NHS and Community Care Act 1990, involve much more sharing of personal health information in order to provide better health care both to individual patients and to populations of individuals. These improvements in the processes of handling health care are being accompanied by improvements in the associated confidentiality, data protection and security measures being adopted within the NHS. The following issues are the most significant at the present time:

Registration

The NHS reforms require that each NHS trust must register its data usage because it is an independent legal entity and it must address these issues directly at trust level, assuming responsibility for its activities. Since it is independent of the region it cannot rely on a region to get it out of financial difficulties arising from computer and legal disasters. Likewise, the removal of crown immunities from the NHS also tends to concentrate the minds of senior management on the issues of risk. All authorities and trusts must have the basic capability of understanding the relevant issues and adjusting their activities accordingly.

Contracting information

A major issue relates to the internal market where purchasers of health care purchase services from providers of health care. This third-party payment system is very similar to private health care arrangements where insurance companies pay for care. However, for the NHS it means that some very basic personal health information needs to be transferred from the providing unit to the purchasing unit in order to implement the correct level of payment. Because this process did not happen before the implementation of the NHS and Community Care Act 1990, the transfers of contract minimum data sets and information about extracontractual referrals has caused a considerable amount of concern and discussion. This issue is now seen as a security issue rather than a confidentiality issue because sufficient information is clearly required for handling and auditing payments but this does not mean that the purchasing unit can be slack about security and allow anyone other than those specifically involved to get access to this confidential information. The Department of Health has issued security guidelines in respect of confidentiality in the contracting environment (Department of Health, 1992a, b). Clearly, the practice of sending open faxes containing personal health information is unsatisfactory and should not happen except in an emergency. The

sender has no information about the location of the receiving fax machine or the availability of someone to handle the confidential information in a secure fashion.

Future developments

As the use of information systems spreads into more and more clinical areas and involves more and more people, it will be necessary to manage the security of information systems in a much more self-conscious fashion than has been the case so far if we are to avoid dangers to NHS patients. Already security issues are surfacing in both the computing and the national press in respect of health information systems. There have been disasters with radiation treatment planning, loss of emergency calls for ambulances and loss of follow-up in screening systems reported during the last year. All of these issues can lead to death or damage to patients and in governmental computing circles these dangers attract serious countermeasures to ensure that the systems are designed, operated and maintained correctly. These pressures are leading to the need for more explicit security to accompany the increasing use of information systems. The following aspects of the situation stand out for the future:

Increasing NHS dependence on information systems. These issues will become worse as the NHS develops more ambitious activities using the available information technology systems and networks to achieve an improved service for delivering health care. As the NHS relies more on its information systems to support its activities, it will need to assess all new developments from the point of view of the security issues and ensure that they are adequately addressed within the design and procurement specifications.

Greater reliance on computer records for clinical care. Clinicians are finding considerable benefits in the use of information systems to support their clinical care. When considering the inclusion of these new tools within their repertory, they must also examine the security issues that need to be addressed. Misinformed, mismanaged, misidentified, mistimed, mislaid, missing, mistaken health care and treatment can lead to patient damage and deaths arising from the information systems. Appropriate security must be included so that these side-effects are kept to an acceptable minimum when considered alongside the benefits derived from the systems.

European data protection and security environment. The EC has issued a draft directive concerning the protection of individuals in relation to the processing of personal data. This document was redrafted in 1992 for further consultation. It is expected that the harmonized European data protection and security environment will involve more security than the existing UK practice. When this is implemented it is likely that there will have to be another round of tightening of NHS data protection and security activities but by then it is hoped that we shall have implemented an effective information systems security policy which will be able to take these changes in its stride.

In addition, it will be necessary to keep track of other EC directives such as those on *The Minimum Safety and Health Requirements for Work with Display Screen Equipment* (European Commission, 1990) which sets standards for visual display units and associated facilities and on *Standardisation in the Field of Information Technology and Telecommunications* (European Commission, 1986) which affects the purchasing of information systems.

Circulation of health records around the NHS and Europe. The security problems will become worse as health records are networked around not only the NHS but also across Europe. Issues of identification, authorization, integrity verification, non-repudiation of receipt and many other security services will have to be invoked within our standards to ensure that these processes are handled in a secure and a safe fashion.

Computer records as the legal health record. Eventually, we shall reach that original objective of the early medical informaticians who sought to provide the clinicians with a better health record than could be provided on paper. This objective has proved much more elusive than was anticipated. When the computer record becomes the legal record, either because it is impossible to find one's way around the paper record or because there is nowhere to store the

volume of paper required to back it up, it will be necessary to establish a number of procedures to ensure that it can produce accurate and up-to-date information; that it is clear who entered what information into the record; that the record has not been tampered with and cannot be repudiated and that it can be produced in evidence in court in a legally acceptable state.

Access to health records within the NHS

The process of obtaining copies of health records was set in train in the UK by the Data Protection Act 1984. Subject access is the generic name for this process and the essential components of this process were developed in connection with the Data Protection Act 1984 which handles computerized personal health information, while another two acts deal with non-computerized personal health information.

The Data Protection Act 1984

The fundamental issues relating to subject access involve an assessment of whether information in the health record is likely to cause serious harm or to disclose the identity of another individual.

Where the data user (person who has registered the data usage) is a health professional his or her judgement on these issues would normally be all that is required, although there may be situations where it would be helpful to seek the views of other health professionals. However, where the data user is not a health professional (i.e. is a health authority or NHS trust) that data user is required to seek the views on these issues of the 'most appropriate health professional' before either supplying information to or withholding information from the data subject.

The Department of Health (1987d) has issued guidance which includes a flowchart designed to indicate the various steps in the process of handling subject access under the Data Protection Act 1984.

What is a valid request?

A valid subject access consists of a written or typed request which includes sufficient information to identify the data subject and sufficient information to locate the personal data specified.

The 40-day period allowed for handling the request starts when the organization has received the request, as distinct from the time at which it has been received within the Data Protection Office. It is important that staff should know what to do with any such request, to avoid having a request lying around on someone's desk or circulating round the internal postal system using up time that may be badly needed later. If the request is being made by another individual on behalf of the data subject, then it will be necessary to identify that individual as well as the data subject and the authority or authorization to receive the personal data requested. There may also be consents from third parties that might be identified in the health record which would, if accepted as genuine and relevant, avoid the need to withhold some information from the subject access procedures, but there is no requirement for the health authority to seek such consent.

Handling requests from or on behalf of children

The handling of subject access from children is very complex and there are a number of difficult issues to address:

1 In England, if the child can understand the implications of his or her request, then he or she can initiate it directly. In Scotland the law is more specific as 'minors' (girls aged 12 and over or boys aged 14 and over) can generate their own requests without any test of understanding, which in specific cases may mean that very young children may understand and very old children may not understand. For younger children ('pupils') the rights are vested in the pupil's 'tutor'.
2 Where requests come from adults or organizations, it is important to establish the legal standing of the adults and the basis on which the request is being made. Essentially, if the child can make his or her own requests then any other subject access request requires his or her consent, which should accompany the request. If the child cannot make his or her own request, the request must, nevertheless, be in the child's interest, not in the interests of some other person or organization. Also, it will be necessary to establish the legal basis on which it is being made.
3 There may be a request for disclosure from the record, as distinct from a subject access request, but this is a clinical issue which should be handled by the clinicians and the administration in the normal way, not via the mechanism of a subject access request. The issues here will be likely to be those of

good clinical practice and current law concerned with the care of children rather than that of the Data Protection Act 1984, although even here it is important for the data protection registration to be kept abreast of current practice in terms of the purposes of the data usage, the data subjects, the classes of data held and the sources and disclosures of that data.

How do you find and obtain all the specified personal data?

A subject access request covers all data which may be held on many different information systems. To help track this down it is helpful to have a list of all individuals and departments with systems indicating the scope of their data.

Who is the 'most appropriate health professional'?

The most appropriate health professional is described in the Health Order as:

1 The medical practitioner or dental practitioner who is currently or was most recently responsible for the clinical care of the data subject in connection with the matters to which the information which is the subject of the request relates.
2 Where there is more than one such practitioner, the practitioner who is most suitable to advise on the matters to which the information which is the subject of the request relates.
3 Where there is no practitioner falling within the subparagraphs above, a health professional who has the necessary experience and qualifications to advise on the matters to which the information which is the subject of the request relates.

What information may be withheld?

The judgements formed by the health professionals are professional clinical views which should be entered into the clinical record for future reference and so that the data protection registrar or a court could verify that the law had been complied with. As much information as possible must be made available subject to withholding the information in the health record that:

1 would be likely to cause serious harm to the physical or mental health of the data subject;
2 would be likely to disclose to the data subject the identity of another individual (who has not consented to the disclosure of the information) either

as a person to whom the information or part of it relates or as the source of the information or enable that identity to be deduced by the data subject either from the information itself or from a combination of that information and other information that the data subject has or is likely to have.

The withholding information that would identify an individual does not apply to health professionals where they are functioning in their professional capacity. The data user is obliged to provide as much information as possible subject to withholding material coming within these closely defined categories.

Obtaining the health professional's advice

It can be difficult getting the most appropriate health professional's advice within the allowed 40 days, especially where that individual is not readily accessible to the data user, but the definition includes allowance for the possibility of getting appropriate advice even where the individual who would be most obviously suitable is not available. It is important to note that the definitions in the health order, the social work order and the access to personal files (Social Services) Regulations Order relating to the Access to Personal Files Act 1987 all define personal health information in the same way and require the issues of 'serious harm' and third-party identification to be advised by an appropriate health professional.

Time limit for providing access

The time allowed for handling a subject access request is 40 calendar days from the time when the organization has received a valid request. The maximum fee for a subject access request is currently £10 for all personal data held under a single registration.

Providing a copy of the record

It may in some cases be helpful or convenient to show an individual the computer record on a computer screen but the subject access procedures require that the individual is supplied with a physical copy of the record which may be typewritten, hand-written or computer-produced. All local codes must be translated into their practical meaning and generally abbreviations should be avoided. The issue is the information held in the record, not what the implications are for the patient arising out of that information. It is generally believed that it is good practice to supply the information to the data subject, indicating that the information available to him or her under the Data Protection Act 1984 is enclosed, without indicating whether or not any information has been withheld in these procedures. It is felt that to indicate that information had been withheld because it was likely to cause the data subject serious harm could do even more damage than supplying it fully in the first place. In some cases the appropriate health professional may wish to hand over the information during an interview but this would have to be done during the 40 days allowed. This is to be encouraged where it is feasible as it could address the implications of the information in the record but this should be addressed during the normal clinical consultations and frequently it would not be feasible or necessary.

Advising the general practitioner

Where the health record is kept by a hospital it might be useful for the information to be supplied to the data subject to be copied to the data subject's general medical practitioner but this should only be done with the data subject's consent.

Administration

The process of handling subject access requests is quite complex because most health authorities do not have an integrated index of their computer-based patient files. It is therefore necessary to search all the systems which might have files relating to the individual concerned. This is time-consuming and the process of obtaining clinical advice can also be time-consuming. However, the volume of requests received so far has been sufficiently small as to allow the process detailed personal attention. Any serious increase in the volume of requests would be likely to need a revision of the approach and the implementation of an information system to assist in handling the processes involved.

Access to Medical Reports Act 1988

This act which came into effect on 1 January 1989, and is concerned with medical reports requested for employment or insurance purposes. It utilizes the same basic concepts as the Data Protection Act 1984 and the associated Health Order. A medical report is a report 'relating to the physical or mental health of the individual prepared by a medical practitioner who is, or has been responsible for the clinical care of the individual'. The act sets up arrangements to ensure that medical reports are not requested unless the individual is notified of the proposal to request such a report and has consented to such an application. It provides that the individual can request to see the report or have a copy of it before it is supplied to the person requesting it, subject only to the medical practitioner withholding information that 'would in the opinion of the practitioner be likely to cause serious harm to the physical or mental health of the individual or others or would indicate the intentions of the practitioner in respect of the individual'. Information can also be withheld if it would reveal the identity of another individual – not a health professional within the meaning of the Health Order under the Data Protection Act 1984, who has not consented to this disclosure. There are a number of not very complex provisions relating to these arrangements and the individual may seek to have matters which 'the individual considers to be incorrect or misleading' corrected or else to have a record of his or her views attached to the report if the medical practitioner is unwilling to amend. The medical reports have to be kept by the practitioner for 6 months and 21 days are allowed for handling the issues of consent. A court can require that any individual failing to comply or likely to fail to comply with the requirements of the act shall comply with those requirements.

Access to Health Records Act 1990

This act provides access to manual health records in a complementary and similar fashion to that provided for in the Data Protection Act 1984, except that there are a number of differences which need to be taken into account. The main difference is that it is not retrospective and there is no automatic right to records made prior to 1 November 1991. This is unlike the Data Protection Act, which does not take into account when a record was made but only whether it is currently 'held'. This difference is there to protect health professionals who may have made

injudicious remarks in their records in the belief that they would never be seen by their patients. There is a small loophole in this blanket exclusion where knowledge of the earlier material may be necessary to the understanding of the subsequent record.

The same period of 40 calendar days has been adopted for the access to be completed but if the patient is undergoing treatment (phrased as: the record has been added to within the previous 40 days), then only 21 days are allowed for the access and the copy of the record must be provided without any fee other than for postage or photocopying. In other circumstances, the maximum fee that can be charged is the same as that for subject access under the Data Protection Act 1984, exclusive of postage and photocopying.

The Department of Health has provided detailed guidelines for handling the requirements of the act in Access to Health Records Act 1990 (Department of Health, 1991). This guidance includes a detailed flowchart to guide the person handling the access request through the various stages of the process. In some authorities and NHS trusts these requirements are being handled by the medical records departments while in others they are being handled by the data protection officer because the processes are so similar.

It is worth noting that under the Data Protection Act 1984, the printed output from a computer system is still subject to the act in respect of disclosure control, even where the original computer record no longer exists because it has been erased. However, there is no subject access to such material under the Data Protection Act 1984. This situation arises in many medical records where laboratory reports may not be kept in computer form for lack of computer storage space. However, access to these results would come under the Access to Health Records Act 1990.

Access to Personal Files Act 1987

These requests arise from a social services department responding to a request under this act and requiring advice on some personal health information which had been made available from a health professional or a health authority, or was believed to have originated from such. On the receipt of such a request the social services authority must request advice from the health authority concerned or from an appropriate health professional within 14 days of receiving the request.

Information systems security

In reviewing the organization's security, the following strategy provides a basis for gradually building up confidence in its security capacity:

Data protection registration

There is an absolute requirement for registration under the Data Protection Act 1984. It is therefore important to ensure that the organization is registered and that its registration reflects current practice.

A top-level information systems security policy

The next step is the development and implementation of an information systems security which describes the organization's requirements in terms of security and which can be understood by all concerned. A top-level information systems security (Department of Health, 1992c) has been promulgated from the management executive as a basis for NHS policy development.

Baseline security

The NHS Information Management Centre has developed a series of basic security measures which it believes should be implemented throughout the NHS. These measures are outlined in *Basic Information Systems Security* (NHS Management Executive, 1992) and they should be installed throughout the organization. They will not provide adequate security for many information systems but they ensure a reasonable foundation for future development.

Small systems security

The Information Management Centre has licensed a CRAMM-compatible methodology (see below) for assessing the security of small systems and this approach provides an easily utilized follow-up to baseline security, allowing one to handle a multitude of small systems, thus clearing the way for serious work on the major systems.

Risk analysis and CRAMM

The process of handling risk analysis is a complex one that requires a systematic approach.

The Central Computing and Telecommunications Agency's risk analysis and management methodology (CRAMM) provides considerable assistance in handling this process so that the security to be installed is not idiosyncratically dependent on a particular consultant providing advice or the information technology representative security who last made contact with the organization. It is a rigorous and demanding methodology which requires training to use and serious attention from senior management, but it can tease out the fundamental security issues facing an organization (Central Computing and Telecommunications Agency, 1993).

System security policies

Each system needs to be governed by a compatible system security policy also based on the conclusions of a risk analysis of the particular environment in which the system operates and which outlines how its security is intended to function.

Security management

Handling security management is a difficult issue because a wide variety of specialists are involved. Their activities need to be coordinated and managed as a whole so that the various specialists understand the implications for information systems security which arise from their activities and how their work needs to be modified to include their contribution to the information systems security environment. Examples of the widely dispersed nature of these include:

1 Fire officer.
2 Security officer.
3 Data protection officer.
4 Works department.
5 Personnel department.
6 Supplies department.
7 Auditors.
8 Information technology department.
9 Line management.
10 Users.

UK Computer Misuse Act 1990

Under the Computer Misuse Act, access is defined as follows:

A person secures access to any program or data held in a computer if by causing a computer to perform any function he:

- alters or erases the program or data;
- copies or moves it to a storage medium other than that in which it is held or to a different location in the storage medium in which it is held;
- uses it;
- has it output from the computer in which it is held (whether by having it displayed or in any other manner).

There are supplementary definitions of use, output, unauthorized access and modification. The act defines three offences:

1 Unauthorized access to program or data.
2 Unauthorized access with intent to commit further offences.
3 Unauthorized modification of the contents of any computer.

Copyrights, Designs and Patents Act 1988

Software piracy involves illegal copying of programs beyond the licence purchased. The tradition of copying programs grew up as part of the automatic security arrangements at a time when computer media were much less reliable and then it developed with groups of users sharing their software via networks or otherwise. However, from the point of view of security, it is important that all software should be legally obtained and used. Illegal copying and use of software is defined in the Copyrights, Designs and Patents Act 1988.

Conclusion

The establishment of these basic aspects of data protection and security constitute the initial steps in beginning to address the issues. The top-level information systems security policy will, if implemented from the highest levels of management, provide the basis on which all the other more detailed work can be developed. The data protection registrations must be in place and monitored and thereafter baseline security can be installed, together with some basic awareness and training activities across the organization, followed by small systems examination of the many isolated systems. Then serious work on risk analysis using CRAMM can be undertaken on some major systems. These are only the first steps but they naturally lead on to the consequential activities required to develop a security culture within the NHS that will allow the NHS to use its information systems with confidence in the knowledge that they are safe and secure.

References

Central Computing and Telecommunications Agency (1993) *CRAMM 1991 User Manual*. CCTA, IT Security and Privacy Group, Riverwalk House, 157–161 Millbank, London, SW1P 4RT.

Chalton, S. Gaskill, S. and Sterling, J.A.L. (1988) *Encyclopaedia of Data Protection*, vols 1 and 2. Sweet & Maxwell, London.

Comité Europée de Normalization (1993) *Directory of the European Standardization Requirements for Healthcare Informatics and Programme for the Development of Standards*. CEN, Brussels (also available from BSI secretariat to IST/35 at NHS Information Management Centre, 15 Frederick Road, Edgbaston, Birmingham, B15 1JD, UK).

Council of Europe (1981a) *Convention 108 for the Protection of Individuals with Regard to Automatic Processing of Personal Data*. Council of Europe, Strasbourg.

Council of Europe (1981b) *Recommendation on Automated Medical Data Banks* R[81]1. Council of Europe, Strasbourg.

Council of Europe (1983a) *Recommendation on the Protection of Personal Data Used for Scientific Research and Statistics* R[83]10. Council of Europe, Strasbourg.

Council of Europe (1983b) *Recommendation on the Protection of Personal Data Used for Social Security Purposes* R[86]1. Council of Europe, Strasbourg.

Council of Europe (1986) *Recommendation on the Protection of Personal Data Used for the Purposes of Direct Marketing* R[85]20. Council of Europe, Strasbourg.

Council of Europe (1987) *Recommendation Regulating the Use of Personal Data in the Police Sector* R[87]15. Council of Europe, Strasbourg.

Council of Europe (1988) *Report on Computerisation of Medical Data in Hospital Services including University Hospitals* R[87]23. Council of Europe, Strasbourg.

Council of Europe (1989) *Recommendation on Computer-Related Crime* R[89]9. Council of Europe, Strasbourg.

Data Protection Registrar's Office (1989a) *Guideline 1. Introduction to the Act*. Data Protection Registrar's Office, London.

Data Protection Registrar's Office (1989b) *Guideline 2. The Definitions*. Data Protection Registrar's Office, London.

Data Protection Registrar's Office (1989c) *Guideline 3. The Register and Registration*. Data Protection Registrar's Office, London.

Data Protection Registrar's Office (1989d) *Guideline 4. The Data Protection Principles*. Data Protection Registrar's Office, London.

Data Protection Registrar's Office (1989e) *Guideline 5. Individuals' Rights*. Data Protection Registrar's Office, London.

Data Protection Registrar's Office (1989f) *Guideline 6. The Exemptions*. Data Protection Registrar's Office, London.

Data Protection Registrar's Office (1989g) *Guideline 7. Enforcement and Appeals*. Data Protection Registrar's Office, London.

Data Protection Registrar's Office (1989h) *Guideline 8. Summary for Computer Bureaux*. Data Protection Registrar's Office, London.

Department of Health (1984) *Guidance, produced under the aegis of the Steering Group on Health Services Information (chaired by Edith Körner). A Report from the Confidentiality Working Group chaired by David Kenny*. HMSO, London.

Department of Health (1987a) *Data Protection Act 1984: Modified Access to Personal Health Information* HC(87)14. HMSO, London.

Department of Health (1987b) *Data Protection Act 1984: Social Work Orders etc: Individual's Right of Access to Information*, HC(87)15. HMSO, London.

Department of Health (1987c) *Data Protection Act 1984: Modified Access to Personal Health Information*. HC(87)26. HMSO, London.

Department of Health (1987d) *Guidance, Data Protection Act 1984: Modified Access to Personal Health Information*. HC(87)26. HMSO, London.

Department of Health (1989) HC(89)29 *Data Protection Act 1984: Modified Access to Personal Health Information*. HC(89)29. HMSO, London.

Department of Health (1991) *Guidance, Access to Health Records Act 1990*. NHS Management Executive, HSG(91)6. HMSO, London.

Department of Health (1992a) NHS Management Executive. *Handling Confidential Information in Contracting: A Code of Practice*, issued with Executive Letter EL(92)60. HMSO, London.

Department of Health (1992b) NHS Management Executive. *Guidance on Extra Contractual Referrals*, issued with Executive Letter EL(92)60. HMSO, London.

Department of Health (1992c) NHS Management Executive. *Information Systems Security: A Top Level Policy for the NHS*, issued with Executive Letter EL(92)60, developed by the NHS Information Management Centre, Birmingham, HMSO, London.

European Commission (1986) *Standardisation in the Field of Information Technology and Telecommunications*. Directive 87/95/EEC. European Commission, Brussels.

European Commission (1990) *Directive on the Minimum Safety and Health Requirements for Work with Display Screen Equipment*. Directive 90/270/EEC. European Commission, Brussels.

European Commission (1991) *Health Informatics: Handling Health Data in Europe in the Future*. European Commission, Brussels.

Griesser, G., Bakker, A., Danielsson, J. *et al.* (1980) *Data Protection in Health Information Systems: Considerations and Guidelines*. North Holland, Amsterdam.

Griesser, G., Jardel, J. P., Kenny, D. J. and Sauter, K. (1983) *Data Protection in Health Information Systems: Where do we Stand?* North Holland, Amsterdam.

HMSO (1987a) *The Health Order*. HMSO, London.

HMSO (1987b) *The Social Work Order*. HMSO, London.

NHS management executive (1988) *The NHS Data Protection Handbook*. Information Management Centre, 15 Frederick Road, Edgbaston, Birmingham, B15 1JD, UK.

NHS management executive (1992) Information Management Group. *Basic Information Systems Security*. Information Management Centre, 15 Frederick Road, Edgbaston, Birmingham, B15 1JD, UK.

7.6 Using data for medical audit

Charles D. Shaw

National guidance

Health departments

UK

Among a variety of proposals for change in the organization of the NHS, *Working for Patients* outlined a plan for the introduction of medical audit (Department of Health, 1989a). This was amplified in the subsequent working paper number 6 (Department of Health, 1989b) and Scottish working paper number 2 (Scottish Home and Health Department, 1989a). Medical audit was defined as 'the systematic, critical analysis of the quality of medical care including the procedures used for diagnosis and treatment, the use of resources, and the resulting outcome and quality of life for the patient'.

England

Health circular HC(91)2 (Department of Health, 1991a) outlined the arrangements which health authorities and trusts were required to make in order to ensure that a framework for medical audit was in place by April 1991. Guidance on implementing medical audit in general practice was issued in HC(90)15 (Department of Health, 1990a).

From 1990, the Department of Health allocated funding to regions for audit according to the number of whole-time-equivalent consultants and on receipt of satisfactory implementation plans. Initially these plans were to specify how audit was to be organized and what resources were needed in terms of information, staff and training (Department of Health, 1989c). Later plans were to specify how audit funding would support postgraduate and continuing education, how hospitals would collaborate with general practice and community services, how the effectiveness and appropriateness of medical interventions would be measured, and how the effectiveness of the audit programme itself would be assessed (Department of Health, 1991b). From 1994 central funding is unlikely to be identified separately for audit unless agreements are reached for regional topslicing.

The standing medical advisory committee, at the request of the Secretaries of State for Health and for Wales, presented a valuable summary of the history, principles and practice of audit which was distributed to every doctor in England and Wales (Department of Health, 1990b).

Northern Ireland

Expanding on working paper number 6 (Department of Health, 1989b), the circular *Medical Audit in the Hospital and Community Health Services* (Department of Health and Social Security, 1990) outlined the functions of the Northern Ireland regional audit advisory committee, also responsible for audit in general practice, and of the four area audit advisory committees. Time required for each doctor was estimated at one-quarter to one-half session per week to take part in a regular audit programme – which should be incorporated in future job descriptions. Guidance on general practice was included in a separate circular. Funding was included in one global allocation for developments under the NHS review.

Scotland

Guidance on Implementation of Medical Audit, based on Scottish working paper number 2 (Scottish Home and Health Department, 1989a), was issued to general managers of health boards and the Common Services Agency in August 1989 (Scottish Home and Health Department, 1989b). Area audit committees were to report to the national clinical resource and audit group (CRAG), chaired by the chief medical officer. CRAG is responsible for determining national audit strategy, identifying and disseminating good practice, coordinating audit at national level and monitoring audit training.

Wales

Draft guidance on implementation in the hospital and community dental service was issued in WHC(90)32 (Welsh Office, 1990). The Welsh advisory group on medical audit (WAGMA) was set up by the Secretary of State for Wales to promote audit nationally, to organize audit of regional and small specialties and to assist the Welsh Office in dissemination of advice to district health authorities and family practitioner committees. WAGMA offered detailed advice in November 1990 on a range of practical issues, including the location of specialty audit, management support, role of audit committee chairpersons and support staff, confidentiality and links to postgraduate and continuing education (Welsh Advisory Group on Medical Audit, 1990).

Medical royal colleges

Many of the colleges and national professional associations have issued advice on the organization and practice of audit within their specialty. In general, these cover:

1 *Purpose of audit*: to identify opportunities and to implement improvement in the quality of medical care, medical training and continuing education, and effective use of resources.
2 *Organization*: responsibility for implementing audit rests with consultant medical staff; effective coordination is required within and between specialties at local, regional and national level.
3 *Methods*: audit should involve the objective peer review of patterns of care, be sensitive to the expectations of patients and other clinical disciplines and be based on scientific evidence of good medical practice.
4 *Issues for audit*: all types of patient, clinical condition and medical activity should be eligible for audit; priorities should be defined locally.
5 *Resources*: medical staff should be provided with the time, data, technical assistance, library support and training required to fulfil the agreed programme of audit.
6 *Records*: the documentation of medical care and of medical audit should comply with defined standards of good practice.

These general statements may be expanded into specifications for defining medical audit or for the purpose of contracts (Shaw, 1991).

Organization of audit

Structure

National

Although Northern Ireland, Scotland and Wales each have a national body to oversee the development of medical audit, in England regional audit committees have no national forum in which to share data, methods and results. Within specialties, this function has been largely absorbed by the medical royal colleges.

Local/regional

Although every doctor and specialty needs to identify primarily with one audit group, arrangements should allow alternative combinations of staff which are appropriate for occasional review of a particular topic or regular discussion of common interests.

The centrally defined responsibilities of local audit committees are to:

1 ensure a comprehensive mechanism and programme for local audit, in which all doctors participate;
2 produce an annual report summarizing local activity;
3 produce an annual forward programme;
4 ensure the confidentiality of audit results relating to individual patients and doctors.

The prime focus for audit is within provider units and many former district audit committees have been reformed to reflect their separation from the purchasers. But the need to share comparable results among a peer group argues in many specialties for a supradistrict or regional forum which, like postgraduate education, transcends local management boundaries. This hybrid of local and (sub)regional audit needs to be explicitly defined between audit committees to ensure that it is comprehensive and adequately supported with personnel, data and finance. It also requires agreement between clinicians and managers on reporting mechanisms and on access to data generated by audit.

Whatever location a specialty chooses for its routine audit activity, regional specialty subcommittees can contribute:

1 Agreement on sharing subjects, methods and results of audit undertaken locally.

2 Agreement on common local minimum data sets, including definitions to be used and routine clinical statistics to be produced.
3 Coordination of specialty training for audit within the region.
4 Liaison with regional advisers and national colleges, faculties and associations.
5 Reporting to the regional audit committee on general issues facing the specialty.

In England, projects of regional medical audit committees have included:

1 Policy on definition of audit, confidentiality, data capture.
2 Advice on the allocation of funds, on audit priorities and on the content of annual plans and reports.
3 Training seminars.
4 Publication of a regular newsletter.
5 Establishment of a regional resource centre.

Integrating audit

Hospital quality improvement and clinical audit

The emphasis on audit in the White Paper was on medical and dental care, yet the same ethical responsibility for self-regulation is shared by other clinical professions which have received much less tangible support. In reality, few clinical activities exclusively involve doctors; arrangements for medical audit should allow for joint review of appropriate topics (such as amputees, stroke rehabilitation, diabetic care) with other professions in the clinical team.

Community and general practitioner services

Community medical and dental services have the same requirements as hospital-based specialties to implement audit. Community-based consultants and some clinical medical officers have integrated their audit activities with hospital departments such as paediatrics or gynaecology, but many community units are underresourced and underrepresented on local audit committees dominated by acute hospital services. It is also important for local audit committees to liaise with Family Health Service Authority-based medical audit advisory groups (MAAGs) and to ensure adequate cover without duplication of activities.

MAAGs coordinate audit among local general practitioners and are responsible for ensuring that all practices take part by April 1992. In England and Wales, a framework for collaboration is provided by cross-representation (often by the two chairpersons) between the local audit committee and the MAAG. In Scotland and Northern Ireland closer liaison is provided by having one group to coordinate audit in both sectors at area level.

The Department of Health specifically encourages joint projects, for example, on locally agreed management policies, referral practices and communication. Although the scope of available data varies between practices, many have a limited diagnostic index which can identify patients with chronic diseases which lend themselves to review (such as asthma, diabetes, hypertension and epilepsy).

Medical education

Teaching of audit

If audit is an integral part of clinical practice, it should eventually be taught by example to students and juniors on the wards. In its infancy, it is a fashionable addition to courses in epidemiology or management – or a course in itself. Some such courses are aimed specifically at junior medical staff, but more are attended predominantly by consultants. Many hospitals offer 1-day introductory seminars on general issues, but do not have the resources to provide practical tuition for individual specialties; this is better organized on a collaborative basis with the help of regional specialty committees and the appropriate national colleges, faculties and specialty associations.

Education as a response to audit

The scope for education to implement change and 'close the feedback loop' is limited by the type of opportunity for improvement which audit identifies. In practice, audit does not often reveal a lack of knowledge or skills, which might be amenable to improvement by education, or indeed a lack of resources; problems more commonly result from the policy of the service or from the organization of the available resources, such as:

1 Lack of policy (e.g. on control of intensive care beds).
2 Deviation from policy (e.g. antibiotic prescribing).
3 Lack of system (e.g. for avoiding redundant clinic visits).
4 Failure to consult (e.g. by juniors prior to emergency surgery).
5 Failure to record (e.g. what information is given to a patient).
6 Inappropriate use or servicing of equipment (e.g. calibration of sphygmomanometers).

Most amenable to educational development are the knowledge and skills of individual doctors. One issue raised by audit in many specialties is the volume–outcome link; in the hands of frequent operators, technical procedures and decisions tend to lead to better results than in the hands of occasional operators. Apart from technical skills, audit may highlight training needs in decision-making and in interpersonal skills such as leadership and communication.

Mitchell and Fowkes (1985) have summarized overseas experience of educational follow-up of audit, and tested it in the UK. Essential ingredients for implementing change include:

1 Explicit definition of policy.
2 Local ownership of definition.
3 General dissemination of policy.
4 Measurement of individual performance.
5 Feedback of results of measurement.
6 Peer review of results and of policy.
7 Explicit agreement on further action.
8 Repeat cycle to show progress.

Audit as an educational tool

Audit offers a bridge between the principles of medicine and personal clinical experience, between patterns of practice and individual patients. It does not supplant bedside teaching or case presentations but it adds a framework for learning and comparing in objective but general terms that converge medical science and clinical practice. For example, audit enables discussion on:

1 *Standards*: review of literature, explication of good practice and criteria for measuring it.
2 *Records*: definition of contents, accuracy and legibility.
3 *Data*: availability and application of statistics in clinical practice.
4 *Variations*: social, epidemiological, clinical and economic factors affecting uptake, process and outcome of services.

5 *Management*: effecting change in individuals and in the organization.

If topics selected for audit are of general interest (not the personal hobby of one individual), if cases reviewed are recent enough to include the current junior staff, and if all doctors take part, then it can be an effective and interesting activity. Consultants responsible for audit should ensure that junior staff are not left to run audit on their own, are not subjected to repeated criticism of record-keeping and are not expected to devote hours to data capture which could be done by audit assistants or other staff.

Audit of the educational process

On general principles, audit of any endeavour needs three elements: a defined expectation, a mechanism for measuring achievement and the means to implement change. Applied to the educational process, this implies:

1 *Expectations*: an agreed strategy for postgraduate and continuing education should define responsibilities, processes and outcome objectives at local and regional level.
2 *Measurement*: accurate, current information and effective monitoring mechanisms should be available to evaluate the educational process. This requires collation of data from each locality on staffing levels, appointments, accreditation visits, educational facilities (activity, supervision, funding) and individual academic and career achievements.
3 *Change*: the regional postgraduate department should be able to influence educational policy and practice at local and regional level through the medical advisory and management structures, and in collaboration with the medical royal colleges, faculties and training committees.

Audit and management

Managers are held responsible for the overall running of hospitals, including the effectiveness and efficiency of medical services; they need to know there is a mechanism for internal quality assurance, to see evidence that it is effective, to agree the resources required and to ensure that effective remedial action is taken when deficiencies are identified. At least, it is essential to agree:

1 Specifications for audit: what it is and how it will be recognized.
2 Structure for audit: links and activities in other units.

3 Managerial input to audit agenda and process.
4 Accountability of audit staff (managerial and professional).
5 Resources provided for audit (time, data, help).
6 Budgetary authority for audit funds.
7 Funding arrangements.
8 Access to data generated by audit.

Data systems designed for resource management cannot be assumed to support audit, or vice versa. The two activities have:

1 Common need for basic clinical data on clinical activity.
2 Common costs for data capture and verification.
3 Common challenges to medical organization and behaviour.
4 Different accountability: audit is primarily professional.
5 Different boundaries: audit may cross management borders.
6 Different end-users: resource management is a tool for purchasers and providers to monitor contracts for services; audit is for doctors to focus on their own clinical practice.

Whether the functions of medical and clinical directors can be combined with chairing hospital or specialty audit groups depends on the support of the medical staff for the individuals concerned.

The inclusion of clinical outcome data in purchaser – provider contracts may be inappropriate, at the current stage of developing indicators. Both providers and purchasers need to be confident of the accuracy, comparability (e.g. adjustment for case mix) and normal distribution of such measurements. Premature inclusion in contracts of outcome data derived from audit may bias or inhibit further audit activity, and be misleading to all concerned.

However, contracts should include requirements for internal audit mechanisms as long as these are defined by specifications agreed by clinicians and managers (Shaw, 1991). This should also ensure that medical audit continues to be resourced through contracts after central earmarked funding ceases in 1994 if there is no further regional topslicing. The intent and organization of internal medical audit (a provider function) should be clearly differentiated from external monitoring of contracts (a purchaser function). Only the general and aggregated results of audit should be made available for the purpose of contracts as evidence that an effective and comprehensive mechanism is in place.

Confidentiality

Clinicians are unlikely to participate fully and effectively in medical audit without some assurance on how the information they generate may be used and by whom. Although audit may be assumed to be in the public interest, specific legal protection of the activity is unlikely in the UK. It is therefore the more appropriate to define codes of practice governing access to and use of audit data by medical colleagues, managers, patients and their representatives.

Interim national guidelines have been issued in Scotland (Clinical Research and Audit Group, 1990) and England (Conference of Medical Royal Colleges and their Faculties in the UK, 1991), and several regions have developed their own policies on confidentiality. General messages among them include:

1 Access to data: levels of access should be defined for all users, and on a 'need to know' basis only.
2 Minutes of audit meetings: should be confidential but assumed to be accessible and thus not identify individual patients or doctors; no other record of meetings should be kept after the meeting which would identify them. Minutes should include:
(a) meeting: date, time, duration, place.
(b) attendance: individual name, grade, specialty.
(c) subjects: general issues considered.
(d) conclusions: reports/action to follow, responsibility for these.
(e) follow-up: date for review of agreed actions, previous meetings.
(f) next meeting: date, time, place.

Audit methods

General issues

Audit should involve the objective peer review of patterns of care, be sensitive to the expectations of patients and other clinical disciplines and be based on scientific evidence of good medical practice. To this end, cases for review would be selected randomly or by previously agreed criteria; patterns of practice, quantified where possible, would be compared with explicit guidelines; and these guidelines, though agreed locally, should be consistent with regional and national advice and with the body of scientific knowledge.

No single approach is universally applicable. Indeed, using a variety of methods is more likely to maintain flexibility, innovation and interest in an audit group. Some methods screen 100% of cases for predefined events which are then subjected individually to peer review; others – the majority – focus on a limited sample of cases which have a characteristic in common (such as a symptom, investigation, treatment or complication). The more common and general methods are outlined here.

Adverse patient events

Adverse patient event or occurrence screening involves the systematic identification and analysis of events during a patient's treatment which may indicate some lapse in the quality of care (Bennett and Walshe, 1991). Screening criteria, aimed at recognizing a particular occurrence, are defined by the participating clinicians but may be applied to individual clinical records by non-medical assistants. For each criterion there is a detailed definition of the occurrences it is intended to identify, together with notes of known exceptions, guidelines on use, examples, and details of the information required about each occurrence. Findings are analysed by the peer group to determine causes and effects which may be used to plan changes in patient management. Generic (whole-hospital) criteria developed in Brighton include:

1 Admission for adverse results or complications of outpatient management.
2 Readmission for complications or incomplete management of problems on a previous admission.
3 Unplanned removal, injury or repair of organ or structure during surgery/invasive procedure.
4 Unplanned return to theatre.
5 Pathology/histology report varies significantly from preoperative/antemortem diagnosis.
6 Hospital-acquired infection.
7 Cardiac or respiratory arrest.
8 Cardiovascular accident or acute myocardial infarction within 48 hours of surgical procedure, or pulmonary embolism at any time postoperatively.
9 Unexpected transfer to higher dependency unit.
10 Neurological deficit on discharge not present on admission.
11 Unexpected death.
12 Evidence of patient/family dissatisfaction.

Clinical indicators

A less focused, more comprehensive approach involves the monitoring of routinely generated data within a specialty in order to identify exceptions or trends which may merit detailed *ad hoc* review. Ideally, each indicator would reflect an agreed policy objective, be routinely and accurately captured and be readily accessible. In practice, despite recent efforts in the NHS to improve the scope, accuracy, completeness and timeliness of data, many hospital doctors are either unaware of what information is available or depressed by its quality. Routine presentation of such data to clinicians, though initially painful, does improve quality and usage. These might include measures – with relevant comparisons over time or place – of:

1 *Workload*: numerical description of cases, e.g. by type, source, site, age.
2 *Access*: measures of availability, e.g. treatment rates, waiting times, non-attendance rates, elective admissions deferred by hospital.
3 *Appropriateness*: e.g. operations out of hours, readmissions, children on adult wards, patients admitted after day-case procedure.
4 *Outcome*: patients discharged home, in-hospital deaths, complications.
5 *Information*: measures of quality (may be by sample study), e.g. cases with final diagnosis coded within 1 week of discharge, records missing at time of clinic visit/admission, delay in letters to general practitioners (GPs), concordance of parallel data systems.
6 *Efficiency*: clinic/theatre sessions cancelled, length of stay (selected diagnoses/procedures), new : old patient ratio, pharmacy costs per ward/clinic, investigations requested, day cases as a percentage of all planned procedures.

Most of these are available from existing data (especially from Körner returns) but need to be collated and refined.

Topic review

Analysis of an agreed topic may be carried out by prospective study or by retrospective analysis of patient records; the latter often reveals inadequacies in recording but is a valuable exercise in providing a baseline for comparison in a later, prospective study. Both approaches involve a systematic review of a large enough sample of similar cases in order to identify, quantify and compare local patterns of practice (Shaw, 1990).

The concept is applicable to surgical and non-surgical specialties, is objective, yields quantitative data and is repeatable – but is very labour-intensive. For this reason, the clinicians may define explicit criteria by which an assistant can extract key information from large numbers of medical records.

The topic should be of general interest (not one person's hobbyhorse, or an exotic rarity) and of high volume, risk or cost or a subject of wide local variation or other concern; it may be a symptom, diagnosis, investigation, treatment, outcome – or just a clinical problem. The simpler and more common the topic, the easier it is to collect data and repeat the audit during the timespan of the junior staff.

The criteria and sample details should be discussed with the audit assistant present in order to minimize later problems of interpretation. The criteria should be about a dozen self-explanatory questions with a numerical or a yes/no answer which can be gleaned from the record. The purpose of these criteria is not to act as a protocol for clinical management but to establish current patterns and to help identify records which may merit individual review; local groups may develop very different ideas which may represent the lowest common denominator on which agreement is achievable.

The assistant then has the often challenging task of finding an accurate and up-to-date listing of patients who had the specified diagnosis and were treated by the doctors concerned within the defined timescale. The next task is to find the records themselves, and not to bias the sample by giving up on the ones that are missing. Abstracting of the records, once found, takes 10–30 minutes per case, depending on the number and complexity of the criteria; multiplied by, say, 20 cases for each of three or four firms, this occupies many hours.

The results then have to be tabulated and presented (ideally with the help of a computer spreadsheet and graphics package) back to the clinicians. They must satisfy themselves that the findings are accurate. Discussion then tends to turn to the choice of criteria, to the interpretation of results and to agreement on action. The audit can be repeated, using the same or modified criteria after an agreed time in order to measure the impact of the changes on patient care.

Examples are given below of common topics which may be applied across the hospital.

Clinical organization

Of 418 consecutive patients attending a general medical clinic in Leicester for follow-up, 27% had appointments in another medical clinic for the same or related problems; 49% of these duplications were due to routine follow-up after an acute admission, 30% due to a second GP referral, and 17% due to cross-referral to another specialist. Many of the patients were elderly, lived over 5 miles away and relied on friends, relatives or the ambulance service for transport – and 70% did not see the need for multiple attendance (Samanta *et al.*, 1991).

Medical records and letters

Clinical guidelines for minimum standards of records have been issued by the Royal College of Surgeons of England (1990); more detailed guidelines for records in general have been issued in Brighton (Bennett and Shaw, 1987); checklists for evaluating records were included in the first audit report of the Royal College of Physicians (1989).

A 3-month study of discharge letters on 89 acute hospital admissions from one group practice showed that a first note was received for 89% after a median delay of 8 days; by then, 53% of the patients had already contacted their GP. A second letter was received on 52% of the patients (median delay 24 days). No letter had been received on 11% of the patients after 2 months (Mageean, 1986).

Therapeutics

Audit of drug usage is valuable both clinically and economically, and data (on choice, route, dose and duration) are generally well-recorded; it also highlights some of the problems of implementing and maintaining change in clinical practice.

Antibiotic prescriptions assessed by medical microbiologists were deemed unnecessary in 28% of cases in a Bristol hospital; after distribution of these results, with written guidelines and advice on the use of laboratory tests, choice of drugs, dosages and routes, a repeat study the following year showed unnecessary prescriptions had risen to 35% (Swindell *et al.*, 1983).

Diagnostic investigations

Audit of the use of diagnostic radiology is indicated by evidence of clinically unproductive routines in many specialties, by potential savings in inconvenience to patients, staff time and hospital costs, and by growing concern over exposure to medical radiation. The joint working party of the Royal College of Radiologists and the National Radiological Protection Board estimated that the current population dosage could be halved without detriment to patient care; the remaining half would still be three times greater than the total of all other manufactured sources of population radiation. Some of this reduction could come from various means of optimizing dosages per examination, but the greater contribution would be in avoiding useless X-rays. At least 20% of X-ray examinations currently carried out in the UK are clinically unhelpful in the sense that the probability of obtaining information useful for patient management is extremely low (Royal College of Radiologists, National Radiological Protection Board, 1990).

The Royal College of Radiologists has now combined findings from a large number of studies on appropriate use of diagnostic X-rays into a pocket book, *Making the Best Use of a Department of Radiology* (Royal College of Radiologists, 1989). Apart from being helpful, especially to juniors, in clinical practice the guidelines may easily be developed into explicit criteria for the audit of current request patterns.

In laboratory medicine the issue of clinical guidelines and a weekly review of records were associated with an immediate reduction in requests for laboratory tests in a medical teaching unit in Cardiff (Fowkes *et al.*, 1986). Average weekly tests per patient fell from 2.0 to 1.1 in haematology and from 4.4 to 2.7 in biochemistry, particularly among repeat requests. The consultants found that formulating the guidelines and discussing them with junior staff was educational and improved their own critical thinking; but the authors wondered whether the impact of the guidelines lay less in their content than in triggering discrimination in the use of tests generally.

A 2-year study of 555 acute medical admissions in Barnsley examined the utility of emergency tests (Sandler, 1984). Only 17% of the 2372 investigations were abnormal and, of these, only one-third helped in treatment and less than one-third helped in diagnosis. The most requested tests – urea and electrolytes – were abnormal in 7% and rarely helpful. Of the patients, 13% had conditions in which a negative result was considered to be of value, but a normal initial electrocardiograph was associated with earlier discharge for patients with chest pain and a normal chest X-ray for patients with respiratory infection.

Random case review

Cases may be selected randomly or by a predetermined system from among the general workload for critical review by doctors not previously involved in the clinical management. Findings can then be presented to the audit group for discussion. Checklists may be used to ensure that each case is reviewed according to an agreed system of questions (Royal College of Physicians, 1989).

The method is easy to use, requiring minimal resources and no numerical data. Many groups find it a useful introduction to more structured discussion of clinical management. But it requires considerable time from the reviewer prior to the meeting, major issues may be missed through the randomness of selection, discussion tends to be subjective and criticism often centres on the inadequacy of the record and thus the junior staff. In many hospitals, one or two audit meetings a year are given to random reviews as a change from more focused analysis of single issues.

Patient satisfaction

Although not an audit method in itself, the assessment of the views of patients and their relatives must be incorporated into the judgements which doctors apply to their work. Formal surveys of patients' views are generally included in the overall quality improvement programmes of hospitals, rather than in medical audit. But audit may scrutinize evidence of thorough history-taking, treatment plans agreed with patients, information given, perceived value of treatment, and outcome measurements expressed in the patient's own terms.

Complaints leading to litigation are increasing and analysis of the underlying causes can provide guidance for avoiding similar events in the future. Failure to communicate, explain or apologize can add substantially to even a relatively minor mishap and become a prime reason why patients or relatives pursue legal redress. Clinical and administrative lessons can also be gleaned from the experience of the defence organizations, and provide food for audit.

Among 55 cases in which litigation followed the management of head injury, extradural haematoma was the commonest diagnosis (Garfield, 1991). The most frequent error was failure or delay of transfer from a general hospital to a neurosurgical unit; treatment was often delayed while awaiting a computed tomography scan despite evident clinical grounds for immediate transfer or an exploratory burr hole. Other errors included:

1 Inadequate records on admission, and on discharge following observation.
2 Failure to ensure or to respond to appropriate nursing observations.
3 Failure of communication between accident and emergency and ward staff, and between doctors and nurses.
4 Lack of involvement of more senior staff by relatively junior admitting doctors.
5 Inadequate and delayed review by senior staff of skull X-rays in the accident and emergency department.

Comparative audit

The confidential pooling of aggregated data, using standard definitions and formats, allows individual doctors to receive feedback on their own performance compared with others working in the same field. This can be simplified with standardized data systems, but the method of production of the statistics is less important than their accuracy; the most effective and reliable data are those collected and contributed by individual clinicians.

Resources for audit

Time

Clinicians

The amount of time recommended by the royal colleges to be set aside for audit varies between a quarter and one half-day session per week according to specialty and to definition – particularly with respect to overlap with other educational activities. In practice, much of the time related to audit, for example in recording and verifying clinical data, is not as readily identified as formal audit meetings.

The participation of individual doctors in audit is, for various reasons, expected by provider managers, purchasers and the national colleges and faculties. Since much of the time spent on audit is 'soft' and less easy to identify, the recording of individual attendance at meetings is likely to become a proximate measure for participation generally. Reasonable attendance will also have to be defined, e.g. two-thirds of all monthly meetings, allowing for emergencies and leave.

Coordinators

The additional work of planning, organizing, minuting and ensuring that appropriate action ensues is generally allocated to one lead clinician for each specialty and, overall, to the chair of the audit committee. Many districts have agreed honoraria or additional sessional payments (commonly one session for a district coordinator, sometimes more) in recognition.

Audit assistants

Audit assistants (also called facilitators, officers, analysts or administrators) can minimize the extra time required of doctors in moving from traditional case review to more formal audit of patterns of care.

The time required to retrieve records and abstract and analyse data depends on a host of local administrative factors as well as on the subject and detail of the audit itself. Experience in the UK suggests that to collect a defined set of 12–15 data requires 15–25 minutes for an inpatient record or 6–10 for an outpatient.

Data

General issues

Audit, workload agreements, service contracts and resource management have placed a new value on the patient records service which in the NHS has traditionally been given low status. Systematic audit emphasizes not only the need to put information into records, but also to get it out – a function for which many departments are ill-equipped. The immediate problems are first in identifying samples of patients with common characteristics, second in finding their records, and third in interpreting their content when found.

Most clinical computing systems in routine use collect only a limited subset of the total clinical record; this allows overall statistical analysis of the variables captured, but the individual patient record remains the prime source of detail when examining a defined sample of cases with a common characteristic. The most basic need is therefore for timely, accurate and complete lists to identify these cases according to the chosen theme, for example, by primary diagnosis, medication, investigation, procedure or complication. A variety of potential sources is available to NHS hospitals (see below) but many have suffered from disuse, underinvestment or lack of awareness of their potential; also, while clinical practice increasingly moves to outpatient care, most clinical data systems continue to focus on inpatients and day-cases.

The likelihood of finding a record is inversely proportional to the size of the hospital and the complexity of the case. The presence of temporary folders on the wards or the absence of records in clinics is a symptom of a common problem which also afflicts audit – and should itself be subject to scrutiny. Since they often represent the atypical cases, it is important to persevere in the search for missing records. The added burden this gives to records departments should be met with funded additional clerical time.

Another unsurprising discovery of audit is that records are often unable to explain what happened to patients and why. Much of this may be attributed to lack of agreed definition, teaching and monitoring of the purpose and characteristics of a good clinical record – another topic for audit.

Sources of clinical data

Apart from the individual patient record, other traditional manual sources may provide information for audit. These include registers in maternity, theatres and the accident unit, and admission books in wards (especially intensive therapy units). If there is no other central record of cardiac arrests, the switchboard may have a log of emergency calls.

The proliferation of stand-alone and linked personal computers (PCs) has improved the accuracy and availability of data for many clinicians. The arguments over whether to take this route in preference to existing standard hospital systems and which package to purchase are beyond the scope of this chapter and have been

well-described elsewhere. The Royal College of Surgeons has given a useful summary of the required characteristics of computers for audit; most of this advice is equally appropriate to physicians (Royal College of Surgeons of England, 1991). Even those doctors who already have PC systems may yet benefit from exploring data from other hospital sources; and those who do not could reflect that their existing hospital system could be equally accurate if clinical input were given the same personal attention as enthusiasts give to their PCs.

Under a variety of titles, the former hospital activity analysis lives on; in each hospital it captures details of primary and secondary diagnosis, complications and procedures from the discharge letter (or note) of every inpatient and day-case. It is therefore able to generate consultant-specific lists of patients:

1 by diagnosis;
2 by complication;
3 by procedure.

But the completeness, accuracy and timeliness of this data rest heavily on the quality of the discharge letter. Even when data entry is accurate, many doctors find that simple reports are slow and unhelpful and more complex ones are unavailable. Errors have also been identified in translating diagnosis and procedure codes into diagnosis-related groups (DRGs). Of 153 joint replacements identified from theatre and ward records in Leicester, 9% of the patients' records were missing; of those available, 24% were considered to have been allocated to the wrong DRG; of these errors, 64% were ascribed to incorrect primary coding and the remainder to incorrect translation (by computer) to DRG (Smith *et al.*, 1991). The commonest cause of incorrect coding is incomplete recording of clinical details.

Many departments have data systems which, though set up for other purposes, may yield valuable data for audit such as:

1 *Laboratory*: many systems are capable of reporting usage profiles for individual firms, specialties or investigations (e.g. lithium assays for psychiatrists).
2 *Radiology*: some record radiological diagnosis, others only the investigation; either could be a source for topic audit or for routine monitoring (e.g. of selected X-rays requested out of hours).
3 *Pharmacy*: most systems can identify stock issues to individual outpatient clinics or to inpatient wards

but not to individual patients; but this can monitor trends in prescribing or offer a basis for audit of individual drugs (e.g. streptolysin, anaesthetic agents, interferon, antibiotics).

4 *Nursing*: systems for measuring patient dependence (and estimating required nurse staffing levels) may provide data on medical management (e.g. patients on full oral diet but receiving intravenous medication).

5 *Maternity*: clinical system well-tended (often by midwives) to offer accurate clinical reports (e.g. episiotomy, caesarean section rate).

6 *Theatre*: management systems record timing, staffing and resources used for individual operations (e.g. implants); they can also identify critical events (e.g. delayed recovery from anaesthesia).

7 *Child health*: usually community-based, but may be able to identify children with selected handicaps, diagnoses or problems (e.g. for joint hospital–GP audit).

8 *Other departments*: e.g. medical photography, cardiology, accident and emergency, paramedical services.

Unfortunately, even though many departmental and hospital systems are capable of answering *ad hoc* or unusual requests, staff are sometimes either unaware of this or do not have the knowledge or time to retrieve the data. Advice on the available data may be sought from the information officer locally.

Sources of additional data

The patient administration system (PAS) is the core of most hospital computer systems, comprising a master index of all patients (and their personal and demographic details) and a range of added modules, usually including inpatient, day-case and outpatient activity, waiting lists and sometimes accident and emergency. From this can be obtained routine reports, including consultant and specialty-specific data on:

1 Bed allocation, availability, occupancy, admissions, transfers, discharges, deaths, length of stay.
2 Day-cases.
3 Source of admissions, destination of discharges.
4 Non-arrivals for booked admission, waiting list.
5 Clinic session numbers, attendances, non-attendances, cancellations, waiting list.

PAS is generally relatively complete and accurate (compared with clinical data capture systems descended from hospital activity analysis), but many hospitals continue to be erratic in their definition and recording of day-cases and outpa-

tient procedures. Doctors whose workload is thus likely to be underrecorded may be particularly concerned to obtain and verify these data. It is also important to ensure that deaths in the community which are notified by the registrar to the director of public health are reported to the master patient index of the hospital.

From April 1991, the NHS minimum data set for ambulatory services (outpatients and ward attenders) has included in each case the identification of GP and consultant, and any procedure performed. From 1993 this will extend to day cases, and will include the patient's NHS number, GP diagnosis, clinic diagnosis and the grade of doctor seeing the patient (Department of Health, 1991c).

Formerly misnamed performance indicators, health service indicators are available for districts in England and Wales and are becoming increasingly accurate and clinically relevant. The data and systems disks are issued each year to hospitals and health authorities, offering a variety of formats for comparing individual districts and regions with the country as a whole. A dictionary of indicators is published by the Department of Health (1990c); many of these relate to resources, but others describe clinical process or outcome, such as:

1 Avoidable deaths (standardized mortality ratios); e.g. hypertensive disease, cervical cancer, breast cancer, lung cancer, asthma, rheumatic heart disease, common surgical conditions (hernia, cholecystitis, appendicitis), Hodgkin's disease, myocardial infarction.
2 Admission rates and length of stay (by age group):
  (a) general medicine: asthma, diabetes mellitus, cerebrovascular accident, ischaemic heart disease, poisoning.
  (b) general surgery: appendicectomy, repair inguinal hernia, varicose vein operation, cholecystectomy, mastectomy.
  (c) urology: prostatectomy.
  (d) paediatric surgery: orchidopexy, pyloric stenosis.
  (e) trauma/orthopaedics: concussion, femoral fracture, joint replacement (hip, knee).
  (f) otolaryngology: tonsillectomy, adenoidectomy.
  (g) ophthalmology: correction of strabismus, cataract surgery.
  (h) gynaecology: prolapse repair, abdominal hysterectomy, cervical biopsy, dilatation and curettage.

Data quality

The responsibility for accurate clinical data should be agreed and shared between clinicians and managers; no amount of investment in technology alone will suffice. Practical local steps might include:

1 Define and monitor minimum standards for clinical records (e.g. adapt or adopt guidelines from the Royal College of Surgeons of England (1990) and the Royal College of Obstetricians and Gynaecologists (Maresh and Hall, 1991)).
2 Define minimum data to be recorded on diagnosis, complications and procedure for abstraction into hospital clinical system.
3 Routinely check that these data are complete and accurate in the discharge note, summary or card from which they will be captured.
4 Explore the scope, accuracy and potential of data already collected.
5 Test the response of sources to *ad hoc* enquiry (e.g. for topic audit).
6 Define and request regular provision of routine statistics.
7 Involve information officer, records staff and coding clerks.
8 Monitor key indicators: some of the criteria used by hospitals to monitor performance of the records service may also be of value to the medical staff, such as:
   (a) percentage of duplicate records on master patient index.
   (b) case notes not delivered to ward 24 hours after request.
   (c) temporary folders still in use after 24 hours.
   (d) computer records without diagnostic codes completed within 4 weeks of discharge documentation being available.
   (e) discharge letters not sent within 7 days of discharge.
   (f) case notes missing from clinic.
   (g) temporary case note folders in clinic.
   (h) GP clinic letters not sent within a week of dictation.
   (i) concordance of PAS and clinical information systems.

Audit assistants

Under various titles, one or more assistants have been appointed in most hospitals in the UK since 1990 to support the medical staff and to avoid the unnecessary use of medical time in audit. Job descriptions vary but the main elements are to:

1 be professionally accountable to the doctor responsible for coordination of audit, who should supervise the allocation of time to individual projects;
2 be bound by an agreed written code of confidentiality;

3 assist with organization of meetings, collation of reports from specialty groups, drafting of annual report and programme, abstracting and presenting audit data, collation of relevant clinical literature;
4 receive initial and continuing training in the organization and methods of audit.

Prime requirements include the ability to work effectively with individual medical staff but with limited supervision; experience of hospital organization and operation; and knowledge of clinical terminology and records. The ability to handle basic statistics and use standard computer software to generate reports is an asset.

The required level of skill, experience and initiative implies a salary at least equivalent to administrative and clerical grade 5. This, and the number of hours required, depends on the activity of the medical staff (particularly in criterion-based audit), the scope of the job description and the availability of clerical support (e.g. for retrieval of records).

Reference sources

Medical library

Apart from information on local activity (described above), doctors need access to information from elsewhere on audit methods, on good medical practice and on comparable results from other hospitals. For most doctors, the nearest reference source is the local medical library; staff time and other revenue should be budgeted to cover additional literature searches, copying, interlibrary loans, subscriptions and acquisitions.

Periodicals

Papers on medical audit now feature in many clinical journals. There is also a growing number of periodicals dealing primarily with audit and related issues (often under the general term, quality assurance), including the following:

Australian Clinical Review: Published quarterly by Blackwell. From PO Box 20, Glebe, New South Wales 2037, Australia.

Quality in Health Care: Published quarterly by the British Medical Journal Publishing Group, BMA House, Tavistock Square, London WC1H 9JR.

Quality Assurance in Health Care: Published quarterly by Pergamon Press plc, Headington Hill Hall, Oxford OX3 0BW.

Network: newsletter addressed to audit support staff/assistants in the UK. From Medical Audit Association, Yorkshire Regional Health Authority, Park Parade, Harrogate.

Medical Audit News: monthly newsletter published by Churchill Livingstone, Longman Group UK, Subscription Department, 4th Avenue, Harlow, Essex CM19 5AA.

References

Bennett, J. and Shaw, C.D. (1987) Guidance on what should be in the clinical medical records for the Brighton health district. *Medical Record Healthcare Information Journal* **28**, 103–110.

Bennett, J. and Walshe, K. (1991) Occurrence screening as a method of audit. *British Medical Journal* **300**, 1248–1251.

Clinical Research and Audit Group (1990) *Confidentiality and Medical Audit: Interim Guidelines*. GRAG/SHHD, Edinburgh.

Conference of Medical Royal Colleges and their Faculties in the UK (1991) Interim guidelines on confidentiality and medical audit. *British Medical Journal* **303**, 1525.

Department of Health (1989a) *Working for Patients*. HMSO, London.

Department of Health (1989b) *Working for Patients: Medical Audit*. Working paper number 6. HMSO, London.

Department of Health (1989c) *Implementation of Medical Audit: Allocation of Funds for the Support of Medical Audit*. EL(89)MB/224. DoH, London.

Department of Health (1990a) *Medical Audit in Family Practitioner Services*. HC(90)15. DoH, London.

Department of Health (1990b) *The Quality of Medical Care: Report of the Standing Medical Advisory Committee for the Secretaries of State for Health and Wales*. HMSO, London.

Department of Health (1990c) *Health Service Indicators Guidance: Dictionary*. HMSO, London.

Department of Health (1991a) *Medical Audit in the Hospital and Community Health Services*. HC(91)2. DoH, London.

Department of Health (1991b) *Medical Audit in HCHS – Allocation of Funds 1991/92*. EL(91)32. DoH, London.

Department of Health (1991c) *Framework for Information Systems: The Next Steps*. Appendix 2.2: Minimum data set, out-patients. HMSO, London.

Department of Health and Social Security (1990) *Medical Audit in the Hospital and Community Services*. DHSS, Belfast.

Fowkes, F. G. R., Hall, R., Jones, J. H. *et al.* (1986) Trial of a strategy for reducing the use of laboratory tests. *British Medical Journal* **292**, 883–885.

Garfield, J. (1991) Head injuries and litigation. *Journal of the Medical Defence Union* **7**, 2–3.

Mageean, R. J. (1986) Study of 'discharge communications' from hospital. *British Medical Journal* **293**, 1283–1284.

Maresh, M. and Hall, M. (1991) *Medical Audit Unit: Second Bulletin*, RCOG, Manchester.

Mitchell, M. W. and Fowkes, F. G. R. (1985) Audit reviewed: does feedback on performance change clinical behaviour? *Journal of the Royal College of Physicians of London* **19**, 251–254.

Royal College of Physicians (1989) *Medical Audit: A First Report – What, Why and How?* RCP, London.

Royal College of Radiologists (1989) *Making the Best Use of a Department of Radiology*. RCR, London.

Royal College of Radiologists, National Radiological Protection Board (1990) *Patient Dose Reduction in Diagnostic Radiology*. NRPB, Didcot.

Royal College of Surgeons of England (1990) *Guidelines for Clinicians on Medical Records and Notes*. RCS, London.

Royal College of Surgeons of England (1991) *Guidelines for Surgical Audit by Computer*, RCS, London.

Samanta, A., Haider, Y. and Roffe, C. (1991) An audit of patients attending a general medical follow-up clinic. *Journal of the Royal College of Physicians of London* **25**, 33–35.

Sandler, G. (1984) Do emergency tests help in the management of acute medical admissions? *British Medical Journal* **289**, 973–977.

Scottish Home and Health Department (1989a) *Medical Audit*. NHS review working paper number 2. HMSO, London.

Scottish Home and Health Department (1989b) *Guidance on Implementation of Medical Audit*. NHS circular 1989(GEN)29. SHHD, Edinburgh.

Shaw, C.D. (1990) Criterion based audit. *British Medical Journal* **300**, 649–651.

Shaw, C.D. (1991) Specifications for hospital medical audit. *Health Service Management* **June**, 124–125.

Smith, S.H., Kershaw, C., Thomas, I.H. and Botha, J.L. (1991) PIS and DRGs: coding inaccuracies and their consequence for resource management. *Journal of Public Health Medicine* **13**, 40–41.

Swindell, P.J., Reeves, D.S., Bullock, D.W. *et al.* (1983) Audits of antibiotic prescribing in a Bristol hospital. *British Medical Journal* **286**, 118–122.

Welsh Advisory Group on Medical Audit (1990) *Advice on the Implementation of the Medical Audit Process in the Hospital and Community Health Services in Wales.* WAGMA, Cardiff.

Welsh Office (1990) *Assuring the Quality of Medical Care: Implementation of Medical and Dental Audit in the Hospital and Community Health Service.* Draft WHC(90)32. WO, Cardiff.

Section 8

Managing in a clinical directorate

Introduction

Hugh Saxton

There must be a beginning of any great matter but the continuing unto the end until it be thoroughly finished yields the true glory (Drake, 1587).

Management has been defined as making things happen through other people. The emphasis here is both on achieving positive results and on the need to do so through other people. In this, as in many other ways, the management process in general has close parallels with clinical management (Table 8.1). Yet management is often seen by doctors as a totally alien subject. There are, it is true, many aspects of general management which would take time to learn if a

Table 8.1 Comparison between the processes of clinical and general management.

Clinical management	General management
1 Define problem	1 Define problem
2 Gather information (history, examination, diagnostic tests)	2 Gather information
3 Formulate management plan with implicit objectives based on diagnosis and available resources	3 Formulate management plan with defined objectives, usually after detailed discussion
4 Organize implementation of plan	4 Organize implementation of plan
5 Motivate patient and others to make it happen	5 Motivate staff to make it happen
6 Monitor progress; alter plan if necessary	6 Monitor progress; alter plan if necessary
7 Record final outcome	7 Record final outcome
8 Review process (audit)	8 Review process

Communication is important at all stages.

doctor wished to become a full-time manager, but as we have noted, this book does not aim to do that. To absorb enough to be an effective part-time manager requires a willingness to learn and to change one's perspective. In spite of the similarities set out in Table 8.1, there are differences, but they are mainly cultural or attitudinal.

To begin with, most medical problems are patient-sized; those in general management tend to involve part or all of an organization – a ward, a department or a hospital. The staff helping the doctor are, on the whole, well-motivated, responsive and relatively few in number: a general manager may have large numbers to deal with and their attitudes are often less positive. The doctor communicates mainly at short range, to patients and close colleagues. The general manager will also have to communicate with and influence part or all of an organization. The general manager has a greater need for long-term planning than most hospital consultants. Above all, the doctor, who can be said to be at the apex of a supporting pyramid, has seldom regarded it as his or her responsibility to run or manage those who support him or her. Once this is included in the consultant's role, the cultural change is under way.

Management ability and the need for a team

The perfect manager, like the perfect doctor, does not exist but, as Belbin has pointed out (1981), a team can often provide the mix of qualities needed. A basic list of desirable managerial qualities may give an idea:

1 The ability to plan and set goals.
2 Leadership: the ability to motivate.
3 Care over details.
4 Breadth of vision; sensitivity.
5 The ability to handle numbers.
6 Persistence; follow-through; toughness.

7 Flair; imagination; flexibility; openmindedness.
8 The ability to communicate.

The consultant taking on a management role should look at such a list and consider where he or she is weakest. This will give an idea of what qualities are needed in the business manager or nurse manager with whom he or she will work. Delegating appropriately is the key to efficient management since it puts the task in the hands of the person best suited to it.

Talking to people – and listening

Doctors sometimes feel uncomfortable when they find that management involves a good deal of talking and listening. The American management expert, Tom Peters, talks about MBWA – 'management by wandering around' (Peters, 1989). He points out that talking to the people in an organization, with whom one does not normally interact, yields ideas and information which can be of crucial value. In addition, talking is needed to keep others informed, to involve them in problems or decisions and to enthuse, motivate or persuade. Sometimes it may be to direct or discipline someone. In this context there are two important points. First, it is a mistake to rebuke or discipline someone for apparently doing something wrongly, without first hearing his or her perspective. It is equally a mistake to chide someone for failing to perform in a particular way, if it has not been made clear to him or her earlier what is wanted.

Above all, the emphasis of this style of management is not on being a director but on being an involver, so that while all in the directorate know who is in charge, everyone feels able to communicate with him or her. The ideas and support that will be given to such a director will be many times greater than those available to an autocrat who takes the title literally.

Functions of a clinical director

Although the title of clinical director is not wholly appropriate, no better one has been found and it has the merit of familiarity. The list which follows is not exhaustive but offers an indication of the scope of a clinical director in current resource management hospitals. It follows from what was discussed earlier that some functions may not actually be carried out by the clinical director, but it is his or her responsibility to ensure that these things happen.

1 Provide leadership, motivation and cohesion.
2 Ensure a high standard of service and patient care.
3 Ensure and promote the formulation of directorate policies and plans, preferable including a 5-year plan. These plans must be compatible with the policies and aims of other directorates. This heading also includes the annual business programme.
4 Create an organizational/committee structure appropriate to the needs of the directorate: everyone working in the directorate should be represented on one or other of its subcommittees.
5 Take responsibility for the budget and related matters.
6 Determine the directorate's information requirements and see that they are met.
7 Develop and maintain a directorate policy on waiting lists, where appropriate.
8 Make arrangements for the recruitment and grading of personnel.
9 Ensure that the training needs of directorate staff are met. Liaise with the medical school over student teaching where appropriate.
10 Ensure that proper audit mechanisms are in place and functioning.
11 Interact with other directorates to promote/maintain/protect the interests of the directorate.
12 Attend hospital management board meetings as required.

Signs of change

It takes time to build a good clinical directorate and, as with most human organizations, continued work is needed to maintain its function and relationships. Some of the more conventional signs that the directorate is well-managed will be:

1 It is clear to everyone who is responsible/accountable to whom.
2 Everyone knows the part he or she has to play in the directorate.
3 Everyone who is interested knows what is happening.
4 Each group has its own committee with a representative on the main directorate committee.
5 There are plans for 1–5 years ahead.
6 The directorate pulls together: people enjoy working in it.

It may be added that there are other significant, if less tangible, signs, for example, the attendance at and relationships within directorate social functions. And to take an example at the consultant level, the non-managerial consultant will say something like: 'The X-ray department are hopeless. I never get the X-rays on my patients in outpatients: it's been like that for years: when I write they just make excuses'. The managerial consultant will say to the directorate business manager: 'There's a problem in getting X-rays to my outpatients. Can you set up a meeting with your opposite number in X-ray and with the Sister in my clinic? Try and identify the problem and see if it can be sorted out at your level. If it can't, set out the salient issues and we'll have a meeting with Dr Röntgen and me there as well'.

Conclusions

Management can be seen as a systematic approach to achieving goals. It is also a conscious and structured way of making the most of the available resources of money, space, equipment, computer systems and people – their time, abilities, energy and ideas. The effective manager will do all this and in doing so will probably be found 'inspiring, politicking, plotting, cajoling, fighting, bargaining, compromising and persevering' (Gabbay, 1988) – a mixture with which, no doubt, Sir Francis Drake would have been familiar.

References

Belbin, M. (1981) *Management Teams: Why Some Succeed and Some Fail*. Heinemann Professional Publishing, Oxford.

Drake, F. (1587) *Dispatch to Sir Francis Walsingham*.

Gabbay, J. (1988) Opinion: inspiring, politicking, plotting, cajoling. *British Medical Journal* **297**, 992.

Peters, T. (1989) *Thriving on Chaos*. Pan Books, London, pp. 423–432.

8.1 Anaesthesia

Robert W. Buckland

Introduction

The management structure at The Royal Hampshire County Hospital, Winchester is based on a system of directors of clinical services with management and budgetary authority with responsibility for an area of the hospital known as the clinical directorate.

The management structure had the full support of the unit general manager, the district general manager and crucially the medical staff committee. This structure, in place by early 1986, predated the resource management initiative (HN(86)34) and has been previously described (Resource Management Initiative, 1989). The principle inherent in this decision was that those whose actions initiate resource expenditure – the clinicians – should necessarily be involved actively in the management of the organization. The decision was however not that clinicians should be involved in the management process but that they should become the managers.

In January 1986 I was chairman of the division of anaesthesia and, with the full approval of my colleagues, became the first director of clinical services (anaesthetics). To survive as a medical manager one must have the confidence and support of the consultants within the directorate. Although it required an enormous amount of time, it was essential to be an active clinical member of the department.

The organizational issues resulting from the change were immense; the first and perhaps most important was the experience of adjusting to being a manager as well as a clinician. It was clear that the evolving role of the clinical director could encourage interference in the clinical judgement of other doctors, but at the same time, it was necessary to promote the idea of consultant accountability for the use of resources.

An example of this conflict arose over the use of isoflurane in place of halothane or enflurane; the unit general manager insisted on a reduction in expenditure and my colleagues insisted on their clinical freedom to use the most appropri-

ate agent. As clinical director I supported both points of view. The policy of virement, whereby money saved within the directorate could be used elsewhere within the directorate, had been agreed by the hospital management board. By a variety of means, including reducing expenditure on locums and a review of the use of circuits and gas flows in theatre, the department was able to fund the deficit and maintain clinical freedom through clinical responsibility.

The clinical director is also a member of the hospital management board. The board became responsible for the management of the unit with executive responsibility for the finances and other resources of that unit. As a clinical director in anaesthesia I was required to balance the needs of my own directorate with a very different role as a member of a board with collective responsibility for the future of the hospital.

At that time I was the chairman of division and carried on both roles. Within a year it was seen to be necessary to separate these roles. As medical audit is necessary to complement resource management, so a clinical chairperson of the department is necessary to complement the clinical director. The separation of the purchaser and provider and the necessity for work agreements has made that separation of roles even more important.

Thus in January 1986 I became responsible for a clinical directorate consisting of the department of anaesthetics, intensive care unit, the day unit, the operating theatre department, the central sterile services department (CSSD), and the theatre sterile services unit (TSSU). This included budgetary and management responsibility for all nursing staff, administration and clerical staff, operating department assistants, porters and medical staff below the grade of senior registrar. I had therefore taken on a commitment to manage several departments, in excess of 120 full-time equivalent staff and a budget of some £2.5m. Five years on it is difficult to understand the enthusiasm engendered at that time and the fool-hardiness of taking on such responsibilities. I would suggest that no anaesthetist would today take on such responsibilities without an absolute guarantee of the enormous support that is required to carry out such a role. We were strongly supported by the resource management initiative and central funding, but no one should underestimate either the task or the support that is required.

Clearly at this stage a project plan was required to put into place a management structure within the directorate and to set up a management process that would enable a busy anaesthetist to cope with this responsibility. It was also necessary to consider what information technology we would require, what information we would require and the issues of quality, people and training.

It has been said, sometimes I suspect by those who feel most threatened, that doctors do not have management skills. My experience leads me to believe that many managers, particularly at that time, did not have management skills. The argument however is futile: we both need to learn from each other and management courses are an essential part of that learning process. Anaesthetists have always taken a leading role in management and administration and I would strongly recommend that full use is made of available management courses.

Management structure and process

The guiding principle within the directorate was that operational management should be devolved to the most appropriate level. It was quickly put in place that each of the various parts of the directorate were managed by a clinician and by a senior nurse. The day unit, for example, was managed by a consultant anaesthetist with a senior sister responsible to him for the operational management of that unit. For the first time they were supplied with financial information and details of expenditure on both staff and non-staff. The same principles were applied to the intensive care unit and to those areas with non-clinical managers, such as the CSSD and TSSU.

It was not possible or desirable that the clinical director should be involved in the operational management of these subdirectorates. The object of this devolution was not only to free the clinical director but also to achieve a feeling of ownership amongst staff of the man-

agement process. People are able to take responsibility and in fact welcome it, since centralized decision-making merely destroys confidence.

It is interesting that with the advent of the NHS bill and the contracting process between provider and purchaser, the process of costing patient care is much simplified by the existence of decentralized budgets. In the old system of centralized budgets based on function it was, for example, very easy to know how many nurses there were and what they cost, but no one had any idea of the breakdown in costs by department.

At an early stage it was agreed that the management structure within the directorate would be based on a tripartite structure with senior nurse manager and a business manager managerially accountable to the director. This I believe to be the key to success, combining business skills with medical and nursing expertise to maximize resource usage without compromising quality of care.

The increase in the scope and work of the department necessitated an increase in secretarial assistance. The post of personal assitant to the clinical director was created on a grade higher than that of the medical secretaries. In my view it is impossible to sustain the post of clinical director without adequate secretarial and business manager assistance. These are posts that cannot be shared with anyone else or promised at a later date; they need to be upfront at the time of appointment.

Anaesthetic departments are organized in a variety of ways and the use of departmental administrators is not new (Horton and Vickers, 1984). Early on in the resource management initiative the appointment of business managers was viewed with suspicion, particularly at the use of the word manager. The often-asked question was: 'What does a business manager actually do'? A colleague, a fellow clinical director, replied, 'She keeps me sane'. Initially the role was not clear but now the business manager is seen as an essential part of the directorate. The provision of information to the clinical director with regard to finance, staff and workload is essential. Regular management reports on such matters as theatre usage, outpatient activity (pain clinic) and a review of activity against contract targets are regularly provided by the business manager.

One of the keys to surviving as a medical manager is to devolve day-to-day operational management to the business manager and the senior nurse manager. In many hospitals business managers are appointed by and accountable to either the unit general manager or the chief executive. I believe such appointments are viewed only as management spies by the directorates in which they work. The business manager should be appointed by and be accountable to the clinical director, although he or she must have appropriate professional links. The same principle should apply to senior nurse manager, with links to the director of nursing services.

Information systems

Information and information technology are both necessary and desirable. It is however important that the management structure is in place before decisions on information technology are made. Early on the directorate bought and installed the Theatreman System and this has been developed to include audit information. The setting up and running of the information technology was and remains the responsibility of the business manager. As I would not know a megabyte from a Big Mac, this was a great relief to me! One of the great difficulties we encountered was in persuading our colleagues to fill in forms during busy theatre lists. Most of this information for management purposes is now collected by the nursing staff, whilst anaesthetists have a clear responsibility to complete those sections pertinent to anaesthetics. The information must be collected and owned by the department to ensure that it is accurate and robust.

Managing the theatres

It was decided from the outset that theatres would be managed by the director of clinical services (anaesthetics). It would be run as a service and, since it represented one of the most expensive resources in the hospital, it was essential that it should be efficient.

As an experiment it was decided to recharge theatre time to the surgical specialties. Initially, run as a paper exercise, it was an attempt to cost theatre time, to monitor theatre usage and plan more effectively.

At the commencement of the financial year, an agreement is reached between the clinical director in anaesthetics and surgical counterparts as

to how many operating lists are required per year to meet their contractual commitments with purchasers. An estimate is made of the number of emergency hours that would be required based on the previous year's activity.

The total cost of running theatres is calculated for both staff and non-staff. Care is taken to exclude those activities within the directorate that do not involve theatres, such as the intensive care, the obstetric department, X-ray or elsewhere. The help of the finance department is crucial in this exercise. Each operating session is charged at a standard rate, which includes all the activities concerned with theatre, such as nurse time, operating department assistants, recovery and anaesthesia. In addition, expensive items (over £25) are charged out to the surgical units concerned.

If sessions are not used or are underused, the charge remains. If, however, a session overruns then a premium rate (+50%) is charged. All emergency cases outside the normal working hours of 8.00 a.m. to 5.00 p.m. are charged by the minute at the premium rate.

If the specialty concerned informs the business manager at least 2 weeks beforehand that the session is not required, then no charge is made and the session is reallocated. The role of the business managers in this process is obvious. The all-inclusive recharge is made easier because these budgets are under the control of the clinical director. It was also agreed with the district health authority that case-costing would be on this basis and timed from start of anaesthetic to time into recovery, thus avoiding arguments about how much time was spent anaesthetizing and how much time was spent operating, and this has not been a subject of debate. I believe this is a sensible compromise, facilitating the costing exercise and, provided that the case mix does not alter dramatically, using standard costs as the basis for pricing activity in the operating theatre will be effective without the necessity for collecting detailed information. Thus we have established what could be called internal contracts between surgeon and anaesthetist and this type of trading account allows the directorates of surgery to know their costs well in advance for inclusion in contracts with providers.

The business manager sends reports to the surgical directorates indicating usage of theatres in terms of numbers of sessions used, late starts, overruns and underruns and details of why any session is cancelled. In addition a financial report is produced by the finance department on the basis of figures supplied by the directorate of anaesthesia using Theatreman information on the expenditure against budget for each surgical specialty.

This system, as can be imagined, is not entirely popular but it is intended to be non-aggressive and does serve to highlight the reasons behind the use of theatres. Underusage may be bad planning, inadequate beds, failure to notify absences or plain bad time-keeping. Overruns may indicate a need for increased theatre time allocation and these topics are then discussed both at the management board and at the theatre users' group. The use of such groups to discuss theatre usage information is strongly recommended (Bevan, 1989). Theatre usage has improved and unit costs have fallen but there is a danger that the pressure on daytime operating has increased the out-of-hours working and in our hospital some teaching lists for surgical junior staff have been lost. It is to be hoped that provision is made for daytime emergency work in line with the CEPOD Recommendations (1987) and that quality is not subsumed by financial pressures. This can only be guaranteed by involving surgeons and anaesthetists in the decision process and why I believe that a doctor is the most appropriate person to be in management control of an operating theatre department.

Budget authority

Too many budgets are no more than financial allocations with responsibility but no authority. This is not acceptable. There is very little flexibility in budgets and this is particularly true of small budgets. One of the advantages of running the larger directorates is the ability to switch monies between cost centres.

In the early days as a directorate, we had problems in keeping good operating department assistants. One of my first tasks was to increase their salaries. I was told it could not be done but persuasion, discussion and budget authority resulted in a substantial increase in their salaries and a workforce that has remained almost unchanged for many years.

Similarly, when an expensive item of equipment needed replacing in the intensive care unit it was done, without letters and endless meetings – the advantage of devolved management. This of course depends on the budget and the prob-lem of replacement of capital equipment remains unresolved and will do so until it is seen as a revenue consequence properly funded through contracts and regional monies.

The other major advantage of budget-holding is the increased capability of arguing one's case with knowledge. This has been highlighted by the issue of waiting list initiatives. The department of anaesthesia has been able properly to cost the implications and insist on adequate funding for staff and equipment before agreeing to take them on.

Budget-holding also brings responsibility and, provided one has been involved in the budget-setting process, this is acceptable and desirable. Many changes have been made to ensure more efficient use of resources and awareness of cost has resulted in changes without undue attack on clinical freedom.

As a manager, one cannot survive without an office, to read the unending documents and to hold meetings. An open-door policy is essential so that you are accessible to everyone, within reason. I was amazed at how many staff – doctors, nurses, operating department assistants and ancillary workers – came along to my office to talk and I am convinced that the most important part of the job is the task of communication.

One of the most stressful aspects of the job was being easily accessible in the operating theatre and it became essential for my sanity to separate clinical and management work into distinct time slots. The administration of anaesthesia is a full-time occupation and it would be so easy to become distracted.

Personnel problems could also be stressful and I made full use of the personnel officer. Those who work in operating theatres are often put under great stress and so often the only people who understand this are those who work on that side of the red line. Essential to the early orientation programme for business managers, personnel assistants and indeed financial directors and resource managers was an invitation to spend time with clinicians in the operating theatre and other areas. These offers were enthusiastically taken up and the feedback from such experience is entirely positive. The difficulty on occasion was to get the 'outsiders' accepted as part of the organization and time is needed to achieve this objective.

The senior nurse manager welcomed the organizational changes and, although now managerially accountable to a clinician, saw this as an improvement. In the past problems in theatre could not be solved with ease, partly because of the large number of people involved. The appointment of clinical directors focused the responsibility on individuals and improved problem- solving.

To survive the culture shock, the clinical director needs many things. An office is essential with devoted secretarial assistance. One must have the time to do the job and the full support of clinical colleagues. One must be entirely honest about objectives, clear about strategy, efficient in monitoring and determined to implement the necessary changes. There are times when one will need a confessor, a role perceived to be necessary in the world of business, even for senior managers. It is very helpful to talk problems through, often with people outside the directorate or even outside the hospital. We have a great deal to learn from our management colleagues and I would suggest that they have as much to learn from us. Management training is essential but will not replace the support of an enthusiastic peer goup.

Those of us involved in the initial pilot sites through the resource management initiative were enthusiasts. Such enthusiasm was based on the belief that the future of acute hospitals is dependent on the willingness of doctors to involve themselves in the task of management. It is essential that as anaesthetists we control the direction of change and only then will we be able to ensure the maintenance of quality of care and the proper use of resources.

References

Horton, J. N. and Vickers, M. D. (1984) Administration in clinical units: experience in a department of anaesthetics. *Health Trends*, **16**, 58–60.

Bevan, P.R. (1989) *The Management and Utilisation of Operating Departments*. NHS Management Executive VFM unit. HMSO, London.

Resource Management Initiative (1989) *Central Consultants and Specialists Committee Evaluation*. Report on the six experimental sites. British Medical Association, London.

8.2 Geriatrics and general medicine

Hazel Penny and David A. Walker

The Huddersfield clinical directorate structure has been developing since April 1990, prior to which the Huddersfield Royal Infirmary (HRI) was a resource management (RM) pilot site. Understandably, as the principal acute service-provider, HRI has led the directorate initiative, but gradually the structure is being implemented district-wide. There are four directorates at HRI. Medicine, surgery and paediatrics/obstetrics/gynaecology cover the bed-holding specialties. Each is composed of medical and nursing staff, the business manager, medical secretaries, medical records clerks and ward clerks. The fourth directorate, known as the provider directorate, is made up of representatives from all supporting departments (pathology, biochemistry, haematology, anaesthesia, radiology, pharmacy, electrocardiography, physiotherapy, occupational therapy, works, laundry, central sterile services department, porters, catering, domestics). The three clinical directorates relate to the provider directorate as purchasers in an internal market which is controlled via service agreements.

This structure was introduced by the unit general manager (UGM) following suggestions from the RM pilot consultants and the agreement of medical staff committee. The number of directorates was restricted to four so that the hospital board, on which directorate chairpersons sit, could be limited to a manageable size (less than 10 was considered appropriate). In preference to all consultants within a directorate attending directorate meetings, the nurse manager and business manager are joined by three consultants to make up an executive directorate, also known as a board. The board consultants are elected by their peers, subject to the agreement of the UGM. The board chairpersons emerge from discussions amongst board members.

Management arrangements prior to clinical directorates (traditional functional hierarchies for most of the staff, and a loose peer-group system of independent practitioners for consultants) have influenced the development of the directorates. The current picture is very much transitional, with general management still some way in the future.

The medical directorate comprises general medicine (cardiology, respiratory medicine, gastro-enterology, diabetes), geriatrics, dermatology, haematology, rheumatology, oncology and genitourinary medicine. The 12 consultants still meet under the old 'cog-wheel divisional' system, chaired by the consultant in post prior to clinical directorates. The divisional chairperson is not the same individual as directorate/board chairperson. Whilst two systems appear to be coexisting, divisional meetings are the only time and opportunity for the 12 consultants to meet and share priorities. Organization at specialty level has yet to be clarified.

The directorate chairperson does not direct other consultants. So far the chairperson's role has been coordinating meetings, facilitating discussion, getting agreement on issues external to, yet affecting the directorate, and monitoring progress towards achieving these objectives. There is a strong leadership element in this role. The chairperson also acts as a representative of the consultant staff on the hospital board.

The nurse manager is appointed by the director of nursing services (DNS) following consultation with the board chairperson. The business manager is similarly appointed by the UGM. The board chairperson does not discuss appraisal, merit rewards or have a truly managerial relationship with these two non-consultant board members. Each retains a line relationship within professional boundaries. A complex matrix structure is, however, developing with responsibilities and relationships crossing over these boundaries. The business manager, for example, is now responsible for organizing and coordinating leave for junior doctors. The business manager has managerial responsibility for all secretarial and clerical staff within the directorate. However, consultants continue to have a close relationship with their personal secretaries, and ward sisters control a significant proportion

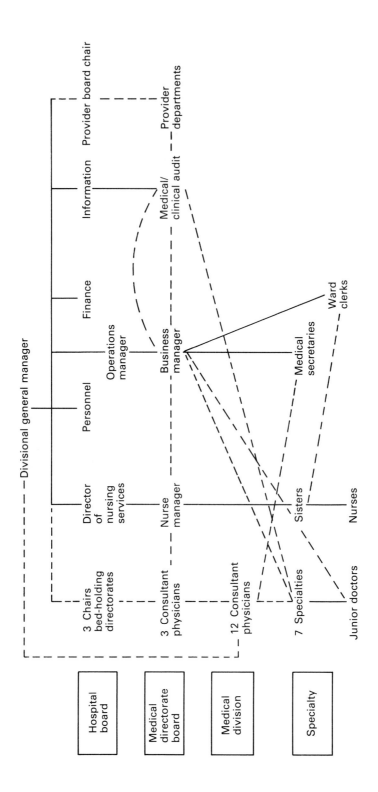

Fig. 8.2.1 Structure and relationships within the acute division of the Huddersfield Royal Infirmary.

of the workload of ward clerks. A scheme of relationships is shown in Figure 8.2.1. Dashed lines denote relationships which are more partnerships with agreed common objectives. It is proposed for board chairpersons that the partnership with the UGM, now referred to as divisional general manager, be backed up by a contract. Individual consultants still have access to the divisional general manager directly, preferably about that consultant's individual service. This has not always been so, but the divisional general manager has sensibly referred non-clinical matters back to the medical directorate.

Many of the dashed lines radiate, quite rightly, from the business manager. Contacts with the financial and information departments are crucial in understanding activity and cost in the directorate, particularly as a baseline for the service agreements with provider departments. Regular contact with individual consultants gives two-way feedback – understanding how a consultant works on the one hand, and on the other hand where that consultant is in his or her appreciation of the development of the directorate. Such insights with a number of professionals are then shared at directorate meetings.

The appointment of nurse manager is recent. However it is the intention that nursing sisters develop relationships within the structure in much the same way as consultants. Team leaders have been appointed for both medical secretaries and medical records clerks and it is proposed that a similar appointment will be made for the ward clerk group. Team leaders have a line relationship with the business manager. They will also provide a focus for developing team relationships along specialties, crossing the boundaries of the individual clerical functions.

The other major area of transition involves the budget. Information on finance is still developing in Huddersfield and so budgetary arrangements are unclear. However, a provisional scheme is shown in Figure 8.2.2.

The bulk of cost flows from salaries. A great deal of work is necessary before relationships, structure and culture are clear as to how a medical directorate board will manage this element of the budget. Changes in the nature of service agreements, from steady-state or block to cost and volume and cost per case may present opportunities for change and moving money around. Medical audit may shed light on clinical practice which need no longer continue or may be replaced by a cheaper alternative. Following such planned creation of spare capacity, the divisional general manager will allow a proportion to remain within the directorate for redeployment. Medical audit may also produce developments which require extra capacity. If spare money has not been generated, either within the directorate or across the hospital, such developments have to be assessed in the light of purchaser requirements via the contract with the

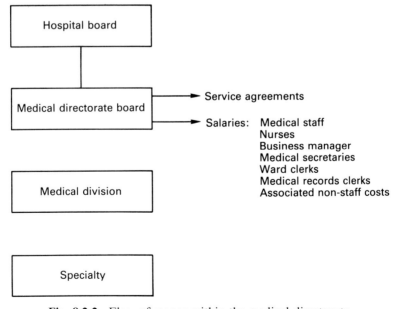

Fig. 8.2.2 Flow of money within the medical directorate.

hospital board. If the development is important to the purchaser – provider contract, some sense of priorities needs assessing at hospital board and throughout the medical directorate.

This overlaps, as do structure and relationships with the culture of the directorate and the style preferred by the chairperson of the board. We have chosen a participative style. So far only consultants, the nurse manager and the business manager have been involved. In the fullness of time, the rest of the directorate's staff will be involved in the process. This style has centred on the medical division. Regular meetings, trying to be open and share, have been supplemented by two 'time outs'. One of these was facilitated by an outside management consultancy; the other, which was devoted to business planning, by the divisional general manager and the business manager. The directorate's achievements to date include:

1 An 83-hour working week for junior doctors, incorporating full cross-cover at house officer and registrar levels between geriatrics and general medicine.
2 A 95% agreement on the 1991–1992 business plan.
3 A 95% agreement on service agreements.
4 Increasing comfort in consultant relationships.

However, some members of the provider departments are uneasy about losing functional budgets and flexibility in managing staff according to hospital-wide demands. Nevertheless, providing services for real internal customers who are empowered by the budget is accepted in the long term. There could be staff changes, either in number or skill mix, in response to the demands of the individual service agreements.

Such arrangements at directorate board level, although discussed and agreed in division, still bypass the crux of the White Paper (Department of Health, 1989) as far as consultants are concerned. Consultants still make most of the important resource decisions, and yet remain unaware of the resource consequences. Information on these is currently aggregated and collated by the relationship between audit assistants and the business manager.

Through relationships, structure and participative style we are gradually recruiting support from consultants for assessing activity and cost at specialty level, through medical audit. Hopefully with skills audit review, SWOT (strengths, weaknesses, opportunities and threats) and full

service reviews, a composite picture of 'what business the directorate is in' can be established. Such a portfolio will have strengths and weaknesses. Dialogue with the purchasers in conjunction with our own marketing activity will help us to decide what will and what will not 'sell'; where we need to concentrate our efforts and where we need to mark time. This process should also highlight service development opportunities and those services which could be phased out.

Achievements have been made during this period of transition. A second geriatric ward has opened on the HRI site, an 83-hour week for junior doctors has been implemented, the consultants within the medical directorate have talked together and shared much more comfortably, and discussions about internal trading with the provider board have started.

The second geriatric ward development at HRI arose following acknowledgment of spare capacity within another directorate. The district management board decided to invest in the second ward and withdraw support for a long-stay peripheral unit, which has now closed.

The 83-hour working week for junior doctors could only be implemented if there was cross-cover between geriatrics and general medicine. Whilst agreements, especially concerning the registrar grade, took some months, the final common rota between the two departments at all levels of junior staff is a major achievement.

It is now much more comfortable to sit round a table with the 12 consultants of the medical directorate. The majority have agreed to an audit of their people management skills. This will lead to a strategy for management development for consultants within the directorate. Attention to human resources in this way focuses on the process of change and not just the outcome.

Internal trading has not been fully implemented yet, but discussions have started. There are many human resource issues involved. Functional hierarchies will change but a lot of attention to the process of change will be required.

Reference

Department of Health (1989) *Working for Patients*. HMSO, London.

8.3 Medicine

John Meecham

To my surprise I have survived as clinical director for 5 years, first in Arrowe Park Hospital and then in the Wirral Hospital NHS trust.

Resource management

The endeavour was triggered initially by the government's initiative, embodied in an official circular (HN (86)34). This was designed to encourage doctors to play an active and responsible part in management. There were other major aims, of course, in seeking to make the best economic use of resources (and hence the label of the resource management initiative) and also the desire to gather information to show whether a measurable improvement in patient care resulted.

Arrowe Park Hospital became one of the six hospitals involved in a study which was originally due to report back in Autumn 1989 before a decision was made whether to recommend the spread of resource management (RM) around the country. In the event, no official report was delivered for two reasons. First, it proved difficult to show that measurable improvement in patient care was directly due to RM, because it was like getting details on a background of continuously shifting sand, although all six pilot sites were firmly of the opinion that such improvement was present and worthwhile.

Second, and more importantly, the government had already made the decision that RM was a success, and had recommended its adoption in many hospitals around the country, before the supposed deadline occurred.

For several reasons Arrowe Park Hospital made a slow start in RM, but rapidly gained ground once started.

At the time of the circular, we still had a traditional divided administration at Arrowe Park Hospital. Hospital administrators climbed up the NHS administrative ladder and controlled the pursestrings, and hospital consultant staff formed the medical board which made proposals and recommendations which were likely to be refused or curtailed on the grounds of expense.

The first positive move towards RM for us occurred in 1987. Dr John Roberts, a consultant psychiatrist, was appointed general manager, and Mr Andy Black (now chief executive officer (CEO) at Riverside trust) was seconded by Mersey Regional health authority to work with him at Arrowe Park Hospital.

Some of us on the consultant staff already felt that a dramatic change in the structure of the hospital administration was necessary. Dr Roberts and Mr Black believed this even more strongly and gradually set about convincing the reluctant and the unconvinced. They set up numerous meetings, varying from one-to-one discussions to groups involving dozens or, at times, hundreds of people from all the different segments of the workforce.

Establishment of clinical directorates

Agreement gradually led to the adoption of a clinical directorate pattern of management, based on the Guy's Hospital model which in turn followed the pattern set by the Johns Hopkins Hospital in Baltimore. Such a pattern has now become commonplace but, at the time, Arrowe Park Hospital was one of the few hospitals around the country which had just taken, or were about to take, the same step. I was the first clinical director appointed, in general medicine. Directors rapidly followed in orthopaedics, geriatrics, paediatrics and other disciplines, eventually totalling 16 directorates, recently trimmed to 13.

We made the decision to have separate directorates for service specialties rather than divide them up into the clinical specialties, and hence established directorates of pathology, radiology and anaesthetics.

On the other hand, paramedical disciplines of physiotherapy, occupational therapy and speech therapy were grouped with the clinical discipline

of rheumatology into the rheumatology directorate, whereas dietetics was included in medicine.

Surgery presented some interesting questions.
The general surgeons were grouped together in
the surgical directorate. It was felt that the
smaller surgical specialties could be submerged if
amalgamated with that directorate, so ear, nose
and throat surgery, ophthalmology, orofacial
surgery and dental surgery were combined into a
special surgery directorate.

Managing the hospital

The clinical directors gather together to form the
hospital council, which is the decision-making
body, in running the hospital as a whole, and in
matters affecting more than one directorate. The
council meets fortnightly with the CEO, finance
director, director of nursing services and quality
and chief pharmacist.

The council elects its own chairperson. Originally we elected the then general manager, Dr
Roberts. However he and Mr Black moved to
new challenges and we are fortunate in now
having another tireless enthusiast, Mr Frank
Burns, as CEO. We elected him chairman shortly after his arrival. I regard that as an important
step and feel it would be a disaster for the CEO
if he was not so elected – though we do reserve
the right to choose someone else if we think it
necessary. I know that other hospitals have made
a different decision in having the CEO sit beside
an elected chairperson.

Managing a directorate

As clinical director I am managerially responsible for what goes on in the medical areas of the
hospital, and for managing the budget (which is
the subject of Section 4.9(b)). I am appointed as
director by the CEO, and responsible to him, not
elected to the office, whether by my consultant
colleagues or by people working in medicine.
However it is clear that the CEO must take
soundings from doctors and nursing staff, for it
is obvious my position would be untenable if I
did not have their approval and support.

The word clinical in the title of director is
confusing for there is no intention to interfere
with the clinical freedom or clinical judgement
of other consultants or their firms. Of course I
expect to discuss practices with them, particularly where costs of drugs or procedures are markedly different, so discussion or persuasion may
cause changes in practice. But if they decide
their present treatment is correct I would not
wish to argue. In the future, medical audit is
likely to make doctors more self-critical, and
publication of simple differences such as lengths
of stay or drug costs may do the same. Discussions leading to protocols of care for specific
conditions may offer a chance to control costs
also. In one way this may produce the best
quality of care at the best cost (in other words
the 'best buy' – not necessarily the lowest cost)
but, on the other hand, we must beware of
becoming bland, regimented or stereotyped.
However, the cost of clinical freedom is certainly
a problem area for the future.

As director of medicine I am supported by a
clinical nurse manager or nurse manager (CNM)
and by a business manager (BM). Most directorates have a similar pattern. In the clinical disciplines the CNM has usually come up a nursing
pathway, and may have been a nursing officer or
senior nursing officer, or more recently have
come from being a senior sister. The CNM deals
with clinical matters related to patients and
wards and acts as manager and reference point
for all matters related to nursing staff.

When first appointed director, and when the
nursing officer in medicine was appointed CNM,
I made a foolish mistake in believing I could do
without a BM. I rapidly realized my error and
corrected it. The BM deals with all non-nursing
staff, especially clerical, administrative and technical, and all matters related to budgeting.

The three of us, director, nurse manager and
business manager, meet regularly every week but
constantly betweenwhiles. Our offices are adjacent to each other so it is the easiest thing to
keep in touch with each other most days, and
certainly several times a week.

I hold meetings of the medical directorate each
month which trained staff of all disciplines are
encouraged to attend. The two managers and I
try to disseminate information from the clinical
meetings and from other sources, and I encourage active participation by all present. Most of
the attenders are trained nurses, by virtue of the
numbers of people in different disciplines on the
wards. But we also have attending senior and
junior doctors, physiotherapists, electrocardiography technicians, pharmacists, dieticians, secretaries, clerical staff and anyone else working in
medicine.

Communication of council information and between disciplines is of crucial importance in running a directorate. Lack of information breeds rumours, and rumours breed discontent. I purposely established directorate meetings to run on an informal basis and feel that it is a major reason for the corporate attitude that is tangible in medicine.

Of course other directorates run meetings of their own. Communication also occurs between directorates at many levels by different groups gathering together. In this way lines of communication occur both vertically and horizontally, when diagrammatically displayed (Fig. 8.3.1).

In describing the situation at Arrowe Park Hospital I should make it clear that I do not claim that this is the only way of running a directorate system, nor that it is the best way. But it is how we have proceeded and it has suited us so far. However it is a dynamic system, not static, and has been modified gradually and no doubt will continue to be so.

Problems superimposed on directorate management

During the last 5 years we have had problems like everyone else in the NHS – reduction in beds, primary nursing, Nursing 2000, 'Achieving a Balance', junior medical staff hours and many others.

Information technology

We realized that we needed better information in pursuit of RM and decided to leap into the next century by installing a hospital-wide computer system. We are now well into the third year of our project to install a patient care information system (PCIS). This starts with patient administration details and communication of orders, requests and requisitions, and the replies, throughout the hospital with terminals in every ward and department. It leads on to programming of

Directorates

Medicine		Orthopaedics		Other disciplines	Meetings across the directorates	
Director		Director		Directors	Council	
CNM		CNM		CNM	CNM meetings	Combined meetings
BM		BM		BM	BM meetings	
Consultants		Consultants		Consultants	Medical staff committee specialty groups	
Junior medical staff		Junior medical staff		Junior medical staff	Junior medical staff committee	
Ward sisters		Ward sisters		Ward sisters	Sisters' meetings	
Nursing staff		Nursing staff		Nursing staff	Nursing staff meetings	
Paramedical staff		Paramedical staff		Paramedical staff	Meetings of various professional groups	
Secretarial		Secretarial		Secretarial	Secretarial meetings	
Clerical staff		Clerical staff		Clerical staff	Clerical meetings	

Fig. 8.3.1 Lines of communication in the directorates. CNM = Clinical nurse manager; BM = business manager.

clinics, waiting lists, operating lists and scheduling of procedures, and to creating a computerized patient record. Through interfaces with other software programs it leads further to scheduling of nurses of appropriate skill mix, creation of discharge notes and letters, coding patients' diagnoses and procedures, the gathering of case mix details, financial details, and therefore to the production of case mix costing information. All this offers massive advantages progressively for the future but has presented problems and challenges in getting staff trained and adaptable, and used to new practices which at first prove time-consuming rather than time-saving.

Trust status

In addition, the hospital became one of the first-wave trusts from 1 April 1991. We therefore have a trust board as another layer superimposed above the hospital council. As the council had become used to the idea of running the hospital, there was the potential for an awkward situation when another layer of authority was imposed. Wisely, any sort of confrontation along those lines has been avoided – the council runs the hospital, the trust board acts as the wise, benign, approving, questioning, cautioning (restraining?), supervising watchdog.

And on top of all these problems, before publication of the government White Paper on trust hospitals, the Wirral district health authority had already decided to amalgamate two large district general hospitals into one hospital on two sites, that is Clatterbridge and Arrowe Park Hospitals. This has been taking place gradually – emotionally over the last 18 months, but actually took place physically at the beginning of April 1992.

How to survive as director of medicine

How have I survived therefore as clinical director of medicine, first in Arrowe Park Hospital and now in the combined Wirral Hospital NHS trust? First, I need the approval of the CEO, and of consultant colleagues and nursing staff in medicine. Loss of any of these would make my position untenable.

Next, I need a good team, and I am indeed fortunate with my CNM and BM, and directorate support.

Next, I need constant access to and advice from educated financial personnel. We have a financial adviser who works under the finance director, attached to every two or three directorates. I could not manage without that help.

Next, I need good information coming in constantly as regards the usage, length of stay, turnover time, drug costs – all related to different wards, or different consultants, or different diagnoses, and attached to nursing or paramedical costs.

Next, I need constant communication, as previously described.

And after that I need a proportion of luck!

8.4 Nursing/obstetrics and gynaecology

Barbara Jones

The special health authority of Hammersmith and Queen Charlotte's Hospitals has a specific role in the NHS as a national centre in medical research and development, with specialist teaching in the care of patients, including those with complex medical problems. It functions as a multidisciplinary tertiary referral centre which requires a range of expert skills.

The obstetrics and gynaecology directorate commenced as a pilot directorate in January 1990, and a process of development and evaluation took place during the first year.

It has a budget of £8m and manages a two-sited obstetric, gynaecology and infertility service, and has a bed complement of 71 inpatient and 14 day-care gynaecology beds and 166 inpatient and three day-care obstetric beds. There is also a large outpatient service on the two sites and an *in vitro* fertilization service. We felt that our vision was to provide a high-quality, cost-effective service, whilst providing training and experience for a wide range of staff. We combine a local general service with a specialist role, providing a national outlook. This equals a complex multispecialty service, of which we are often the sole suppliers, particularly in the diagnostic field and future management of pre-eclampsia and fetal medicine. The obstetric service delivers approximately 5800 babies per year in the two hospitals and also provides a community midwifery service.

Membership of the directorate
Members of the directorate are as follows:

1 *The clinical director*, who is the professor of obstetrics and gynaecology and is based in one hospital.
2 *The deputy director*, who is a consultant obstetrician and gynaecologist and is based in the other hospital.
3 *The business manager*, who is the assistant general manager of the clinical services division and is largely responsible for the future planning of the service.
4 *The financial adviser*, who provides the information on patient activity and budgets.

5 *The nurse and midwife representative*, who manages the midwifery and gynaecology service with nursing, midwives, clerical and other support staff. These staff total about 300 in the two hospitals. She started with 16 middle managers to supervise and manage the diverse aspects of the service, which include community midwifery. She currently manages the largest slice of the budget, which is £6.3m, and the largest number of staff, and reminds her colleagues on the directorate of this fact from time to time.

All the members of the directorate are strong people managing their own part of the service and budget and we have found that we need to meet twice monthly and this frequency remains to date.

Nearly 2 years on, we are all accountable to the clinical director for the business of the directorate, but the business manager and myself relate to the divisional general manager – clinical services, for our personal development. When the directorate began, it was a new post and role for me, and my early understanding was simply to manage the midwifery and nursing service. I quickly began to realize that my role within the directorate was a much wider one, with more responsibility than I at first thought, but with an equal input to all the decisions. It was an ideal opportunity to change and develop the service and the people in it and, in particular, to look at the middle management structure which was overadministered and undermanaged.

I was warned by a nursing colleague to be wary of the business manager as he or she would have no understanding of nursing or midwifery skills and would be keen to reduce staffing levels and save money. However, he has proved to be supportive and has acquired a knowledge of nursing and midwifery practice. Indeed, the combination of his academic knowledge and my practical experience has proved to be advantageous in the directorate's development. As it transpired, I had to be wary of my medical colleagues and needed to increase their knowledge of skill mix and staffing requirements and especially the unique role of the midwife.

Our directorate works by a consensus approach with group decisions which provide team-building opportunities and produce a collective response.

This approach does not mirror nursing decision-making as nursing is a hierarchical system, which means that any nurse member of the directorate must be aware of this change of role in the decision-making process within the directorate system.

Practical achievements

1 The directorate has appreciated a view of nursing at a higher level and there is now a corporate ownership of nursing and midwifery ideals.
2 The members of the directorate were also members of a working group, along with two paediatricians, which carried out an examination of the future of the obstetrics and gynaecology services within the special health authority. This considerably helped the directorate team to gel as a group, meeting frequently in order to produce a document for the special health authority's final decision.
3 The policy of ward-budgeting and devolving these budgets down to the middle managers has given them authority and greatly improved their development.
4 A new nursing and midwifery management structure was implemented which has produced a stronger middle management team. It has also placed the right people in the right jobs with abilities to get the job done.

Lessons learnt

I consider the directorate structure to be a good one as it works well by giving us financial accountability and marries our different interests. It can be advantageous for nursing and midwifery as it provides the opportunity for implementing change and developing the service in the direction in which nurses wish it to go.

Strengths, weaknesses, opportunities and threats for nursing in a directorate

Strengths

The nursing and midwifery profession has a unique role in using both clinical and managerial skills and can often provide the understanding to bridge any gaps between these two influences.

Weaknesses

If strong nurse and midwifery leadership is not evident in the group, the nursing developments and ideas will be overridden in favour of medical or financial ones.

Opportunities

These can be many and the ability for nurses and midwives to grasp these and use them to promote nursing and midwifery to their advantage is the true test. Nurses must put patients and their needs first and be articulate enough to present these views.

Threats

The threat is to have weak nursing representation in the directorate and therefore a return to a dictatorial management style which produces little or no advances in service or nursing development.

The directorate system presents challenges for nursing and midwifery and therefore new skills are required. I consider myself to be a senior manager with a nursing and midwifery background.

New skills required for nurses

1 To provide a bridge between clinical and managerial skills within the group.
2 To be able to participate fully in the broader role of the senior nurse in the directorate.
3 To provide strong leadership in order to articulate the needs of the specialist nursing role.
4 To develop skills in managing other groups of staff and an understanding of their different roles in the NHS. This requires an understanding and knowledge of the jobs of auxiliaries, secretaries, ward clerks, etc.
5 To be prepared to develop within the directorate and be able to forward-plan.
6 To develop good budgetary skills on a larger scale. This means the ability to implement change in order to make a budget flexible and adaptable to service improvements. If the budget is overspent it requires

excellent management skills to create savings whilst maintaining service provision.

7 To maintain a sense of humour – after all, work can be enjoyable if you want it to be!

The directorate style of management provides opportunities for nursing and midwifery to develop in a way which gives the senior nurse control over its direction and makes good sense for the safe and continuing future of nursing and midwifery.

Doctors at present do not have the skills to manage large groups of staff: nurses and midwives do. By the same token, business managers rarely have the clinical knowledge to supplement their managerial skills. Nurse managers act as an agent to enable these groups to communicate effectively.

Nurse management within the directorate is about advancing into leadership and not retreating into narrow professional boundaries.

8.5 Obstetrics and gynaecology

Peter Jackson

Introduction

The key to having doctors who will survive as medical managers is to recruit the right ones in the first place. This is a fairly basic principle, though in most cases the selection of a medical manager is a rather haphazard process. Certainly at the onset of the resource management initiative, few hospital doctors had received any extensive management training. The best that most had achieved was a brief introductory course on management of the NHS which they had attended as a senior registrar or early in their consultant days. There had been no formal teaching of management skills at medical school or during the junior training appointments. The selection of medical managers therefore depends very much on the assessment of an individual's potential rather than proven success in terms of qualifications. This has on many occasions provided a bonus in that the doctor coming into management is faced with a whole new set of challenges. If the right person is selected and approaches the task enthusiastically, the challenges will be found to be exciting and stimulating. A fresh mind will be of considerable benefit to the organization.

I was the first clinical director for the directorate of gynaecology, paediatrics and obstetrics at Huddersfield Royal Infirmary, one of the original resource management pilot sites. Prior to this I had been a consultant in obstetrics and gynaecology at the hospital for nearly 10 years and the question, which must be asked by many doctors selected for management roles, is – why me? None of our directorates had formal elections but there was a general canvassing of opinion and debate leading to the emergence of a name. In my case I was already the chairman of the old cogwheel-style division of obstetrics and gynaecology and was a known enthusiast for the resource management initiative. To my colleagues therefore I was an obvious choice and I commenced with the reassurance that I had their full support.

The reasons for individual consultants wishing to become clinical directors fall into three main categories – power, ability and duty. Certainly some enter management because they perceive that it will give them a position of power within the organization. There is, of course, also the converse, in that they wish to prevent someone else having that degree of power over them. Second, they may enter management because they consider themselves to have the skills and ability to make a good job of it. All things are relative and perhaps this should be phrased as the ability to make a better job of it than the existing managers. Third, there are those who do it because they feel it is their turn or they are pressurized into doing it by their peers. There may well be a mixture of motives but the concept of doing the job on the basis of 'Buggins's turn' must be firmly rejected.

Selection methods must be devised within each institution that will enable people with the correct management skills to be chosen. Moreover, selected candidates will only be able to succeed if they have the respect and confidence of their medical colleagues. They sit in an uncomfortable role of trying to manage when their position is really one of first among equals. Getting a consultant colleague to change his or her practices can be a delicate and at times a difficult task. Finally, the candidate must be someone who can work well with the general managers and can command their trust and support. The clinical director can only be appointed with the approval of the unit general manager. To have innovative ideas and make progress, a fine balance must be struck between choosing someone with few fresh ideas who will simply be a 'yes' person to the unit general manager, and someone whose ideas are so different from the general aims that there will be conflict leading to stagnation.

Achievements

Survival as a medical manager is dependent very much on believing that one is doing a worthwhile job. Achievements are the rewards that maintain the enthusiasm; without them the frustrations become destructive of morale. As a consultant involved with management, my major achievements have often been as a result of having a catalytic effect on bringing about change within the organization. It is hard to quantify change in cultural attitudes; however there has been a major breakdown in the 'us and them' attitude between the clinicians and managers. All consultants within the directorate now accept that they have both professional and managerial responsibilities. We have regular management development meetings within the hospital where clinicians and managers come together for a sharing of ideas. This cross-fertilization of information helps to improve understanding on both sides. Increasing the knowledge about the running of all aspects of the organization has been a key element in the development of change.

The most dramatic change has been the overwhelming commitment to audit. From the medical point of view we have devoted one half-day per month to a formal structured audit meeting. The main drive has been to produce a quality service and each month recommendations are made to improve medical care. The concept however is more widespread and throughout the directorate we have worked to push the idea of total quality care. This means that there is constant attention to achieving good quality at all levels. The message has been that doing the job well results in good-quality medicine which will be cost-effective. If quality care is not given then there will be more complications, more returns to theatre, longer lengths of stay and more readmissions – all of which mean the use of more resources and inefficiency. Of course it also means more complaints from patients and less job satisfaction for the staff. By carrying out regular clinical audit, doctors have therefore taken many steps which have led to an improvement in efficiency. Areas that have benefited have been a reduction in preoperative lengths of stay by greater use of preadmission clinics, more day-case surgery, reduction of postoperative stay and fewer laboratory or radiological investigations. These are all measures of process and I would like to be able to state that outcomes have also improved. However, this information has proved much harder to obtain than we originally imagined. We had no outcome measures of any real value before resource management so there has been nothing with which to compare. More-over, we have had problems with coding, case mix and recording severity of disease, which have delayed the development of outcome measures. There is, however, now a realization of the importance of this information and clinicians are working on the residual problems.

The integration of nurses, midwives, clerical workers and all other personnel within the directorate has been a slower and more difficult task. Nevertheless we have put on regular 'road shows' within the directorate to keep people informed of the changes and have kept repeating the message that everyone needs to be involved. Devolution of authority has certainly helped to improve the efficiency of the directorate in many ways. The delivery suite sister has stopped having a cupboard full of size 8 gloves, which are rarely used, and now keeps a realistic supply. One of the secretaries suggested a scheme for batching letters to general practitioners, with a considerable saving on the number of envelopes used. The antenatal clinic clerks reviewed and improved the appointment system to reduce patient waiting times. These changes have all come about because we have successfully created a culture where people are thinking along quality lines and trying to improve the service in their own area. We have moved away from the concept of coming to work to do a job the way it has always been done with no real ability to make changes because of a highly bureaucratic organization. People are now encouraged to put the customer first and are given the authority to alter existing practice.

We have certainly not got everything right first time but the ability to make mistakes and learn from them is an important part of management. Perhaps our biggest disaster was in moving towards patient-held antenatal notes. The concept seemed excellent – greater involvement of the patient with her care, more information available to her general practitioner, less paperwork and so on. It apparently works well in many parts of the country but not in Huddersfield! The patients we sampled before starting the scheme were keen but once it became reality they were less than enthusiastic. They did not like other members of the houschold reading their medical details, they did not like carrying their notes around as they were cumbersome and some became anxious about the consequences of losing them. We learnt from this experience and have now gone back to a traditional, albeit modified, maternity cooperation card.

Problems

The role of a medical manager is not always easy and an essential element in surviving is being able to overcome the problems. The greatest problem has been in establishing both the role of the clinical director and the authority of the directorate. Admittedly this is probably more of an issue for the initial clinical directors and will improve as time goes on. Moreover in Huddersfield we made a gradual transition from a divisional cogwheel system to a directorate model. This evolutionary approach has had many advantages but the greatest disadvantage has been that at times elements of both systems have overlapped. Consequently it has been relatively easy to undermine the role of the directorate by using alternative management channels. A clinical director has to work hard to ensure that all the issues are channelled through the directorate. If this cannot be achieved the directorate system will lose credibility and the medical manager will become disillusioned. There is certainly no satisfaction to be gained from being in a role where you are held responsible for the administration of part of an organization without having real authority. This is a lesson that has been a hard one to learn by some general managers who can be slow to let go of their power.

The image of the medical manager role can also lead to conflicts. First, at a personal level managerial decisions will have to be made which conflict with professional values. This raises the question – am I a manager or am I a doctor? Second, what image do I portray to my colleagues? Do they see me as a management stooge and someone who cares more about the balance sheet than about patients? At first the role felt somewhat isolated; in Huddersfield we have only three clinical directorates giving a relatively small peer support group. As time has gone on things have improved and we now have subdirectorates, with the result that more consultants have become involved in management roles. Moreover as the first set of clinical directors are replaced, the number of consultants with an understanding of the role of medical managers is increasing. The ex-clinical director is an important resource of information and can provide vital support for his or her successor.

A major problem is time. In Huddersfield we elected to take on an extra two sessions to carry out the duties of clinical director. This however is an underestimate of the true commitment. There is still far too much bureaucracy in the health service. Both the amount of unnecessary paperwork and the amount of time spent to no value in committee meetings is considerable. For this reason support is a vital issue in helping the medical manager to survive. Each directorate has a business manager and a nurse manager who are invaluable in seeing to the day-to-day administration. We have tried to keep formal directorate meetings to a minimum and indeed most issues are best resolved by informal person-to-person contact as soon as possible. Time management is important and if it is not handled well can result in the development of stress. Being a medical manager is not a role for the faint-hearted: even the robust need to be alert to the problem of stress.

The nursing profession and particularly midwives find it difficult to distinguish professional and managerial roles. The nurse manager on our directorate has a background in paediatric nursing which does not help her credibility with midwives, though perhaps the problem area would be paediatrics if she were a midwife. In theory her background should be unimportant as she is there for her managerial skills. If the directorate takes a management decision it is not unknown for this to be regarded as a professional matter which is taken to the director of nursing services who can countermand the directorate instructions. A recent example arose when the postnatal ward complained of being short-staffed and we carried out a review of duties undertaken by the midwives. One of these duties was to carry each baby on discharge to the front of the hospital and hand it to the mother when her transport home arrived. This took the midwife away from the ward for about 15 minutes and with 3000 deliveries per year this represented a loss of human resource of 750 hours. However, when the directorate suggested this practice could be stopped it suddenly became a professional issue and was blocked by the director of nursing services. Negotiations are ongoing!

Training is a further issue in helping the survival of a medical manager. Again there is a time factor. How much training should you give a doctor for a 2- or 3-year role as a clinical director? If doctors are to have short-term management roles then it is more productive to have some personnel within the hospital who have the appropriate skills who can be called on by each directorate as and when necessary. Most medical managers devote time to learning management skills by reading and attending courses or lectures. However, this will compete with ongoing medical education. No matter how well-intentioned we are, the amount of time spent reading medical journals or on study leave related to our specialty will suffer. The balance will be further swung towards management commitment from clinical commitment where clinical sessions are dropped to take on a role in management. In some cases doctors will see their future career having a permanent management component and will wish to drop most or all of their clinical sessions. This is, at present, an unusual and somewhat courageous move. Consultants in general hold a position of high status within the organization and their credibility as a manager may depend on their skills as a clinician. Would they lose this status and credibility if they withdrew from their clinical role?

Conclusion

The involvement of doctors in management is essential to the provision of an effective health care system. In order to survive in this role the medical manager must have sufficient authority to achieve real benefits. To do this there will have to be a major commitment in terms of time and training. Factors that will aid survival will be establishing a clearly defined role in the management structure of the organization and creating adequate administrative support. There will be tangible successes which will boost morale. However, many of the benefits result from the medical manager's leadership skills in taking the organization along the pathway towards providing an improved service. It has to be accepted that these cultural changes will be hard to quantify.

Those medical managers who do survive have a responsibility to their successors. Ideally, successors should be selected in good time so that they can undergo suitable management training. In our directorate they would spend at least a year as a member of the directorate to become conversant with its role, aims and objectives. There will then be a smooth transition, ensuring that the authority of the directorate is maintained. The presence of a suitable successor will depend on how much appeal the post creates. The clinical director should aim not only to survive but to be recognized as a success and by bringing enthusiasm and excitement to the post will be an encouragement to colleagues considering the role of medical manager.

8.6 Pathology

John Stuart

A clinical directorate (Board of Laboratory Medicine) was established by Central Birmingham Health Authority in the spring of 1989 following an external review of laboratory services by the management consultants Peat Marwick McLintock. Their review highlighted the fragmented nature of the existing laboratory service and recommended the formation of a management board chaired by a director of laboratory medicine with responsibility for some 350 staff and a budget of £5.7m (excluding medical salaries and equipment).

The Peat Marwick McLintock report was strongly supported by the district general manager and the health authority proceeded with the appointment of a part-time (3 days per week) director of laboratory medicine. Four part-time (2 days per week) discipline directors (clinical chemistry, haematology, histopathology and microbiology), each supported by a full-time laboratory manager, were also appointed from existing consultant staff. No additional consultant sessions were funded to offset the loss of consultant time to the laboratory service and no budget was allocated for training in management for either the directors or managers. The board was supported by a full-time implementation officer (business manager) for its first year, by a financial adviser, and by a personal assistant to the director of laboratory medicine.

The board had management responsibility for the 'policy and planning of all the district laboratory medicine services'. Laboratory staff, however, remained professionally accountable to heads of departments, who retained responsibility for employing staff via hospital personnel departments; refilling of vacancies required the approval of the discipline director. Consultant pathologists became managerially accountable to the appropriate discipline director who, in turn, was accountable to the director of laboratory medicine. The latter reported directly to the district general manager.

The establishment of this clinical directorate predated creation of the NHS internal market by 2 years. The board was seen nationally as an important management initiative that stimulated the formation of laboratory directorates in other health authorities. On 1 April 1991, the internal market was created, Central Birmingham Health Authority fused with the adjacent South Birmingham Health Authority, and a new chief executive was appointed to the combined authority. Hospital units within the new authority, although not yet applying for trust status, were expected to function more independently than hitherto. As a consequence, the board of laboratory medicine was dissolved and its budget divided amongst the hospital units.

This exercise in laboratory management provides a number of important lessons for clinical directorates in general, as described below.

Management of staff in the directorate

The extent to which a director has responsibility for direct management of staff will vary between directorates according to the human resource functions that are retained by hospital personnel departments. In the case of the board of laboratory medicine, which was a district-wide directorate, there was originally an opportunity to bring together all the personnel function for some 350 laboratory staff in five hospitals. The recruitment, induction and performance appraisal of such a large staff would have required dedicated personnel staff for the directorate. This was not possible but would have had a unifying effect on laboratory medicine which would have been highly desirable had the district-wide approach been maintained. The directorate, managing a budget in excess of £5m, would then have functioned as a small hospital unit.

When a directorate comprises a specialized workforce, as in laboratories, there is benefit in customizing the human resource strategy for that staff. Useful strategies might include a school recruitment programme for laboratory staff, use of block advertisements, a policy of holding vacancies until the summer recruitment drive, a standardized induction programme with a strong emphasis on safety at work, and a performance appraisal scheme oriented towards professional needs. A coordinated system of staff development and appraisal can be highly effective in a laboratory environment, as it is possible to set detailed criteria for performance that make the appraisal objective rather than subjective (Stuart and Hicks, 1991). These strategies are more difficult to implement if the personnel function is divided between several hospitals within a health authority.

Organization of staff in the directorate

A large directorate will have many tasks that compete for the limited time of the clinical director and support staff. The natural response is to form subcommittees but there is widespread disenchantment with health service committees, which are often considered to be a forum for communication rather than action. There may be a statutory requirement for certain committees such as those concerned with accreditation, audit or safety but, in clinical directorates, most committees can be replaced by temporary task forces (Stuart and Hicks, 1991).

Task forces can be used to give direction and purpose to the directorate and develop its strategic plan. A task force should be small (not more than 5–10 members), have a short life span (not more than 3–4 months) and be allocated a clearly defined task that can be achieved in that time. Once a short report for the directorate has been prepared, the task force is automatically disbanded. This has the great advantage that its members are free to participate in other groupings for different tasks. If a task has not been successfully achieved, then a new group of individuals with a slightly different remit and a different leader is often successful in achieving a fresh approach.

Task forces usually comprise a mixture of grades of staff whose leader need not be the most senior; often it is preferable to choose a younger individual who has the time, interest and motivation to achieve the task. The clinical director can act as a facilitator if required and should monitor progress; the latter should be more than the occasional vague enquiry as to progress and should include agreed milestones when feedback is to be made. The use of junior staff as team leaders fosters a sense of involvement in the staff who quickly appreciate how difficult it is to plan good strategy and implement change. Their own management skills then start to develop.

The task force report should be circulated to all members of the directorate to disseminate information, to involve all individuals in planning the development of the directorate, and to lay the groundwork for implementing change. Individuals appreciate better the need for change when they can see the whole picture and can understand the reasons behind difficult decisions.

Almost all the activities of a directorate are suitable for the task force approach, but each task force should be established as a specific initiative of the directorate to address a specific problem of high priority. Examples in laboratory medicine included the on-call service, specimen transport, disposal of laboratory waste and staff recruitment.

Time commitment of the director

Clinical directorates of this size are time-consuming and carry substantial budgetary and human resource responsibilities. They require the time commitment and intensity of effort that a professional manager would bring and cannot therefore be considered as an addition to the work of a busy full-time consultant. Adequate sessions must be allocated to the job and the vacated clinical sessions should be taken over by others. Clinical director posts are temporary assignments, often of 3 years' duration, and there must be a clear plan for return to clinical work at the end of it.

Doctors as a profession are highly responsible, have a strong work ethic and readily become overcommitted. They often find it difficult to prioritize because clinical tasks have to be done and it is not easy to be selective. Management requires a different approach with an emphasis on strategic planning, determining priorities, negotiation and managing change. Some doctors find the transition to be stressful, particularly when they have to deal for the first time with difficult colleagues who do not readily accept that their own departmental interests are not the same as those of the directorate. The combination of simultaneous clinical and managerial responsibilities can be particularly stressful and the director may feel there is insufficient time to do either job properly.

The new director must therefore look for things to stop doing to create capacity for the new task, remain aware of the risks of becoming overcommitted, and focus on selected tasks of high priority. The words of Peter Drucker (1990) are particularly relevant:

> The first step toward effectiveness is to decide what are the right things to do. Efficiency, which is doing things right, is irrelevant until you work on the right things.

Training in management for the director

While good management requires both common sense and interpersonal skills, it is naive to assume that doctors do not also require to learn some of the skills of professional management (Stuart and Hicks, 1991). Doctors should not accept a clinical directorate if the health authority does not offer management training. In addition to teaching specific skills, such management training enables the doctor to understand how a manager thinks, while the contact with other clinical directors allows one to talk over potential solutions to management problems. The beneficial effects of management training also include the development of problem-solving skills and the ability to implement change more effectively.

A part-time clinical director requires the support of a business manager or equivalent, plus secretarial sessions. Adequate support from hospital personnel and finance departments is also needed to facilitate the work of the directorate. The director, however, must have sufficient basic training in management to work effectively with such managers and to understand the principles of personnel and finance management.

Appointment of clinical directors

A directorate is unlikely to be successful if there is not general support for the director. If the director is elected by the members of the directorate, there is the risk that management may be unhappy with the nominee. Equally, if the director is appointed by management, the directorate may be unhappy with the appointee. Great care is therefore required over the selection process so that members of the directorate unite behind, and have a sense of ownership of, their director.

Conclusion

It is greatly to the credit of clinical directors that, despite a lack of formal training in management, they can rise to the challenge of running a successful directorate. Their professional background and the interpersonal skills that develop from dealing with patients provide a strong foundation on which to build management skills. Many graduates from business schools in the USA are perceived to lack such a foundation (Deutschman, 1991). The board of laboratory medicine of Central Birmingham Health Authority did much to develop a cohesive strategy for laboratory medicine, despite the conflict that subsequently arose between a unified district-wide directorate and a competitive unit-based structure. More than 50 task forces completed their work over a 2-year period and thereby provided an invaluable basis for the future direction of the pathology disciplines. The benefits of this will survive the political *volte-face* of the 1991 internal market.

References

Deutschman, A. (1991) The trouble with MBAs. *Fortune International* **15**, 119–127.

Drucker, P. F. (1990) *Managing the Non-Profit Organization*. Butterworth-Heinemann, Oxford.

Stuart, J. and Hicks, J. M. (1991) Good laboratory management: an Anglo-American perspective. *Journal of Clinical Pathology* **44**, 793–797.

8.7 Paediatrics

Cyril Chantler

A paediatric clinical directorate

Most of the important points in introducing a clinical management structure apply to all clinical directorates irrespective of specialty, though obviously there are individual differences. The interdirectorate relationships have to be considered. Within paediatrics there are two important associations, one with obstetrics and the other with the community. The relationship with both needs to be discussed in detail early on and clear management and staff accountability should be established. As an example, with obstetrics, it is important to determine which group will be responsible for the special baby care unit or neonatal intensive care unit, how the unit will be staffed and to which directorate the staff will be accountable. Similar considerations apply to other services and other staff that are necessary for the satisfactory functioning of the paediatric directorate.

There are few isolated children's hospitals left in this country because it is increasingly difficult to justify the high running costs and undercapitalization of such hospitals. Where a children's hospital is established in a district general hospital or teaching hospital then it is necessary for the paediatric directorate to ensure that adequate facilities are available throughout the hospital for children, either managed directly by the paediatric directorate or bought in from other directorates or departments. An internal accountancy system to ensure that bought-in services are properly costed is essential and, like any purchaser, the paediatric team has the right and the responsibility to ensure that such services are provided in a way which is appropriate to children and to an appropriate standard. Such arrangements however are simply an extension of the more general arrangements within general management and indeed at Guy's Hospital now the clinically based directorates increasingly receive the income from the contracts that they have made with commissioners and are then responsible for paying their share of the overhead costs of the hospital. They also pay for the services that they subcontract within the hospital, be they in operating theatres, in the anaesthetic department, in pharmacy, in therapy services, medical equipment and supplies and in the various investigative departments such as pathology and radiology.

The relationship between a paediatric directorate in a district general hospital and the community paediatric services is complex (Chantler, 1990a). Various models have been suggested and are being piloted and it is too soon to draw general conclusions. Paediatricians are attracted to the model whereby the community paediatric services and the hospital services come under a joint management so that, for the children at least, health services are provided either by primary care from general practitioners or secondarily from the combined hospital and community service. This model has the advantage of improving continuity of care and should encourage, if properly applied, the provision of services in the community rather than in the hospital. The problem in the past, however, has been that the needs of the acute hospital tended to dominate and lead to hospital services developing at the expense of community facilities. For this reason some community staff have preferred to maintain their own management structure but in this event it is vitally important that the hospital directorate and the community directorate work closely together. This can be facilitated by joint appointments and managerial responsibility for district community paediatricians. In my view, however, there will be an increasing move to joint hospital – community units and the dominance of the hospital will be reversed by the purchaser insisting on the promotion of care in the community rather than in the hospital.

Practical problems (Chantler, 1990b)

Frustrations

A major frustration for the doctor in management is the feeling that responsibility has been transferred without adequate authority for its fulfilment. It is thus vitally important to ensure that the organizational structures are correct before accepting the commission. A further frustration concerns the inadequacy of the financial and budgetary arrangements. The difficulties inherent in the process do need to be understood and clinical directors corporately, acting through the hospital management board, need to argue for the introduction of adequate systems with the maximum amount of decentralization commensurate with the corporate good. The latter point is important because, whilst tensions inevitably exist between the decentralized clinical directorates and the central hospital administration, none the less, it is in no one's interest for the hospital as a whole to overspend and when it does it is inevitable that the problem then has to be transferred to those who spend the resources, namely the clinical directorates. To coin a phrase, there is no way that the foot can be healthy if the heart has stopped beating.

Interdirectorate relationships can also lead to tensions because directorates tend to fight each other for resources to promote the services of their own patient groups. This can result in healthy competition with resources being allocated to those with the best case within the confines of contract. On the other hand, such competition, unless managed within carefully devised rules and policies, can lead to great difficulties. It is the job of the top management to regulate these arrangements and ensure collaboration between the different groups. The groups themselves have to be prepared to negotiate and compromise but in this respect a hospital is no different from any large business. Certainly such conflicts in our experience have been much more productive than the conflicts that used to exist between different professional groups and particularly between doctors and administrators.

Quality

The drive to improve the quality of the service to patients is imperative if the NHS is to survive. Indeed, the recent reforms were partly stimulated by increasing evidence that the NHS was treating patients as charitable cases who should be grateful for what they received (Toynbee, 1984). Quality again means considering efficiency and effectiveness and will only be achieved by all who provide the service, irrespective of professional discipline, working together. There are many examples of good and bad practice available. We used to be plagued with an appalling outpatients service where up to 10% of the notes were unavailable at any one clinic, patients were kept waiting and brusqueness and rudeness to patients were all too common. The introduction of the clinical decentralized management system enabled the staff – doctors and nurses and reception staff–to sit down together and work out how to provide a better service. The 42 staff who used to work in central records were decentralized so that large clinical groups were able to employ their own receptionist and clinic preparer. The introduction of an outpatient computer system enabled this individual to be responsible for all bookings of clinics and to act as the receptionist in each outpatient session. The results have been dramatic. In my own outpatients in the last year there has not been a single case of a set of notes being missing when the patient has been seen. Most of the notes contain the results of investigations and, if they are not available, they are easily obtained through the computer at the time of the clinic. In a recent survey 96% of the patients were seen within half an hour of their appointment time. The important point is that quality can only be achieved from the bottom up, not from the top down.

Time

A common argument is that doctors do not have the time to be involved in management. I have come to the conclusion that the argument should be reversed; they do not have the time not to be involved. It is worth asking how much time is spent in committees and whether the effort is productive. Using your own and others' time efficiently is an essential part of management. Much can be achieved using the telephone, by being rigorous about reading and only keeping essential material, by not being overbureaucratic about recording minutes for meetings, by stating when a meeting will end as well as when it will start, by avoiding continued minutes on the agenda, and by delegation. Time spent in determining operational policies is seldom wasted and a well-organized clinical service releases time and resources for caring for patients. Management time can often be created outside clinical sessions. A small point concerns secretarial time. A good clinical secretary will spend a great deal of her or his time organizing activity, including consultations, rather than writing letters. Some discipline regarding what is essential in a clinical letter and what is not is important. In my experience, many who complain of lack of secretarial assistance write extremely long letters that nobody reads.

Listening

It is only too easy to become overwhelmed with administration and to spend management time bound to a desk. It is important to be available to listen to everyone's views and a good way is to set aside definite times in the week to be out of the office. A good ship's captain spends a great deal of time walking around the ship, which is similar to the old adage, 'The best manure is the farmer's feet'. Dealing with mail efficiently and promptly is important and Oscar Wilde's dictum 'Never put off till tomorrow what you can put off until the day after' does not work for management.

Decisions and leadership

A good manager has to be decisive but not all decisions will be correct and there is often no harm in admitting mistakes and trying again. A good decision will command support amongst all those who have to implement it and they should have been involved, as far as possible, in considering the nature of the problem and helping to formulate the solution. Often a properly led discussion will produce an obvious decision, but at other times competing priorities will preclude such an outcome. The decision then has to be made but will usually be carried through with

enthusiasm as long as those who have to implement it have been consulted. Leadership implies that those who are led are prepared to follow. The clinical director who loses the support of other staff in the directorate, particularly professional colleagues, can hardly continue in office. Checks on the possible abuse of authority are important and the British system of all consultants carrying equal authority in their professional lives is too important to discard. Management is essentially about persuasion rather than command.

Incentives and motivation

The old NHS made it very difficult indeed to reward good performance with a financial benefit, though there is evidence now that the introduction of trusts is changing this. Financial recognition is important, particularly for many staff in the NHS who are inadequately remunerated. For professional staff, however, motivation often comes in different ways, not least by having responsibility and authority and the opportunity to improve service, whether it be to patients, to teaching or to research.

It is important to ensure that all members of the organization understand their role and know to whom they report and their performance should be reviewed formally and regularly to provide motivation, advice and help. Setting personal objectives on a regular basis and discussing them with the person to whom you are accountable and with the people who are accountable to you is a useful discipline.

References

Chantler, C. (1990a) Paediatricians and the new National Health Service. *Archives of Disease of Childhood* **65**, 357–360.

Chantler, C. (1990b) How to be a manager. *British Medical Journal* **298**, 1505–1508.

Toynbee, P. (1984) Patients and the NHS. *Lancet* **1**, 1399–1401.

8.8 Psychiatry

Rafeek Mahmood

The directorate of psychiatry sees its responsibility as developing and delivering a psychiatric service within the resources available to the residents of a district and making every possible attempt to encourage all members of the directorate to feel part of the decision-making process.

Psychiatry has a special relationship with other statutory and non-statutory bodies such as general practice, social services, voluntary bodies and the independent sector.

To ensure the success of our aims a very close working relationship has been established with community organizations such as Mind, Alzheimer's Society, Schizophrenia Fellowship and advocacy groups.

Communication is the strength of our directorate, involving all professional groups concerned in the delivery of care. The collaborative effort made by the directorate to involve all organizations responsible for the delivery of care reflects our perception of the whole approach.

The clinical director is appointed by the chief executive following discussion with colleagues, and is managerially accountable to him or her and takes full responsibility for devolved operational management. All staff in the directorate are ultimately accountable to the clinical director. Operational management is wholly a directorate duty.

Management at the Wirral Hospital devolves total decision-making to the staff. The clinical directorate is a small unit of management led by the clinical director, supported by a business manager and a clinical manager.

This structure means that staff no longer owe allegiance to their professional groups; there is a definite and deliberate breakdown of professional tribalism. Staff loyalty is to the directorate rather than to individual professions. Staff relate to the directorate and to corporate objectives. The process of consultation and decision-making occurs within the directorate. The directorate draws its strength and authority through empowering other members to make decisions (Table 8.8.1).

There were a number of factors to overcome to ensure the success of the directorate. Locally, psychiatry is delivered from two hospital sites. The first task which faced the directorate was to promote a sense of identity within the directorate. Second, we needed to develop clear lines of communication and make available a forum for discussion on various topics. Third, it was necessary to develop a sense of accountability away from the traditional line management within each profession to accountability to a directorate which is involved both in decision-making and delivery. Finally, it was important to help towards an effective culture change and the development of individual skills within the directorate.

Table 8.8.1 *Psychiatry activity 1991–1992*

Senior medical staff	11.00 (persons)
Junior medical staff	11.00
Nursing staff	183.00
Administration and clerical	18.90
Paramedical	4.00
Total	227.90

Number of outpatients
12 192

Number of inpatients
1529

Number of consultants
10

Number of beds
Clatterbridge
    60 General acute
    10 High-dependence unit
    25 ESMI
Arrowe Park
    40 General acute
    10 High-dependence unit

Budget
£4 527 651

It is important to realize at this stage that this account is a snapshot of the present situation. Management structure is constantly changing and evolving. As a directorate we have seen various patterns of communication change with the maturity of the directorate. To ensure proper communication, we have tried to involve as many of our staff as possible in executing various objectives from our own directorate objectives.

A number of small interdisciplinary task forces, which are time-limited and goal-set, formulate a policy which is discussed once within the directorate, then relayed to the executive body – the clinical director, business manager and clinical manager. The decision and action taken are based on discussion and consultation. There are no permanent groups that meet regularly, but rather a flexible arrangement bringing in different people and different disciplines for differing tasks. The fact that decisions are made at ground level and the staff are able to see the results of their discussions and decisions fairly rapidly has made for a new perception of Management.

Figure 8.8.1 shows the lines of communication adopted by the directorate of psychiatry. Although at first glance this may seem cumbersome, in practice we have found that a clear structure for communication, with specified dates and times, allows the staff to be up-dated as to various matters occurring within the directorate or within the whole hospital. Furthermore, topics that staff feel they would like to discuss in a wider forum are addressed within various meetings.

All business is conducted within these groups. Staff are encouraged to discuss professional issues with the professional bodies but, as far as issues of management and service delivery are concerned, these are only to be discussed and decisions made within the directorate.

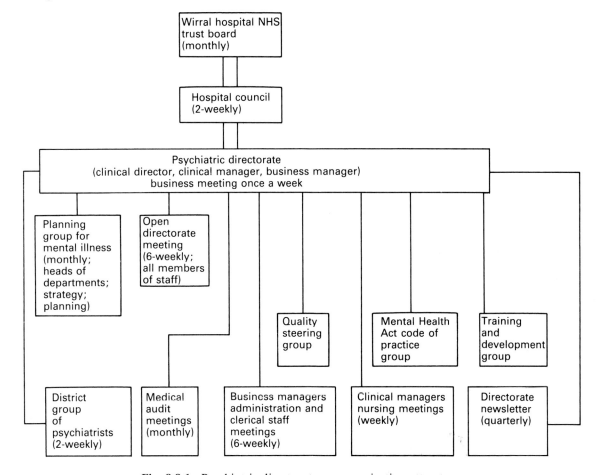

Fig. 8.8.1 Psychiatric directorate: communications structure.

The directorate is required to provide a business plan in January/February. This is reviewed and budget-setting exercises are carried out based on the developments or otherwise suggested by the directorate. Before the business planning stage, a series of discussions take place within the directorate looking at the future. A plan for 1, 2 and 5 years is formulated. We see this as an opportunity to develop a genuine strategy for mental illness and begin to cost the exercise well in advance.

Out of the business plan and budget-setting exercise, directorate objectives evolve, with very specific issues discussed, such as marketing, public relations, service quality, contractual issues, clinical efficiency, financial targets and human resource issues. The directorate objectives are partly drawn out of the corporate objectives and are partly specific to individual objectives for the clinical manager and business manager. There is an individual performance-related bonus for achieving certain objectives for both the clinical manager and business manager. Before referring the directorate objectives to the chief executive it is essential that these are discussed within the directorate in the widest possible forum, as there are implications both for individuals and for the directorate as a whole.

Once directorate objectives are agreed, a final meeting is arranged with the chief executive, the finance director, the director of nursing and the human resources director.

In this instance it is worthwhile spending some time looking at the role of the chief executive. It is essential that the chief executive manages the clinical directorates at arms-length. Delegated management must be a reality and the lack of 'interference' in day-to-day management of the directorate only strengthens that directorate. Operational management is wholly a directorate responsibility. Strategic decisions are made within the directorate but discussed at directorate reviews and not dictated by an executive committee: they stem from the very wide base of a mature directorate structure. Within the Wirral we have had a true change of traditional management style and the devolvement of management to a directorate team.

At this point it may be important to use an example to illustrate a process and a structure, starting with a vision and ending with a change in clinical practice.

Discussions have taken place within psychiatry for a number of years regarding sectorization. The Wirral has a population of 350 000 and traditionally psychiatric services were delivered from two hospital sites by two groups of psychiatrists working in north and south sectors. To deliver a more responsive service, it was thought better to subdivide the Wirral into three sectors, based on social services and the Family Health Service Authority's (FHSA's) boundaries, forming teams of two acute adult psychiatrists, one psychogeriatrician and one child psychiatrist, each with his or her own multidisciplinary teams.

Although the idea was acceptable, no progress was made. An interdisciplinary project group was set up, which became known as the steering committee, to discuss the principle. Small task forces were devolved from the whole of the directorate. Small groups with a very specific remit to evaluate and gather information were formed. These groups studied populations, looked at needs and assessed them, followed through current 1991 census data and looked at geographical sectors. Collaborative work was carried out with social services and the FHSA. For the first time the Wirral population was studied from the point of view of needs and the totality of our resources were looked at with the aim of devolving these resources to the most needy sectors.

Eventually an 'away day' was organized to bring all the relevant information together and a decision based on collated information was reached. A consultative document was produced which was discussed within primary care, social services and the planning group for mental illness (which involves voluntary bodies, the independent sector and various interested bodies). The outcome of this short planned project, managed by the directorate and owned by the staff, will ensure the success of 'home-grown' changes in practice.

Throughout the process the directorate enabled, facilitated and motivated, but kept in focus the vision of a truly community-based psychiatric service and was able throughout to give informative advice.

The clinical director spends an average of three sessions per week in directorate work. The support and commitment of the directorate team are invaluable; total and honest delegation is essential. As has been mentioned previously, the fact that the directorate team meets regularly once a week (and has discussions and communicates with the majority of staff once every 6 weeks) ensures the commitment of the 214 staff members.

The job of the clinical director would be impossible without the support and encouragement of the body of consultant colleagues, as well as the support of all members of the directorate. It is important that the chief executive allows decision-making to be a directorate business and avoids traditional management interference in the directorate.

8.9 Radiology

James D. Laird

The theory of managing an imaging department is quite straightforward, just like the theory of riding a bicycle. In both cases, the practice is somewhat different. In theory there are a considerable number of things which should assist imaging department management. The most important is a clear tradition of active administration with leading participation of radiologists. Management theory sees the need for a clear structure with appropriate definition of responsibility and authority. Most radiologists believe this exists in imaging departments (even when it doesn't). The theory also requires an understanding of the product produced and the resources used in doing so. Again in imaging departments, the product is usually clear (although it should be stressed that the report and *not* the images is the final product). Imaging departments have recorded throughput in some form (radiographic units, patients examined, or Körner units) for many years. Increasingly the resources used to produce this output have been defined. The number of radiologist sessions, radiographers, clerical staff and films used are now defined and recorded by most imaging departments.

Therefore, unlike clinical areas, imaging departments have been used to some form of direct management and have the infrastructure and information to assist this.

This is the theory. The practice, as any radiologist will tell you, is different. Radiologists have usually not been trained in management. Superintendent radiographers, in contrast, usually have had specific management training. On occasions, this can lead to conflicts. However, the more usual effect is that a senior radiologist is nominally in charge of a department, but the superintendent radiographer is the effective manager. For example, many radiologists never see the budget statements for radiographic staff, X-ray films or maintenance and leave control and responsibility for this entirely to their superintendent radiographer. In most cases, this is much more than simply delegating authority.

There have been other problems due to the legacy of the remarkable financial system used in the British NHS up to the 1991 reforms. Capital for equipment was not regarded as part of the resource used in the production of images and their subsequent reports. Thus there was no penalty for the underuse of expensive equipment or for the unnecessary purchase of replacements.

However, the biggest gap between theory and reality is the status of individual radiologists within the organization structure. The theory requires a defined and recognized management structure. The reality is that all consultants are equal (although, like George Orwell's pigs, some consider themselves more equal than others). Management becomes more consensual than hierarchical in style and colleagues must be led not driven.

Management of any large and complex structure has many requirements. In non-hospital terms, imaging departments are the equivalent of quite big commercial undertakings. Many have multimillion pound budgets and employ large numbers of staff. All are very capital-intensive, possessing often several million pounds worth of imaging equipment. Active management is therefore not just important, but vital.

It is possible to divide management problems in imaging departments into three large groups – management structure, information and quality.

Management structure

At first glance it would appear that most imaging departments are run by some form of specialty committee. The exact form may vary, but it is usually composed of all radiologists plus some senior radiographic staff.

It is chaired by a radiologist and often, quite mistakenly, he or she is perceived as being fully in charge of the department. Indeed, he or she may share this delusion. The reality is, as indicated earlier, that responsibility is divided (not delegated).

The superintendent radiographer usually manages all the radiographic and darkroom staff. He or she will normally do so with little reference to the chairperson of the committee. This relationship is rarely spelt out and so consequently exists in a very ill-defined form, just waiting for a crisis to expose it as a problem.

The specialty committee is very unlikely to consider activity or financial figures on any regular basis. It thus differs fundamentally from a board of management. The committee members do not regard themselves as bound by committee decisions. When individual consultants feels their interests are threatened they often believe they can ignore committee decisions with impunity. There have been some positive aspects however. Most such committees have usually considered and prioritized requests for replacement equipment. Individual important changes in the functioning of departments have been debated and agreed. In the past the most useful function of such committees has been the dissemination of information.

If this is the current practice, the implementation of management theory would require a series of quite radical changes.

As already indicated, management should be based upon a clear and universally understood structure showing exactly where authority and responsibility reside. A starting point is to define the scope of the department itself. For example, it is necessary to define which staff belong to the department. Clearly radiographers belong, but what about porters and clerical staff? As a general rule, staff who work exclusively for a department should be made directly responsible to its management. There will be other employees such as domestic staff who are few in numbers and perform only a specialist service. It is better to think in terms of a service agreement defining a level of quality and provision at an agreed cost.

Along with the definition of staff employed by the department goes a similar task for functions performed and equipment used. Custom and practice will almost certainly have laid down a framework for any existing department. It is necessary to review this and define the full extent of the department and its services and responsibilities. This can be a useful exercise, identifying problems with neighbouring services, for example.

Once it is clear who and what are to be managed, the next task is the definition of how. There

are a fairly wide variety of management models. However, there are certain basic principles. There is a need to provide both strategic planning and operational management. Strategic planning will decide the intermediate and long-term future of the department. Given that all consultant and senior radiographic staff have a vested interest in this and the former a relative veto over action, strategic planning requires a large and representative group. Proposals for action and plans for approval can be constructed by small groups, but any long-term strategic policy must be endorsed by a larger committee.

Operational management is concerned with the day-to-day running of the department. There are a very large number of tasks which are not vital in themselves, but need to be dealt with in order to keep the service running. This sort of management task is the function of a small group ultimately responsible to the large departmental committee.

All this may sound common sense. However, in the past many departments were merely administered and not managed. Operational management in some form has usually occurred. Strategic planning has, at best, been uncoordinated and, at worst, non-existent.

There needs to be a fundamental review of the objectives of the department and any related problems. Such an analysis can be expected to produce radical changes, for example, using equipment for many more hours per day, employing part-time staff, or extensively reorganizing work patterns. A major characteristic of a managed department is that it can respond quickly and effectively to external change. Once a strategic plan has been adopted it is necessary to monitor progress at regular intervals. Usually this will entail monthly reports to the larger (or departmental) committee. In the context of the NHS reforms strategic planning is necessary to allow contracts or service agreements to be negotiated. Regular progress reports will therefore deal with activity figures within contracts. The reports will also have to deal with finance to see that the department is living within its projected budget.

In principle therefore the structure can be a simple one. There should be an executive team headed by a consultant radiologist. The team should include the superintendent radiographer and a business manager if such a post exists. The team needs to be small. It should meet on a very regular basis (once or twice a week).

This team is responsible for operational management and for guiding a larger departmental committee in the realms of strategic planning. It should be responsible to the departmental committee containing all consultant radiologists and other senior professional staff.

It should be remembered that a clinical director or chairperson of the departmental committee will also be responsible to the central hospital management for the efficient running of the service. This double level of responsibility needs to be understood as it can lead to conflict. An imaging department will have its own set of priorities, but ultimately this must fit into the overall objectives of the hospital.

Management structures are easy to define. Management processes working in these structures are much more difficult. (It is all too easy to set the structure up and find it does not change anything.) Processes can be assisted by written definitions. It is therefore very useful to define the roles of any committees and of all the key players. Getting all concerned to debate these definitions is also helpful. The objective is to produce the required clear outline of all the management processes, lines of authority and areas of responsibility. In doing so it is vital to gain active or tacit acceptance of all, or at least a large majority, of the consultants on the departmental committee.

Management information

There is a long tradition of imaging departments gathering figures to measure activity. In the past, information gathering has been at the behest of the district, region or Department of Health. Very often the production of activity statistics is seen by imaging departments as an unnecessary chore. The figures so produced have been unused by anybody and indeed in some cases so inaccurate as to be useless. Occasionally radiologists have attempted to support the case for more staff or equipment by reference to these activity figures.

All too often regions and districts have found reasons to ignore the statistics they themselves demanded. All this is changing. Departments now need information to manage internally and usually this is more detailed or different in type from that required by regions and the Department of Health.

If we look at the management of imaging departments it is clear that we need a number of types of information. It is important to measure output, but we must also look at the resources used to achieve this. Thus we can break down information requirements into two large groups – measures of output and of resources used.

Output activity figures

A very important management aspect of output measurement is the production of information which will help control the use of resources. It follows from this that simple statistics such as the total number of patients examined will not be sufficient. The total number says nothing about the complexity of each examination or the cost of the equipment used. The Department of Health introduced Körner statistics as a means of improving measures of output. The Körner statistics group output of X-ray departments into six types. Examinations in each group are supposed to be roughly similar in the use of resources. With only six groups, it is clear that each covers a broad range of examinations using different types of equipment and often with dissimilar demands upon staff. However, on the positive side, Körner statistics have the advantage that every department in the UK already gathers them.

At the other end of the spectrum of information-gathering it would be possible to list each type of examination and record these separately. This would prove very time-consuming and wasteful of clerical staff (and paper).

So in the UK, the starting point must, at present, be Körner statistics, but every department should give thought to improving local use of these.

Improvements can be achieved by creating subgroups of examinations using the following types of criteria:

1 Same major piece of equipment used.
2 Roughly similar use of radiologist and radiographer time.
3 Roughly similar use of consumable items.

Clearly, these groups can vary from department to department (depending, for example, on availability of equipment). The number of groups should be kept as small as possible. In management terms each group is meaningful. It takes roughly the same amount of resources for every examination within the group. This type of measurement of output takes some time to develop, yet it is important not only for internal management, but also for clinical contracts, service agreements and calculating costs.

Procedure costs

There are two approaches to the calculation of the costs of imaging procedures. The first of these is referred to as a top-down approach. In this the total cost of the imaging department is worked out. (Most hospitals already make this sort of calculation.)

A formula is then worked out to apportion all the departmental costs on to the output activity figures. For example, a weighting factor for each Körner group may be used. This will apportion the total departmental costs to all the Körner groups and thus to each individual examination.

This approach is fairly straightforward. It allows a cost to be calculated for each examination and, at the same time, ensures that the total costs of the department are accounted for. Unfortunately, it also hides inefficiencies. For example, if a piece of expensive equipment is used very little, this fact is completely concealed and the cost is buried in every procedure cost.

The second method of calculating procedure costs can be called the bottom-up approach. This requires the true cost of the procedure to be calculated. This can be achieved by recording a sample of each type of procedure, showing the number of minutes of radiographers' and radiologists' time, the equipment used and consumable items. Quite a lot of calculation is required as the cost per minute of each grade of radiographer and radiologist must be worked out. Also the total cost of the equipment must be converted into a cost per minute. All these sorts of calculations require the help of the hospital finance department. If the examinations have already been grouped to record output, samples of each group rather than each examination are all that is necessary. Obviously adding together the costs of all the procedures will produce a figure much smaller than the real cost of running the department. The difference is an overhead, a *pro rata* portion of which must be added to each procedure.

The great advantage of this more complicated process is that is shows just what is happening in the department. For example, it will illustrate any equipment that is being underused (and in so doing can load the cost on to the few procedures actually performed upon it). It is also possible to add up all the time spent upon procedures for each grade of radiographer and subtract it from the total time available. This gives some indication of capacity to increase the workload. For these sorts of reasons, the bottom-up approach is superior to the top-down approach, but it does require a lot more effort to achieve.

Measures of resources used

Traditionally imaging departments have seen the control of resources as completely separate from output. This has produced some quite astonishing features. As already mentioned, equipment is seen as being controlled completely separately from everything else. This means that very expensive equipment can be purchased and grossly underused. In industry or private medicine, expensive equipment is used 18 or more hours per day in order to recover the capital cost. In the NHS, far too often, such equipment is used on a nine-to-five basis only.

An extension of this problem is that equipment tends to be replaced on a historical basis – a screening table is often replaced by a more modern version of the same thing. With changing patterns of work, it is important to decide at a very early stage what the department most needs. Replacing equipment becomes a very different matter when the cost must be justified by improvements in quality, throughput or major reductions in repair bills. The future will demand effective management linking the control of resources very tightly to output. This will require radiologists to rethink completely the control of equipment.

Staff

Most departments will receive information about staff in post and their costs. Such statements will cover radiographers and darkroom staff. However, it is important to ensure that they also cover all other staff who are exclusively employed in the imaging department. Having agreed with the hospital the type and variety of staff employed by the department, any budget figures must reflect this.

Control of this budget is much more than just living within a fixed allocation of money. Regular examination of the skill mix is important.

For example, would radiographic helpers take some of the drudgery out of radiographers' work (and also cost less)? Information about staff should also cover their professional training. It is an important aspect of management to ensure that appropriate and adequate training is given to *all* grades of staff.

Equipment

In order to work out capital charges for equipment, information is required on the initial and annual costs of each major piece of equipment. The hospital may choose to control this information centrally or to delegate some of the responsibility to the imaging department. The advantage of the latter approach is that it brings home the real cost to the department. In any case, the use of procedure costs (including an element for capital charge) will have the desired effect of linking equipment cost to output.

This will cause radiologists to question the concept of automatic replacement of equipment at intervals. Equipment becomes more likely to be bought to achieve a specific outcome (improvement in technique, throughput or cost).

Service agreements

One of the great management problems of imaging departments has been the inability to control demand while constrained by a fixed financial allocation.

With the NHS reforms and the onset of clinical contracts, departments have a chance to get away from this strait-jacket. In order to do so, they need to produce service agreements with clinical specialties. In essence these are agreements to provide imaging procedures up to a certain level for a fixed amount of money. This means that departments would have real budgets, i.e. an allocation of money to produce a specific number of procedures. (Real budgets are in sharp contrast to the traditional cash allocation. With a budget the priority is to achieve an outcome. With a cash allocation the priority is to live within it.) While clearly this is a desirable

state of affairs, quite a lot of work is necessary to set up the agreements. Activity figures must be available for past years to allow comparison. Procedure costing must be in place. It must also be possible to divide the costs of procedures into fixed and variable elements. (If a department performs a barium meal there is a certain cost. However, if the meal is not performed, the saving is very much less as the equipment and staff will still be a cost to the department.) This concept is very important to imaging departments as it protects against unrealistic savings demanded by clinical areas.

Service agreements must be negotiable with each clinical area. There must also be a clear understanding of the volume and appropriate mix of procedures to be supplied. The volume, in practice, should be allowed to vary within certain limits (for example, ± 5%).

This is to allow for the variations in clinical activity brought about by alterations in the mix of cases treated. (Fairly small variations in workload should be within the capacity of departments to absorb.)

Agreements should specify what will happen with excessive over- or underdemand by any clinical specialty. It is reasonable to think in terms of saving variable costs. In summary, it is likely that most departments will gradually develop service agreements. The effects of this will have profound implications for the way departments are managed.

Computers

Considering the sheer complexity and volume of information now required to manage an imaging department, the use of computers appears essential. Activity analysis, monitoring of service agreements, procedure costing and asset registers all require computer assistance.

There are now a large number of radiology management systems on the market. The other features such as procedure costing and asset registers are only just beginning to appear. It is perhaps important to stress that most systems should communicate with the other hospital computers. Life is much easier if a radiology management system can get information from a patient administration system or send any required information to the finance department automatically and electronically.

Quality

It is all too easy to be lulled into the belief that the main task of management is to deliver a product at as low a price as possible. This is completely to ignore the vital element of quality.

One of the most important lessons from private industry is that consumers do not buy solely on price and indeed quality is one of the most important factors. This means that imaging departments need to be managed to deliver the highest possible quality at a reasonable price. Quality can be considered in three major areas – response time for a report, patient satisfaction and image and report quality.

Response time for a report

The ultimate objective of any request for an imaging procedure is the delivery of an expert report to the clinician concerned.

There are a number of key events in the conversion of a request into a report of a procedure:

1 Reception of request by department.
2 Waiting time for procedure to be performed.
3 Sorting time for films (including location of previous films).
4 Reporting and typing time.
5 Time to dispatch (including method of dispatch).

All departments try to control these events, but where many fall down is the absence of any routine monitoring process. Management of a department should receive regular reports of the waiting list and waiting time for all procedures. It is also worth checking that there is no delay in making the appointment, leading to a concealed increase in waiting time.

It is worth trying to monitor the average delay between the taking of an X-ray film and the radiologist reporting it. In many large departments, there are significant problems with the location of previous films, leading to a delay in reporting.

After dictating a report the radiologist often feels that his or her work is complete. Consequently the typing and dispatch of reports and films are neglected. There should be as short a delay as possible in typing reports.

It is absolutely no good performing an examination very promptly if the report is sent by internal or external mail and takes several days to arrive. It is part of a quality service that reports are delivered as quickly as possible. Means of delivery therefore need to be examined and controlled.

Patient satisfaction

The NHS is only beginning to become patient- (or consumer-) oriented. For years departments were run to suit staff, not patients (many appointment systems were designed to prevent radiologists having to wait between examinations, rather than keeping patient waiting time to a minimum).

It is vital to consider each patient as an individual (and usually a very frightened one). It is helpful if all staff wear name badges and introduce themselves to each patient. Departments now need to consider the waiting areas and waiting times for patients. Indeed, there are very many aspects where departments should be viewed from a patient's perspective to identify problems.

Some form of survey of patient satisfaction is well worthwhile. Surveys should however lead to improvements. They should not be regarded as interesting pieces of research.

One important area is the extent of communication between radiologists and patients. Surveys have shown that patients value being able to talk to and question the radiologist. They are generally very keen to know what has been found on their X-rays. Good patient communication should be part of departmental policy and actively encouraged.

The essential element is to encourage all staff to become more sensitive to patient needs. This is a continuous task. It requires special training for reception and telephonist staff. It will be helped by group discussion of radiologists and radiographers. This whole area requires a planned approach and a recognition of its importance. Fortunately most hospitals have now recognized this and quality in patient care is a widely discussed topic.

Image and report quality

Fundamental to the services of any imaging department is the production of very good quality images. This must not be regarded as an automatic result in an otherwise well-managed department. There must be a clear strategy to ensure the production of optimum images and there must also be internal monitoring on a regular basis. Such a strategy should embrace a very wide range of features. Recruitment policy and in-service training are important.

Regular monitoring of performance of equipment (especially film processors) should also occur. There should be some internal system for the routine identification of film faults and the correction of errors.

The most important single message is the need for a carefully planned and comprehensive approach to film quality.

The quality of procedure reports is harder to control. At present this is best achieved by regular clinical meetings with individual specialties or units. Some internal disciplines can also be helpful. It is useful to insist upon every report having a one-line summary or conclusion. It can also assist if interesting or doubtful cases can be identified in any computer system and so reviewed at a later date.

The linking of clinical data through the new case mix systems available in some hospitals promises the possibility of comparing X-ray findings with pathological or discharge diagnoses. This sort of review of report accuracy or relevance is some way off, but is likely to develop as integrated hospital computer systems spread.

Conclusion

Surviving as a medical manager in radiology is not easy. There are many facets of management and most of them seem to be required for imaging departments.

The two essential features are the support of fellow radiologists and the assistance of good professional staff, especially the superintendent radiographer. It is, however, becoming ever clearer that the success of departments in the future will be inextricably linked to the success of their management.

8.10 Surgery

Ron Parker

It is hard to overestimate the potential for change that the new form of management of clinical services brings to the NHS. We are in the midst of a quiet revolution. From a situation in which management decisions were often made by non-clinicians outside the hospital, we have moved to one in which they are made by clinicians near to the patient.

The clinical directorate type of structure is central to these changes and I will illustrate this by reference to the surgical directorate in which I work at Walsgrave Hospital in Coventry. The function of this directorate is to manage the surgical services on a day-to-day basis, to plan for the future and to relate to other parts of the unit in order to provide a complete service.

For effective directorate activity there must be maximum devolvement of power down to it, consistent with the smooth running of the whole organization. This is a difficult step for many general managers to take as it implies a loss of power. Once taken, however, it is clear that it empowers many other people and leaves the general manager free to concentrate on more strategic issues. The loss of control over significant decisions, a control which often dilutes and delays action, is more than offset by the power gained in running a lively and active organization.

At the same time as devolution of power, there must be a clear understanding of the boundaries of a directorate's activities, including limits to the level of decision-making and action that can be taken, and rules of financial virement. The boundaries may need to be renegotiated from time to time; there is no fixed pattern. Lack of clarity leads to frustration, stop – go activity, overlap of activities with those of other directorates or of the unit and gaps in service provision.

My directorate includes general and ear, nose and throat surgery, the department of anaesthesia, associated wards, virtually all of the theatres, including the day unit theatre and the endoscopy suite, together with a variety of smaller departments and functions. It has a budget of approximately £10m per annum. The budget is totally devolved to the directorate with the main guideline being to remain within it. There are some broad virement rules. Hiring and firing of personnel is also a directorate function with support from the personnel department of the trust. The medical contracts are handled by the personnel department because of the skills required which are common to all directorates. The directorate senior nurse deals with nursing personnel matters and advises on nursing.

The clinical directorship is a key post and is occupied by one of my consultant general surgical colleagues. All the directorate posts in this trust were appointed by the general manager, with the agreement of their peers. In other units the medical staff elect directors but the appointment requires the support of the general manager. In any event a director needs to have credibility with both parties and needs to have a genuine interest in management. Some previous experience and ability in management are obviously a great help but the demands of the post are great, and further management training and personal development will be required. In Walsgrave Hospital trust, each director is supported by a business manager and a senior nurse. This triumvirate, together with some secretarial support, and with advice and support from the trust, comprises the management of the directorate.

One of the central needs of a directorate is to bring together its members into one team. There is little place for tribalism and internecine warfare in the business of providing better care for patients. A good starting point is to try and articulate a common vision. Each of us has an internal set of standards and a sense of direction in our professional lives. These are usually surrounded by powerful feelings and we are embarrassed to talk about them. We assume that they are commonly held and shared, but this may not be so and we may each be on a slightly separate path. When we talk to other disciplines about this, the divergence may be even greater. To work out a common vision or set of values or an agreed mission statement can help to build the team. Another approach is to do this by way of discussing individual plans for the directorate or problems we have experienced. Doctors seem more comfortable with this approach and this is the one that we have informally adopted. As a team enterprise, if taken increasingly seriously, this will lead to a common vision statement. In the meantime we share the mission statement of the trust and agree with them a set of objectives for our directorate.

Conflict and disagreements inevitably occur between colleagues in all staff groups and these are dealt with at directorate level by the appropriate member of the triumvirate; ultimately it is the director's responsibility. This requires skills over and above those usually held by doctors. So often colleagues in hospitals in which I have worked have adopted a competitive attitude to each other: this can cause considerable friction. The skills shown by doctors in their relationships with patients, when confidentiality, caring support and unconditional positive regard are used, have to be transferred to the organizational level. All members of the team respond well to praise and understanding and badly to undermining criticism. If carried out well, this activity improves teamworking; done badly it is destructive.

Out of directorate discussions about service provision naturally follow outline business planning and forward planning. These have yet to be fully developed in our directorate but a full day meeting of all of the directors in the trust and of an adjacent hospital have begun to develop the direction for our planning for the next 10 years. These will be eventually tied up into definite plans, including business plans. Contracts are mostly held with Coventry district purchasing authority. They are block contracts and are developed in collaboration with the directors and the directorates. Cost and volume contracts are being developed. A similar process will be used with individual fundholding general practices.

Quality care is a central issue in the NHS. In Coventry the purchasing authority conducts regular quality reviews of our services. Although the questions are clustered around the elements of the Patients' Charter, they do extend much more widely. In addition, the medical audit process regularly reviews our surgical performance. Discharge summaries are typed using a word processor attached to an Apricot computer and the diagnoses are coded using Metabase. These provide morbidity and mortality data on broad case mix categories as a basis for the audit process. Walsgrave trust is a HISS site and in due course other arrangements will be made for coding. The audit meetings are chaired by a rotating chairperson who has read all of the discharge summaries. Considerable ingenuity is used here in checking for oddities or an unusual length of stay, which may throw light on unrecognized problems.

The audit process is mostly used as an educative one, and to help us modify patient care. We are not yet regularly feeding useful information into the directorate or the trust managers, which will help to change the organization and how it performs. Since it is claimed that some 70% of problems with patient care are institutional rather than down to the individual doctor, we have obviously yet to realize this opportunity to change the organization. A natural step from medical audit is to move into clinical audit, involving other clinical staff and other disciplines. We have not yet carried out this step. Patient surveys of our services are highly supportive of our efforts, as usual. The patients are not involved in service planning, apart from the lay members of the trust board.

In a rapidly changing world, organizations which do not respond become increasingly irrelevant. The devolvement of power in the NHS is changing its management structure from a vertical centralized one to a flat and flexible one. The interaction of clinical staff with patients and the patients themselves have become central to management activity and not peripheral. This can tap into the powerful idealism of all clinicians, releasing rich creative activities and providing powerful motivation to the organization. Directorate-type structures are an important component of this and we have certainly felt some of these differences in my directorate.

8.11 Surgery

Peter D. Wright

Survival as a medical manager in any specialty, be it medicine, surgery or a service specialty, depends upon such a person having a clear understanding of the relative roles of the clinicians within the specialty, of his or her own role both as a clinician and as a manager, and the role of the management structure within the hospital or other medical community in which he or she is operating. To uphold this role satisfactorily clinical directors clearly have to have the confidence of their colleagues, both as a clinician and also as a manager, at the same time as maintaining confidence within the management of the hospital as a whole so that they can represent not only the views of their colleagues as a specialty but also work with them to manage effectively the element of the hospital service lying within their sphere of influence. This role has become particularly important since the 1990 legislation introducing a payer – provider relationship into the provision of the clinical service. This has placed much more significance upon the effectiveness with which a clinical unit is managed.

The appointment of a clinical director

The appointment of a clinical director in any specialty is a crucial stage in the development of effective management. In the NHS of the past there was a high degree of consensus management with the distinct ethos among the consultants that they were there to treat patients and others were there to manage and provide the circumstances which allowed them to offer the treatment that they felt appropriate: that there was a clear divide between the management and the clinicians. This scenario developed before there was any concept of cash limiting and was associated with the belief that clinicians, in making their decisions about the care of patients, should not have to consider the financial consequences. In this environment the role of the senior consultant flourished: it was a purely

professional leadership role, usually fulfilled by the most senior consultant in the specialty, in the hospital or on the ward. Although this had a significant role in the aspects of the clinical management of the ward and of teaching and training of the juniors, there was no significant part to play in the effective management of resources either within the unit or a hospital. With the development of resource management, the role of a clinical director or clinician in administrative charge with more defined responsibilities became essential. Indeed, even if the changes related to the payer – provider relationship had not been introduced, it was clear as resource management progressed that a much clearer management role would be required from clinicians if resources were to be utilized effectively. An understanding of this evolution is necessary amongst a group of clinicians if a successful clinical directorate system is to be introduced, because the clinicians from among whom a clinical director is to be chosen have to understand and accept the reasons for the change if it is to be successful.

In the initial days of clinical management there tended to be a rotational clinical head of department who would fill the post for 2 or 3 years and then stand down in favour of the next colleague in line. In this the clinicians were appointed to fulfil a democratic role in which they were representing their colleagues rather than managing them. This has now changed; the need for clear identification of specific management accountability, as opposed to professional accountability, has meant that the clinician has to be appointed by the hospital board but after consultation with the colleagues within that specialty. Then both the position of the person holding the post and his or her role are understood and accepted by both sides. If the clinical director were to be imposed without any form of consultation with the specialty, the nature of the relationship is such that it could be extremely difficult to manage the specialty effectively. They could be working against the opposition of a significant number of colleagues who in fact had significant *de facto* control over the budget that the clinical director was supposed to be managing. Underlying many of the anxieties among clinicians is what is perceived as a potential threat to clinical freedom imposed by such direct managerial involvement by clinicians. It is only by demonstrating that such involvement enables a specialty within a hospital to develop in the direction that it chooses with much more freedom that clinicians will gain confidence and maximize the benefits that such devolution in management can deliver.

The role of the clinical director

The work of a clinical director is difficult as it involves treading a difficult tightrope between clinical accountability, the director's own clinical activities and those of colleagues, and management accountability for the effective management of the specialty.

To manage effectively, a manager must have something to manage. In effect this means that he or she must be in a position to manage and be accountable for the budget for those things within the unit that he or she can control. Since the introduction of contracting for care, a clinical director is responsible not only for making sure that the work of the unit is effectively covered by contracts so that there is a sufficient income to sustain the clinical work, but also needs to be in a position to ensure that those contracts are delivered. In addition to this, there is a responsibility to identify new developments and their implications for contract development in the future. To do this effectively a clinical director must have real control over those aspects of the budget that influence his or her ability to attract clinical work and deliver the care that has been agreed. This means that aspects of the hospital budget that have previously been under the control of middle management, such as nursing and pharmacy, have to be devolved to the specialty so that they can be directed to the best effect. To fulfil these roles effectively, good management support is necessary, preferably in the form of a specialty manager devoted solely to the discipline which a clinical director is managing. This role is crucial as it allows a clinical director to continue with as much of his or her clinical activity as possible whilst managing the unit. The specialty manager

is responsible for collating all the data to enable the clinical director to take the necessary decisions and to do the necessary ground work to ensure that the decisions of the specialty are implemented. It is very important that the clinical director continues to have an active clinical involvement in the work of the unit because if he or she is allowed to become too distant from the routine clinical work, his or her credibility with colleagues will fall and he or she will be unaware of many of the important facets of the day-to-day working of a surgical unit – this could make the difference between success and failure. However, much of the work of managing a specialty takes time. It is difficult to identify specific times within the week when management will occur and others when it will not, as many of the decisions have to be made on a day-to-day basis. Over the course of a week the total time involved in management may be one, two, three or even more sessions, depending upon the size of the specialty and the problems involved. However, these do not all occur at once and much of the work is done on the basis of talking to colleagues and other managers over lunch, over coffee or in the corridor and it is by many of these informal *ad hoc* meetings that the real management work is done, ensuring that not only are decisions taken but that they are also implemented effectively.

Relationships between clinicians

The changes of management ethos have led to different relationships between consultants. Management within a hospital grouping is different from that which might occur within industry where conformity with management decisions can be enforced much more rigorously. In any group of consultants there is a more sophisticated and complementary relationship in that they all depend very much upon each other in providing a comprehensive service. Where many of the decisions which have a real impact upon the utilization of the resources are the matter of a professional judgement, life could be made very difficult for a clinical director in bringing to bear the full force of management without being shown to be both professionally and expensively wrong. This means that there has to be inevitably an element of consensus management in certain aspects of the specialty management. Many of the uncertainties among clinicians about being managed by one of their colleagues are removed by the clinical director being meticulous in involving colleagues in the decisions made within the specialty, so that they have a sense of ownership. Then they are not marginalized and left to feel that important decisions are being made behind their back. If this latter situation is allowed to develop, a clinical director is likely to find that the period of tenure is rather short. Conversely, in a unit where the consultants have been actively involved in the management process and understand the reasons why decisions are being made, effective management becomes much easier and quite challenging issues can be faced and resolved. As part of this exercise formal meetings do need to be held among the consultants, usually with the involvement of the specialty manager, and if appropriate with specialist trainees so that they can understand as they come through the training system the importance of the involvement of clinicians in management and would be appropriately prepared for when they take up consultant posts of their own. Such meetings do need to have formal minutes circulated so it is quite clear what has been agreed and what has been understood. This is an opportunity when the full financial documents and other relevant papers related to the specialty can be circulated among one's colleagues. This ensures that they can peruse them and discuss them in a more formal setting and their views can be clearly understood and recorded. Keeping such matters open and above board significantly improves the effectiveness of the management of a specialty and allows those colleagues with specific clinical interests to be appropriately involved in their development and progress.

Management of the purchaser–provider relationships in surgical practice

The evolution towards a payer – provider relationship has had more impact in the surgical specialties than or many others, particularly as much of the waiting list work is related to surgical specialties. Although initial contracts have been block contracts in most districts, they are rapidly evolving and becoming much more specific and procedure-related. To manage effectively in this environment it is important that the clinicians are actively involved, through the clinical director of a specialty, in first establishing what contracts have been agreed and second, making sure that they are delivered. The consequences of this have a major impact on how a hospital will be run and the relationships between surgery and other specialties within a hospital.

In, for example, general surgery, when a contract is agreed between a hospital and a health authority for delivering an agreed amount of general surgery, a commitment is taken on by the clinical director that care will be delivered in an appropriate time at an appropriate quality. To be able to undertake such a commitment, a clinical director has to be able to identify and control all those facets of the hospital service which have a significant impact upon his or her ability to deliver the contract. In real terms this means that, for example, if a vascular surgeon has a contract for management of patients with vascular disease, a significant amount of that work will depend upon the investigation of patients with procedures such as angiography and transluminal angioplasty. It is not advisable for a radiologist independently to have contracts with the district for angioplasty without the involvement of a clinician, for the reality is that the clinician, who is a vascular surgeon, will hold the contract for the provision of vascular services. Part of that cost, agreed with the district, will include the angiographic services delivered. This has a number of benefits, in that when a contract is agreed with a specialty it will come with an agreed amount of money for provision of the necessary service, for example radiology, so that at least there is some predictability for the radiologists as to the amount of angiographic services they are expected to provide for the agreed number of vascular patients over a given period of time. This concept fosters a philosopy which involves various primary contracts between clinicians and health authorities by providing services and a number of subcontracts within a hospital between the primary contracting clinicians and the various service departments. A further example of this occurs with the management of operating theatres. It would be very difficult to envisage a circumstance where a clinician could agree a contract to deliver a surgical service and not have a significant degree of control over the management of that service, right from admission, through the investigations, through the operating theatre, to recovery facilities and ultimately in the outpatient clinic. In the light of this the management of operating theatre facilities has had to take a much higher profile in the management of a surgical specialty.

One of the major changes that has occurred with the introduction of a payer – provider relationship is that it has tended to move the entire emphasis in the organization of hospitals and the subdepartments within them away from a climate whereby the successful running of a hospital, operating theatre or radiology department could be an end in itself. In the new environment it has to be much more responsive to demands from purchasers and other pressure groups who demand a greater degree of flexibility. The hospital, the specialties and the service departments within it have to be sensitive to changes in demand both in terms of numbers of patients and types of investigations and treatments required. When a clinical manager has responsibility for budgets within his or her control – the largest element of which would be nursing – and can control both of ward nursing and theatre resources, together with the other ward facilities. This allows a much wider perspective of the needs of the specialty as a whole, both in terms of the available nursing skill mix and its distribution. There is then much more freedom to enable staff to work more flexible hours and have a much greater corporate identity within the specialty, which is then reflected in the quantity and, more importantly, the quality of care offered to the patient.

These greater responsibilities for clinical managers do, however, carry, in addition to the accountability for management, a significant degree of accountability for the quality of the environment in which it is providing specialty works, as well as for maintaining both morale within the specialty and appropriate career management and advice, not just for the medical members but for the other specialist groups within the team.

The management of changing relationships within the specialty in a hospital

A significant problem related to the recent developments in NHS legislation and funding has been the anxieties induced by change. Whether

or not a change is for better or for worse, the very fact that a change is occurring makes people feel uncertain and insecure. As part of the development of change, staff at all levels have to be involved and kept informed about the reasons for change and about the aims that such a change are designed to achieve. As the ability of clinicians to influence the development of their specialty is becoming clearer in the new climate, enthusiasm is increasing. One of the major changes that has occurred is the ability for clinicians to identify areas within their specialty which require development and to be in a position to negotiate with the purchasers those developments which are desirable and the agree appropriate funding through the contract process, enabling the changes to be implemented. An example of this is where a specialty identifies an extension and improvement of facilities such as an open-access endoscopy service or a non-invasive vascular imaging service, which is a clear improvement in the quality of service offered, but would involve cost in terms of purchasing the capital equipment and personnel. Under the new climate the costs of such services can be identified very accurately and discussions entered into with the purchasers working with that hospital. Then an agreement can be reached as to whether or not such changes are acceptable; if so, how much they cost and the increase in contract price that would be appropriate to cover these costs. If the contract is agreed funding the increase in cost per case, then with money following patients, the change can be introduced much more quickly than under the previous systems.

The progress of such developments within a specialty will give clinicians confidence about looking forward, making them much more positive about developments in important aspects of quality of care. Many issues that relate to improvement in clinical care are also related to quality and an active and discriminating purchasing authority is very happy to enter into such discussions with clinicians to introduce changes devoted to improving service. Within a hospital, however, competition can develop for scarce resources such as beds, operating theatres and outpatient facilities. As the changes progress and the clinical manager becomes much more entrepreneurial, these problems are likely to increase. Methods have to be derived for open discussion between specialties about the choices between the various developments that are to be made, with an acceptable method of resolving differences. As the demand for medical care universally exceeds the number of beds available and the amount of care that can be provided, and it is necessary initially for the purchasers to prioritize the order in which they wish various groups of patients to be treated. In addition to this, decisions may require to be made in the hospital about allocation of resources, such as operating time and beds. A forum is needed where all the clinical directors meet so that these issues can be discussed openly and an agreed decision can be made between the board and the various clinical directors as to the priorities for clinical care on the basis of how facilities can be allocated to obtain the maximum effect from the resources of the hospital.

Survival as a medical manager is not helped by the current political situation where change may be started or stopped depending upon the political climate prevailing nationally. However, it is to be hoped that whatever environment we operate in, money will continue to follow patients. If this is the case, clinicians must maintain the best clinical facilities possible to treat the patients under their care. An active role of clinicians in the management of those resources can only improve the effectiveness in which those resources are managed. To fulfil such a role will involve balancing the demands of the professional and the management influences. To do this effectively, good communications are of the essence, – not just talking but listening to what others are saying, not only in management but also within the various professional groups in a specialty so that any anxieties that are developing can be allayed and the quality and quantity of service to patients are maintained at a high level.

8.12 Theatre

Ann Naylor

For $4\frac{1}{2}$ years from summer 1986 as theatre manager to all theatres in the acute unit in Basildon and Thurrock health authority, my responsibility was the operational management of theatres, with a particular emphasis on efficient utilization within budgetary limits. All non-medical staff in the theatres were managed by me with day-to-day issues delegated to nurse managers. The unit has two hospitals, 8 miles apart, and until recently each had an accident and emergency (A&E) department, an intensive treatment unit (ITU) and a full range of specialties, both emergency and routine. One hospital had four theatres staffed and utilized for all but one session per week while at the other hospitals four theatres were staff and utilized for three-quarters of their capacity and there were two rarely used minor-op theatres separate from the main theatre.

During the past year, major changes have taken place. First, A&E and ITU have been rationalized to one site; second, we have changed the management through a clinical directorate structure, and third, a new dedicated day surgery unit has been opened, including two new small operating theatres.

Each of these changes has had a major impact on medical and non-medical staff and working practices throughout the unit and in particular on the staff in my clinical directorate, which now includes theatres, anaesthetics, ITU and day unit.

A major part of my responsibility as theatre manager has been managing the budget, but even now the budget is not sufficiently accurate nor timely enough to provide meaningful management data without an efficient management information system. After the appointment of a business manager to the directorate, financial information and management of the budget have improved, and as the role of business manager expands into all areas of the directorate, it has become easier for me to cope with a wider area of responsibility as clinical director and to contemplate the enormous growth in the scope of the role.

Management of non-medical staff in the theatres has been through the site theatre superintendents directly to me as theatre manager and this is still the pattern as clinical director. Thus I have overall responsibility for hiring and firing, grievance, conduct and capability, etc. My involvement in selection and interviewing has been for selected groups of staff, as required, with emphasis on senior grades, plus grades where there have been difficulties with recruitment, retention and turnover of staff.

In the past the introduction of ideas for re-profiling the workforce has been initiated by me but has tended to become stuck between personnel and payroll and negotiation with staff. With the arrival of the business manager, many payroll and some personnel tasks have been lifted from me and together as a directorate we have been empowered to implement some projects. For instance, it has been possible to put into action a plan to recruit and train operating department assistants (ODAs) and by negotiating conditions and terms outside Whitley Council rules to retain NHS (trust) employees and remove agency ODAs over a period of time. Such a project has benefits to the staff group involved, benefits to the whole workforce in gaining greater commitment from the ODAs as direct employees, and benefits to the directorate in saving commission on agency fees. It also fulfils a promise made long ago to staff and not accomplished until the appointment of a business manager, and also of a personnel officer with particular responsibility to the directorate.

When portering in one hospital was contracted out several years ago, the opportunity was taken to remove routine theatre portering from the specification for tender. In this way the porters became theatre staff with increased self-esteem, responsible to theatres, based in theatres and with an intense loyalty to theatres, their nurses and their doctors. By negotiating with them for an element of flexibility and productivity, we were able to offer to them a slightly better deal than that offered to them by the outside contractors had they remained included in the tender. When the second hospital portering contract was won in-house, it was quite a surprise that the porters wanted to come into the theatre staffing rather than remaining in the pool. The attraction has been a regular paypacket rather than the pay deal involving bonus pay. Negotiations with the unions were a formality as staff had obviously made their own choice and were happy. More recent changes have involved further changes for porters who are now employed as nursing auxiliaries. With the advent of NVQ qualifications it is hoped that we can offer some training and career progression and obtain a greater flexibility in function of staff groups.

Objective setting and competency evaluation by appraisal of staff are essential to ensure the best utilization of personnel and to plan future developments. As clinical director I am subject to IPR, as is my business manager and as are my senior nurse managers in the theatre. The ideal would be to have a database of skills and experience of all staff, but at present this is done as a paper exercise with emphasis on assessment of performance and feedback, together with agreement of job objectives and training needs. Managing change in nursing presents a great challenge. The theatre nursing staff are used to the fact that the theatre manager has not been a nurse and have gradually become accustomed to the separation of the managerial and professional roles. Until recently, professional support to nursing staff has been given by a director of nursing services. As a second-wave trust, this type of support now comes from the nurse on the trust board. However, expansion of my theatre manager role to that of clinical director of the larger area has exposed weaknesses in nurse management and it will not be possible for the clinical director and business manager to deal with separate nurse managers for each area of the directorate. A new post of senior nurse manager to the directorate has recently been appointed.

It is essential to gain acceptance that, in the world of the clinical directorate, standards must be set and protocols must be agreed and shared by the nurse manager, clinical and director business manager. In particular, risk management protocols must be understood by all, especially since complaints and any legal matters will now be managed in the directorate by all three team members. Reprofiling issues will be costed by the business manager and evaluated as they are tried. It is no longer acceptable for a nurse to say

'we have always done it this way', or 'I don't think it will work' – changes in practice will now be estimated, subject to a pilot study, and then re-evaluated. By this means, changes in staff numbers and skills mix can be achieved with general acceptance. Multiskilling, the advent of the operating department practitioners (ODPs) and the introduction of NVQs for ODPs and other grades are all areas requiring this type of approach.

As a secondary provider of services to the contracting-provider surgical units, it is essential to maintain good communications and to be responsive to demands made by alterations in practice and developments in medical technology. Since the whole trust operates within financial constraints, it is useful if areas of proposed expansion are included in directorate business plans and hence in the trust business plan. There is a constant need to attract and support our customers – the surgeons – with technology and trained staff, while maintaining standards and ensuring the safety of our consumers – the patients.

Managing change with consultant medical colleagues has been relatively straightforward despite many changes in practice and emphasis. As theatre manager empowered to make changes in theatre utilization, combined with a unit-wide acceptance of the clinical directorate structure, transition has been simplified. A group of theatre-using directorates now meets regularly, as recommended in the Bevan report, to agree necessary changes. The change in culture has been effected in an atraumatic fashion due to the leadership of our unit general manager and to the establishment of management through a board of clinical directors. Resources are managed by those who spend them and there is a genuine understanding that funding is finite.

The experience of being theatre manager and now clinical director has altered my professional (and personal) life. I am paid for two additional sessions and relieved of two theatre sessions but management spreads into my free time and takes at least 15 hours per week. To cope with additional demands, I have attended regular training programmes in-house and at various and other venues and management training centres. For me it has been good to vary the courses and lately these have been supplemented by well-led in-house training with visiting contributors specifically selected for the needs of our board of clinical directors. Our unit believes in working collaboratively with clearly defined shared objectives. Working at our clinical directorates' seminars with our trust executive, relationships are developed and links between directorates and other managers are being forged as a network on which we can all build for the future.

By being involved in a supportive, cooperative managerial structure, it is possible to move from being an operational theatre manager to being a strategic clinical director able to assist and direct staff in my directorate during times of continuing change.

Section 9

A review of management theory

9.1 Perspectives on management

John Hassard

Introduction

In this section we offer an introduction to management thought. The section is arranged in three main subsections. In the first we describe landmark contributions to management theory, discussing the approaches of scientific management, human relations, sociotechnical systems, contingency theory and corporate excellence, and the impact of their ideas on the practice of modern management.

In the second part a sociological perspective is used to explain the role of management within modern society. We analyse managerial work in terms of theories of the industrial society, the separation of ownership from control, the managerial revolution and the technostructure.

The chapter concludes by describing the main theoretical frameworks used to interpret management and managerial work. We outline principles of the *functionalist*, *action* and *radical* approaches to the study of management.

Part 1: A brief history of management thought

Antiquity

Although management research has greatly accelerated in recent decades and although modern management thought dates primarily from the early 20th century – with the work of Frederick Taylor and Henri Fayol – there has been serious theorizing about management and organization since time immemorial. Ideas on organization date from antiquity, with formal principles of management being found in the records of the Egyptians, the early Greeks and the ancient Romans (Lepawsky, 1949).

Indications of the importance of organization in the bureaucratic states of antiquity are found in Egyptian papyri extending as far back as 1300 BC. Similar records exist for ancient China, with Confucius's parables containing numerous practical suggestions for efficient public administration.

In ancient Greece the Athenian commonwealth, with its councils, courts, officials and public administrators, offers an early and sophisticated example of functional management. The claim by Socrates that management represents a skill separate from technical knowledge is extremely close to modern interpretations of the management function.

In ancient Rome, also, the existence of the magistrates, with their functional areas of authority, indicates a scalar relationship characteristic of organization. It is often claimed that the main strength of the Romans – and the reason for the success of the Roman Empire – was their ability to *organize*. Through systematic delegation of authority, the city of Rome expanded to an empire with an efficiency of organization never before seen.

The church and the military

Other early influences on modern management practice were the Catholic church and the military.

It can be claimed that the Roman Catholic church has been the most effective formal organization in the history of western civilization. The longevity of its administrative life has in large part been due to the effectiveness of its management techniques. Amongst these techniques are the development of the hierarchy of authority with its territorial organization, the specialization of activities along functional lines and the effective use of the staff principle. It is surprising that, for centuries, the successful employment of the staff principle by the church had virtually no influence on other formal institutions (Mooney, 1947).

Some of the most durable principles of administration can be traced to military organizations. With the exception of the church, no other form of organization has been forced, by problems of managing large groups, to develop formal organizational principles. The history of military organization has been devoted to improving techniques of leadership and human resources management. Maintaining an organization culture which fosters morale and commitment has always been a primary goal.

Military organizations have also long made use of the staff principle. Notable exponents of this were the French army of 1790 and the Prussian armies of the 19th century. The management practices developed by the latter – based on the integration of specialist functions with auxiliary services – have been copied not only by other military organizations but also by modern enterprises.

Forerunners to scientific management

Accounts of modern management theory commonly commence with the work of Frederick Taylor (1856–1917). The reason for this is Taylor's claim to have developed the most effective management control system of its day – the scientific management approach to industrial organization (Rose, 1975). However, although Taylor's work represents a paradigm in the development of work methods, certain earlier figures also made notable contributions to what might be called a scientific approach to administration.

Boulton and Watt, for example, the developers of the steam engine, in their management of the Soho Engineering Foundry devised many sophisticated management control systems. In the management structure, Watt was in charge of administration and organization while Boulton dealt with sales and commercial activities. Among the management techniques they developed were market research and forecasting, machine layout in terms of work-flow requirements, production planning, production process standards, and standardization of product components. In the accounting area, Boulton and Watt developed detailed statistical records and advanced control systems whereby they could calculate the costs and profit for each machine manufactured and for each department. In the human resources area, they devised both worker and management training programmes, work study and payment by results based on work study and sickness benefit systems.

Charles Babbage, the British mathematician, was another important figure in the history of scientific management. Although most famous for his invention in 1822 of the difference machine, a mechanical calculator which formed the basis for accounting machines nearly a century later, his main contribution to management was his book *On the Economy of Machinery and Manufactures*, published in 1832. In this book Babbage established himself as a mathematical management scientist. He developed a sophisticated analysis of the economies of division of labour, and devised scientific principles to govern a manager's most efficient use of materials and labour.

Despite his mathematical approach to management, Babbage did not overlook the human element in work organization. Like Taylor, three-quarters of a century later, Babbage claimed there should be a mutuality of interest between the worker and the capitalist. Babbage argued for a system of profit-sharing in which workers could share in the success of the factory as they contributed to its increased productivity. The suggestion was for workers to receive a fixed pay rate depending on the nature of their work, plus a share in profits, plus bonuses for any suggestions which led to increased productivity. Babbage's main interests, however, were not in the broader areas of management but in areas of accounting, engineering and incentives, based on principles of specialization and productivity-linked rewards.

Frederick Taylor and scientific management

It is Frederick Winslow Taylor who is generally acknowledged as the founder of scientific management. In fact, probably no other individual has had a greater impact on the development of management thought. Taylor's experiences as an apprentice, a labourer, a foreman, a master mechanic, and then the chief engineer of a steel company gave him an excellent opportunity to understand contemporary problems of work organization and to see opportunities for improving the practice of management.

Taylor's main concern was to increase efficiency in production – not only to lower costs and raise profits, but also to effect increased pay for workers through increasing their levels of productivity. Practical experience had taught him that higher productivity was possible without unreasonable effort on the part of workers. For Taylor, low productivity stemmed largely from ignorance on the part of both management and workforce. This ignorance arose from the fact that both management and workers did not understand what constituted a fair day's work and a fair day's pay. Managers and workers were too concerned with how they could divide the surplus that arose from productivity and not enough with increasing the surplus so that *both* owners and employees could accrue more reward. Taylor saw productivity as the key both to increased wages and increased profits, and he believed that the application of scientific work principles, instead of traditional practices and rule-of-thumb methods, would yield this higher productivity without undue expenditure of effort on the part of labour.

Principles of scientific management

In Taylor's most famous work, *The Principles of Scientific Management*, published in 1911, he explains the fundamental principles of the scientific approach to organization and management. Taylor lays down four 'great underlying principles of management'. These concern:

1 The development of a true science of work.
2 The scientific selection and progressive development of the worker.
3 The bringing together of the science of work and the scientifically selected and trained men.
4 The constant and intimate cooperation of management and men.

The basis of scientific management was systematic observation and measurement of tasks. The most frequently quoted example of this is Taylor's development of the 'science of shovelling'. Taylor insisted that, although shovelling is a simple task, the analysis of the factors affecting shovelling is quite complex. The scientific analysis of shovelling involves the determination of the optimum load that a 'first-class man' can handle with each shovelful. For this, the correct size of shovel to obtain this load, for different materials, must be established. Workers must be given a range of shovels and told which one to use for a particular task. They must then be placed on an incentive scheme which permits first-class men to earn high wages in return for high production.

The need for maximum specialization, and the removal of all extraneous elements in order to concentrate on the focal task, is fundamental to Taylor's thinking. He claims these principles can be applied to management too. For Taylor, the work of a factory foreman is composed of a number of different functions – for example, cost clerk, time clerk, inspector, repair boss, shop disciplinarian – and he considers that these can be separated out and performed by specialists responsible for controlling different aspects of the work and the workers. Taylor calls this system functional management and likens the increased efficiency it brings to that obtained in a school where classes go to specialist teachers for different subjects, compared with a school in which one teacher teaches all subjects.

In order to put these ideas and principles into practice Taylor and his followers developed a set of mechanistic work analysis techniques. To ascertain what a fair day's work was, and to help find the 'one best way' of doing any given job, time-and-motion study was carefully applied. Similarly, various reward schemes based on output were used in an attempt to increase productivity, to ensure that workers who produced were paid according to their productivity, and to give workers an incentive for performance. These techniques were necessary to make the philosophy of scientific management work, founded as it was on improving productivity, on giving workers their best opportunity to be productive, and on rewarding workers for individual productivity.

It is also true that these were often used by companies to increase labour productivity without providing high rewards, quality training or managerial cooperation. Few managements were willing to operationalize one of Taylor's basic tenets: that there should be no limit to the earnings of a high-producing worker. Taylor felt that incentive schemes which specified limits to potential earnings would inhibit the 'mental revolution' in which both sides 'take their eyes off the division of the surplus and together turn their attention towards increasing the size of the surplus'. The failure of corporate management to implement scientific management in full meant that the philosophy came to be associated with worker alienation rather than welfare. During Taylor's lifetime bitter controversy arose over the alleged inhumanity of the system, which was seen to reduce workers to the level of efficiently functioning machines.

In fairness to Taylor, even though he does seem overly preoccupied with shop floor efficiency, he probably never envisaged such crude exploitation of his ideas. Contrary to much sociological analysis, it can be argued that throughout Taylor's written work runs almost a humanistic theme. When viewed as a product of its time, Taylor's work can be seen as somewhat idealistic. One of his main arguments was that the interests of workers, managers and owners could and should be harmonized. Taylor constantly emphasized that managers should design work systems that allow employees to perform to their maximum abilities.

Disciples of Taylor

Taylor's ideas were formalized and developed in practical terms by a number of disciples. Most notable amongst these were Carl Barth, Henry Gantt, and Frank and Lillian Gilbreth. Barth is regarded as Taylor's most loyal and orthodox follower. For many years he was a close colleague of Taylor's, working for him at both the Bethlehem and Midvale steel companies. During most of his later life Barth operated as an independent scientific management consultant. Being an accomplished mathematician, he developed many mathematical techniques and formulae that made it possible for Taylor's ideas to be put into practice.

Gantt was another close colleague of Taylor's. A mechanical engineer, he joined Barth and Taylor at the Midvale Steel Company in 1887. Gantt remained with Taylor until 1901, when he formed his own consulting engineering firm. Although he strongly advocated Taylor's ideas and did much consulting work on the scientific selection of workers and the development of incentive bonus schemes, he was more cautious than Taylor when selling scientific management methods. Although like Taylor he emphasized the need to develop a mutuality of interests between management and workers, in so doing he stressed the importance of an appreciation of systems on the part of both workers and management, rather than a strict separation of planning from execution.

As a developer of management techniques, Gantt is best known for work on graphical planning. His main interests lay in the analysis of time and costs for management control systems. This led to the development of the Gantt chart, which is still in wide use today and was the precursor to related techniques such as PERT (program evaluation and review technique).

However, the most celebrated of Taylor's direct followers was the husband-and-wife team of Frank and Lillian Gilbreth. A building contractor by profession, Frank Gilbreth had been interested in the systematic elimination of wasted movements independently of Taylor's work. In his building firm he used work study to reduce the number of a bricklayer's movements from 18 to five. In the process he claimed to have doubled the bricklayer's productivity with no greater expenditure of effort. Given the success of such experiments, Gilbreth's contracting firm gave way to consulting on the improvement of human productivity. After meeting Taylor in 1907, he synthesized his ideas with Taylor's in order to put scientific management on a more practical footing. One of the most important developments to emerge from this relationship was the development of 'therbligs' (cf. 'Gilbreths'), or the symbols which form the basis for work study.

Frank Gilbreth was assisted in this work by his wife Lillian, who was one of America's earliest industrial psychologists; she received her PhD in the field in 1915. After her husband's untimely death in 1924, she carried on the consulting business and throughout her long life – which ended in 1972 at the age of 93 – became widely acclaimed as the 'first lady of management'. Lillian Gilbreth's work on human factors psychology complemented her husband's interests in efficiency to the extent that the Gilbreths' approach to scientific management became one in which the psychological needs of workers were considered part of the search for the 'one best way'. For the Gilbreths it was not simply the monotony of work that caused dissatisfaction, but rather management's lack of attention to workers' general psychological welfare.

Henri Fayol and management principles

For our own topic of research, *managerial work*, the founder of management theory in this area is the French industrialist Henri Fayol. Although we have little proof that management scholars, either in the UK or the USA, knew much about Fayol's work until the 1920s or even later, his insightful observations on the principles of general management first appeared in French in 1916, under the title *Administration Industrielle et Générale*. This work, although consistently reprinted in French, was not translated into English until 1929, and even then it was printed by the International Institute of Management at Geneva, with only a few copies being circulated outside the UK. Indeed, no English translation was published in the USA until 1949 (Fayol, 1949), although Fayol's work was brought to the attention of some American management scholars in 1923 through a paper translated by Greer, which was later incorporated in a volume edited by Gulick and Urwick (1937). As a consequence, in North America students of management in the first half of the century did not generally have the advantage of Fayol's analysis. It is regrettable too that many of the leading figures who worked on the development of management principles, such as Sheldon, Mooney and Barnard, show little evidence of being familiar with Fayol's work.

In *General and Industrial Administration* Fayol writes as a businessman reflecting on the management principles he has observed through experience. To this end, there is no attempt to construct a grand theory or logical philosophy of management. None the less, such is the authority of Fayol's work that his observations are cited constantly as benchmarks for management practice.

Fayol suggests that all aspects of industrial activity can be divided into six categories:

1 Technical (production).
2 Commercial (buying and selling).
3 Financial (use of capital).
4 Security (protection of property and persons).
5 Accounting (including statistics).
6 Managerial (planning, organization, command, co-ordination and control).

Arguing that principles for the first five activities are well-documented, Fayol devoted most of his book to the analysis of the sixth.

The book comprises observations on managerial qualities, general principles of management and elements of management. Fayol differentiates between principles and elements by reserving the former term for rules and the latter for functions.

From a modern perspective, Fayol's work on *qualities* seems dated. Put briefly, he argues that a manager must possess good *physical*, *mental*, *moral*, *educational* and *technical* capabilities.

Above all, the manager must have superior *experience*, which he or she can only gain from a thorough knowledge of the work proper.

Fayol recognizes that the relative importance of managerial ability increases as one goes up the hierarchical ladder, becoming the most important skill for senior executives. For his time, he notes also a need for *principles* of management and for management teaching, and he deplores the lack of the latter in technical institutions. Fayol argues that managerial ability should be learnt in the same way as technical ability, initially in the school and later in the workplace. Conscious of the lack of a well-grounded theory of management, he set about early in the 20th century to provide one.

In devising his theory, Fayol stresses that principles of management must be flexible rather than absolute; they must be usable regardless of changing circumstances. Based on his business experience, Fayol cites 14 principles of successful management. These can be summarized as follows:

1 *Division of work.* Fayol means that form of specialization necessary for the efficient deployment of labour. He applies this principle to all forms of work, managerial as well as technical.
2 *Authority and responsibility.* Fayol considers authority and responsibility to be related: the latter is the corollary of the former. Authority is a combination of both official (deriving from the manager's position) and personal (psychological, sociological, cultural) factors.
3 *Discipline.* For Fayol, discipline is 'respect for agreements which are directed at achieving obedience, application, energy, and the outward marks of respect'. Effective corporate discipline requires competent superordinates at all levels.
4 *Unity of command.* Employees should receive orders from one superordinate only.
5 *Unity of direction.* Each set of activities with the same goal must have one head and one plan. As distinct from the fourth principle, this relates to the organization of the body corporate, rather than to personnel. Fayol did not mean to imply that all decisions should be made at the top.
6 *Subordination of individual to general interest.* If the two are in conflict, management must reconcile them.
7 *Remuneration.* Reward systems should be fair and afford the maximum possible satisfaction to employees and employer.
8 *Centralization.* Fayol means the extent to which decision-making authority is concentrated or dispersed – essentially the degree of centralization of authority.

9 *Scalar chain*. This is basically the hierarchical chain of superordinates which defines the authority structure. Fayol argues that this chain should be short-circuited when to adhere to it scrupulously would be dysfunctional.

10 *Order*. The principle assumes a natural arrangement of both things and people. Fayol differentiates between two forms of order – *material* and *social*. He follows the adage of 'a place for everything (everyone) and everything (everyone) in its place'.

11 *Equity* – the notion that employee commitment will be gained through a combination of justice and kindliness on the part of managers.

12 *Stability of tenure*. Fayol outlines the problems and costs of unnecessary labour turnover. He argues that it is both the cause and the effect of bad management.

13 *Initiative*. On suitable occasions, managers should sacrifice personal power and let promising subordinates exercise initiative. Initiative is the wellspring of innovative planning and a source of job satisfaction for the intelligent employee.

14 *Esprit de corps* – an extension of the principle of unity of command, but placing greater emphasis on the need for teamwork and the importance of communication in achieving it.

Concluding his discussion of these principles, Fayol stresses that he has not tried to be exhaustive. Instead he describes only those principles he has had the most occasion to use. He feels that a formal specification of principles is necessary if a robust theory of management is to be developed.

Finally, Fayol suggests that the *elements* of management are its functions, and that these are *planning*, *organizing*, *commanding*, *coordinating* and *controlling*. Much of Fayol's analysis is given to an examination of these functions, for which he claims a universality of application across business, religious, political, miltary, philanthropic and other organizations. He argues that since all forms of organization require management, it is necessary to develop a general theory of administration.

The sociology of management

At approximately the same time that Taylor was developing scientific management and Fayol was working on administrative management, leading sociologists were producing ideas which would have a profound effect on our understanding of managerial behaviour. Three sociologists in particular were generating ideas relevant to a *social systems approach* to management and organization.

The first of these was the German social economist Max Weber, whose analysis of government, church and the military led him to conclude that hierarchy, authority and bureaucracy lie at the heart of all formal social organizations. The second was the French sociologist Emile Durkheim, who in *The Division of Labour*, originally published in 1893, developed the idea that social groups, through constructing their own systems of values and norms, control human conduct in organizations.

The third, and for social systems theory most important, figure was the Italian social philosopher Vilfredo Pareto, who in *A Treatise on General Sociology*, published in 1916, developed the idea of society being a complex structure of interdependent units – basically, a social system containing numerous subsystems. Central to this treatise was the idea that social systems seek equilibrium when disturbed by outside or inside forces. Above all, Pareto argued that social *values* cause a system to seek an equilibrium when so disturbed. For Pareto, it was the duty of a society's ruling élite to provide the leadership necessary to maintaining the social system in state of equilibrium.

The social being: Elton Mayo and the Hawthorne experiments

The ideas of Weber, Durkheim and notably Pareto are important in that they influence the social systems approach to management behaviour. In particular, their ideas inform the perspective which underpins the most extensive set of sociological investigations yet carried out in industry – those at the Hawthorne (Chicago) works of the Western Electric Company by Elton Mayo (1933), Fritz Roethlisberger and William Dickson (1939) or the research generally referred to as the Hawthorne studies.

Before Mayo's involvement at Hawthorne, the US National Research Council had, between 1924 and 1927, carried out ergonomic research on the relationship between levels of illumination and other conditions and worker productivity. On discovering that, when illumination was either increased or decreased for a test group, productivity improved, the experiment was about to be aborted as a failure until Mayo and his Harvard colleagues reinterpreted the findings from a sociological perspective.

In the research by the National Research Council, changing illumination for the experimental group, modifying test periods, shortening workdays and varying incentive schemes did not explain changes in productivity. Mayo and his colleagues then came to the conclusion that other factors were involved. Put simply, they found these factors in the *social relationships* of work groups. Altering levels of illumination, up or down, resulted in increased productivity because the members of the experimental group began to consider themselves as special and important. Improvements in productivity were due to social factors such as morale, good relationships between group members and a supportive style of management.

The results of the Hawthorne studies suggested that the industrial being is a social being and that business management is not simply a matter of matching machinery and methods but also of integrating these with the social system to realize a complete sociotechnical system. The main contribution of the Hawthorne studies was a heightened profile for the use of behavioural science in management and a greater awareness that managers operate within a social system. Although many writers before Mayo and Roethlisberger recognized the importance of human factors, what the Harvard team did was underscore the need for a much deeper appreciation of social and behavioural forces in the workplace.

Chester Barnard and the functions of the executive

If one were to choose the single most influential analysis of managerial work it would almost certainly be *The Functions of the Executive* by Chester I. Barnard, published in 1938.

Barnard, while an executive of national standing (he was president of the New Jersey Bell Telephone Company from 1927 to 1948), was also a first-rate scholar who was influenced by Pareto, Mayo and other faculty members at Harvard, where he sometimes lectured. In the style of mainstream Harvard sociology his analysis of managerial work is a social systems one. Barnard argues that the chief task of executives – by which he meant managers in general – is one of maintaining a system of cooperative effort. He attempts to analyse the functions of the executive from a perspective which, simultaneously, seeks to comprehend the reasons for, and nature of, cooperative systems. A brief analysis of *The Functions of the Executive* will explain how this is achieved.

The analysis develops from the proposition that the physical and biological limitations of individuals lead them to cooperate. The very act of cooperation in turn leads to the establishment of cooperative systems in which physical, biological, personal and social elements are present. Barnard argues subsequently that for cooperative systems to continue through time they must reproduce only those subsystems which are efficient and functional.

For Barnard, any cooperative system can be divided into two parts – organization, which includes only the interactions of individuals within the system, and other elements. Organization can in turn be divided into two forms – formal organization, which is a set of consciously coordinated interactions which have a common purpose, and informal organization, which means those interactions without a common or consciously coordinated purpose. Formal organization cannot persist unless there are individuals who can communicate with one another, are willing to contribute to group action, and have a common goal. Similarly, every formal organization must possess a system of functionalization so that people can specialize, a system of effective incentives that will induce people to contribute to group action, a system of power which will lead group members to accept the decisions of executives, and a system of logical decision-making.

From this analysis, Barnard distils three basic functions of the executive in formal organizations:

1 The maintenance of communication through a scheme of organization.
2 The securing of essential services from people in the organization.
3 The formulation and definition of purpose.

The executive must integrate the organization as a whole and find the optimum balance between conflicting forces and events. Barnard argues that to make the executive effective requires responsible leadership. To achieve this, Barnard suggests, 'Cooperation, not leadership, is the creative process; but leadership is the indispensible fulminator of its forces'.

The human relations movement

From the early 1940s, the works of Mayo, Roethlisberger and Barnard served as exemplars for a great many behavioural scientists taking up research into management and organization. These researchers are generally referred to as members of the Human Relations Movement, whose central message was that attitudes towards workers may be more important to efficiency than such material factors as rest periods, illumination and even money. Given the great interest in behavioural science approaches to management, especially during the 1950s and 1960s, only a few scholars from this movement will be referred to here (Burrell and Morgan, 1979).

The movement saw contributions from both sociologists and psychologists. The main contributions from human relations sociologists came from work on groups, cultural patterns, group cohesiveness, goals and objectives. Major figures associated with this work were E. Wright Bakke (1950), Melville Dalton (1959), George Homans (1958), Daniel Katz and Robert Kahn (1950), Philip Selznick (1966) and Peter Drucker (1949).

Psychologists likewise contributed to our understanding of management through analysis of the sources of motivation and satisfaction, the nature of leadership and the pressures for organizational change. Amongst those producing works on these subjects were Chris Argyris (1964), Warren Bennis (1966), Robert Blake and Jane Mouton (1964), Frederick Fiedler (1967), Frederick Herzberg (1958), Harold Leavitt (1958), Rensis Likert (1961), Abraham Maslow (1960) Douglas McGregor (1964), Leonard Sayles (1959) and Ralph Stogdill (1961).

These writers argue that individuals bring more to the workplace than just their labour: they also bring a range of social and psychological needs. Managers must understand this because individuals and groups are their prime concern. These writers also stress that an effective manager is a leader, and that understanding how leadership emerges is central to understanding management itself.

Of those mentioned above, perhaps the highest profile has been given to the contributions by Maslow and Herzberg on motivation, McGregor on management style, and Drucker on goals and objectives.

Maslow's main contribution is his need hierarchy theory of motivation. Maslow postulated that everyone has five basic needs which are constituted in an hierarchical form. In ascending order, starting with the most basic, the hierarchy comprises:

1 Physiological.
2 Safety.
3 Social.
4 Esteem.
5 Self-actualization needs.

The need hierarchy theory includes a number of assumptions. One is that lower needs (physiological, safety) must be satisfied before upper-level needs (esteem, self-actualization) are sufficiently activated and begin to energize behaviour. A second assumption is that, once a need is satisfied, it no longer serves as a motivator. Thus a person whose need for food is basically sated will then move on to a higher level (safety and then social) of the hierarchy. A third assumption is that, in most cases, a number of needs affect the behaviour of an individual at any one time. A fourth is that there are more ways to satisfy higher-order needs than lower needs. The theory also postulates the relationship between need satisfaction and motivation, holding that only unfulfilled needs energize behaviour, and that in the case of equal-need strength, the lower-level need must be sated first.

One of the most popular but controversial theories of motivation is that of Frederick Herzberg. Originally based on research among 200 engineers and accountants, it is commonly referred to as the two-factor theory of motivation or the motivation–hygiene theory.

In their research, Herzberg and his colleagues sought to examine the relationship between job satisfaction and productivity. Using semistructured interviews, they asked their respondents to recall a time when each felt good about his or her job and a time when he or she felt exceptionally negative about his or her job. From the results, the researchers concluded that motivation derived from two sets of factors. The first, associated with positive feelings about the job and related to the content of the work itself, they called motivators. Illustrations included achievement, recognition, the work itself, responsibility, advancement and growth. The factors in the second set, which they labelled hygiene, did not bring about satisfaction; they simply prevented dissatisfaction. These factors were external to the work itself. Illustrations included company policies, supervision, interpersonal relations, working conditions and salary.

Herzberg and those who support his theory believe that hygiene creates a zero level of motivation. If employees are given such factors as good supervision, adequate salaries and a chance to interact with their peers, this will not create motivation, but will only prevent dissatisfaction. If they are given factors such as recognition, increased responsibility, and a chance for advancement and growth, this will result in motivation. Thus the two-factor theory sees satisfaction and dissatisfaction as separate and distinct concepts.

A popular extension of human relations theories of motivation was the theory of management style and leader behaviour proposed by Douglas McGregor. McGregor postulated that managers act according to one of two sets of assumptions about subordinates. One set of assumptions, called theory X, is found in association with the traditional directive style of management. Managers who subscribe to theory X assume the following:

1 Most people have an inherent dislike of work and will avoid it if they can.
2 Because they dislike work, most people must be coerced, controlled, directed and threatened or they will not put forth adequate effort towards the achievement of organizational objectives.
3 Most people prefer to be directed, wish to avoid responsibility, have little ambition and want job security above all.

In contrast, managers who subscribe to theory Y assume the following:

1 The expenditure of physical and mental energy is as natural in work as in play.
2 External control and the threat of punishment are not the only means for bringing about effort towards organizational objectives. People will exercise self-direction and self-control in the service of objectives to which they are committed.
3 Commitment to objectives is a function of the rewards associated with their achievement.
4 Most people learn, under proper conditions, not only to accept but to seek responsibility.
5 The ability to exercise a high degree of imagination, ingenuity and creativity in the solution of organizational problems is widely, not narrowly, distributed.

Theory Y managers emphasize integration of subordinates goals with those of the organization. But this is not to say that theory Y leaders are never directive. As originally introduced by McGregor, this theory X/theory Y view of management style describes a continuum. Even at the extremes of the continuum, some behaviour typical of the other extreme will be observed.

A popular writer on management, many of whose works are influenced by the human relations ideas of Maslow and McGregor, is Peter Drucker. Although the topics of Drucker's many books are divided almost equally between socioeconomic and management analysis, it is for work in the latter that he is best known.

In *The Practice of Management* (1954) he outlines the basic principles behind the management strategy which is most closely associated with his work, management by objectives (MBO). The MBO approach stemmed from his work as a consultant with General Electric, the experience of which formed the basis for Drucker's book *Concept of the Corporation*. On studying General Electric he reported how each manager was responsible for a profit centre and given specific targets to achieve – 7% return on sales and 20% return on investment. He also described the absolute manner in which these objectives were applied, with any failure to meet objectives resulting in job loss. Since it is the bottom line of profitability that determines business success, Drucker feels that organizational goals should be divided into objectives which are clearly assigned to subunits and individuals. Only by such a system of management by objectives can it be ensured that each link in the chain of responsibility functions in the prescribed manner.

Throughout his MBO and other writings on management Drucker is keen to emphasize – like Peters and Waterman below – that the key to productive organization lies in the manager's handling of human resources. For Drucker, superior business performance is a function of ordinary employees achieving extraordinary goals and objectives.

Systems theory

An awareness of work organizations as systems has led to a more logical understanding of the management process. In describing the emergence of systems analysis we have noted Pareto's contribution to *social systems* thinking and the influence of his work upon the Human Relations Movement. However, there are other landmark influences we must cite in the development of systems approaches to management. The most important of these are the school of sociological thought known as *structural – functionalism* and the rise of an interdisciplinary *general systems theory*. These are key influences upon what is now the dominant paradigm of organizational theory and behaviour, the *open-systems* paradigm (Silverman, 1970; Burrell and Morgan, 1979; Clegg and Dunkerley, 1980; Reed, 1985).

While not a management scholar, the Harvard sociologist Talcott Parsons has a place in management history. Parsons is the key figure of structural – functionalism, the theory of sociological analysis which underpins the open-systems approach to management and organization.

Parsons' main contributions to organizational analysis are found in two theoretical articles in *Administrative Science Quarterly* (Parsons, 1956), and in some remarks on the internal processes of organizations in his book *Structure and Process in Modern Societies*, published in 1960.

In the *Administrative Science Quarterly* articles, Parsons expands a theory of organization from the principles laid down in his book *The Social System* (1951). Parsons defines organization in functionalist terms and suggests that: 'primacy of orientation to the attainment of a specific goal is the defining characteristic of an organization' (Parsons, 1956). This analysis highlights the goal-directedness of subunit behaviour, and how subunits in differing ways adapt to changing circumstances. Parsons points out that, while an organization's functions can be seen as subunits of larger environments, these functions themselves possess layers of subunit activity; for example, individual, group and departmental behaviour. The basic problem for organizations is therefore to integrate functions from one level to the next. Indeed, for the structural – functionalist this is the basic problem which confronts all social systems.

Parsons argues that organizations are situated at the cultural – institutional level of social analysis, and that as such one of the main tasks for the systems analyst is to define the goals and values of formal organizations. The systems analyst must determine the values associated with differentiated functional contexts, for in line with another of Parsons concepts – the *central value system* – organizational goals must be legitimated by organizational values which in turn must be consistent with societal values. Organizational goals are judged according to whether they make a legitimate contribution to the functional requirements of the total social system. While the organization places its goals above the goals of the subsystems which comprise the organization, its own goals must in turn integrate with those of the wider society. Only when values and normative patterns are congruent are they able to regulate processes through which the functional needs of the system are satisfied.

In *Structure and Process in Modern Societies*, Parsons moves towards an internal consideration of organizations. This he achieves through the differentiation of three subunit levels – *technical, managerial* and *institutional*. Parsons develops a critique of Weber's analysis of formal principles of hierarchy and argues that to define organizations in terms of fixed pyramids of authority is too simple. He suggests there are qualitative breaks in line structures, and that these can be understood in terms of different technical, managerial and institutional levels.

Parsons describes the *technical* level as the basic level at which the work is organized. This is where the general goals of the organization are translated into actions appropriate to their accomplishment: it concerns the processing of both people and materials. The main constraint at this level is the functioning of the technology.

The *managerial* level is concerned with the organization's administration. Its function is to obtain the resources required by the technical level and to act as intermediary between the technical system and the organization's clients. In practical terms, Parsons is referring to the concrete actions of administrators, managers and executives.

Third, Parsons develops the idea that, through the integration of goals and the central value system, organizations engage in activities which are functional for society as a whole. At the *insitutional* level we see attempts to ensure concord and uniformity between the organization and the wider social system. The institutional level mediates between the technical and managerial levels and the wider society: its role is to integrate the organization with its environment.

Although we have noted that Parsonianism has had a great influence on the open-systems perspective on organization, we must qualify this. In a direct sense, the impact of structural – functionalism was relatively short-lived, with the only major empirical study being Selznick's (1966) account of the Tennessee Valley Authority. We would argue, however, that the amount of related empirical work is not a reliable indicator of the influence of the approach, for structural – functionalism is important in laying the *conceptual* foundations of the open-systems perspective.

Indeed, in the late 1950s many structural – functionalist sociologists began writing as systems scholars of organization (Burrell and Morgan, 1979). Academics who had developed equilibrium models in sociology recast their analyses as open-systems theories of administration. As Mayntz (1964) notes, grafting structural – functionalism on to the field of organizations was decisive for the development of an open-systems orthodoxy in administrative science.

The second major conceptual influence on the development of the open-systems approach to organization was the founding of an interdisciplinary *general systems theory*. The origins of this approach lie in biology and physics, the most influential scholar being the biologist Ludwig von Bertalanffy (1961); although for management studies the work of Kenneth Boulding is important.

Put briefly, general systems theory stresses the similarity of systems processes occurring in many different forms of relationship. Whether we are analysing a machine, an organism or an organization, it suggests we document relationships between the supply of resources (input), the conversion process (throughput), and the production of an object or objects (output). It is the manner in which the parts are shaped by the process as a whole that is the central focus of study.

In recent decades, one of the principal signs of the ascent of the open-systems approach has been its hegemony within the pages of management textbooks, and most notably in textbooks of the 1960s and 1970s. Amongst the best-known textbooks expounding an open-systems approach are those by Johnson *et al.* (1963); Katz and Kahn (1966); and Koontz and O'Donnel (1976). In these books, the synthesis of ideas from structural – functionalism and general systems theory produces an image of the organization as an interdependent set of phenomena striving to accomplish a common goal. These textbooks argue that, in achieving its overall goal the organization interacts with and exists within a specific environment, with this interaction signalling that the organization both influences and is influenced by its environment. As the organization recognizes this environmental relation it is seen as being a more or less open system. The quality of this relation allows managers to discuss the exchange of inputs and outputs, which in turn enables them to determine the organization's system boundary. Organizations as systems are structured in a way that part of the output becomes an input, this process giving rise to the concept of feedback. For the open systems analyst, it is through feedback that organizations monitor progress and behaviour.

Sociotechnical theory

While structural–functionalism failed to inspire many direct studies of organization, open-systems theory has been more successful. In contrast to the closed-systems modelling of Mayo, Roethlisberger and Barnard, systems analysts from the 1950s onwards have conducted empirical analyses which take as the focus of study the commerce between the organization and its environment. Here it is the boundary relation between the organization and its environment that is important, and specifically the issue of how this relation should be managed.

Writers associated with such work are often linked with the *sociotechnical systems* and *contingency theory* approaches to management. Of these, the development of *sociotechnical systems* closely reflects the history of systems theory in general: we see movement from closed to open forms of analysis. The term sociotechnical system is derived from research by members of the Tavistock Institute of Human Relations (London) into production systems design. In particular, it is derived from a study by Trist and Bamforth (1955) into the introduction of the long-wall method of coal-getting in the northwest Durham mines in England. This study described how a new mechanized and mass-production-oriented method of coal-getting replaced the traditional hand-got method, and how in the process this involved a revolution in the forms of work and social systems within the mines. Being informed by psychoanalysis and Gestalt theory as well as systems theory, the analysis portrayed work relations in terms of tensions between social and technical forces. The work group was not depicted as exclusively a social group or a technical group, but rather as an interdependent sociotechnical system. It was argued that the work system of the colliery should be interpreted as fields of social and psychological forces, the balance being influenced by the relationship between technical and human factors. Like the Hawthorne studies model, this perspective is underpinned by the assumptions of an equilibrium model, although one owing debt to Gestalt theory – and in particular Kurt Lewin's (1951) field force theory – as much as Paretian mechanics. In the Trist and Bamforth study, the technical change brought about by the long-wall method was perceived as disturbing the social and technical equilibrium of the hand-got system, with the adverse reactions of the colliers representing evidence of this disturbance.

Open sociotechnical systems analysis

Although advancing a systems theory appreciation of work relationships, the Durham study has been criticized for adopting a closed-system approach based upon a mechanical equilibrium model. In contrast, Tavistock research from the mid 1950s onwards has stressed the sociotechnical concept as 'an open rather than closed system theory, especially as regards the enterprise – environment relation and the elucidation of the conditions under which a steady state may be attained' (Trist et al., 1963). This doctrine suggests that:

> considering enterprises as 'open socio-technical systems' helps to provide a more realistic picture of how they are both influenced by and able to act back on their environment. It points in particular to the various ways in which enterprises are enabled by their structural and functional characteristics ('systems constraints') to cope with the 'lacks' and 'gluts' in their available environment. Unlike mechanical and other inanimate systems they possess the property of 'equi-finality'; they may achieve a steady state from differing initial conditions and in differing ways. Thus in coping by internal changes they are not limited to simple quantitative change and increased uniformity but may, and usually do, elaborate new structures and take on new functions. The cumulative effect of only coping by *internal* elaboration and differentiation is generally to make the system independent of an increasing range of predictable fluctuations in

its supplies and outlets. At the same time, however, this process ties down more and more of its capital, skill and energies and makes it less able to cope with the newly emergent and unpredicted changes that challenge the primary ends of the enterprise (Emery and Trist, 1960).

Since the mid 1950s – and drawing upon the structural – functionalism of Parsons, the general systems theory of von Bertalanffy, and the field-force theory of Lewin – the sociotechnical concept has been incorporated into an open sociotechnical systems approach to management, a perspective which draws upon organismic rather than mechanical analogies.

The classic expression of this perspective is A. K. Rice's (1958) study of work redesign at the Jubilee Calico Mills, Ahmadabad, India. In this research Rice explicitly adopts the model of the firm as a living organism: the organization is seen as open to its environment; it maintains itself by exchanging materials and goods with its environment; it imports capital, raw materials equipment, etc. and exports finished goods, dividends, pollution and so forth. If the organization does not engage in such commerce it is assumed not to be adapting to its environment and thus to be in danger of extinction.

Rice's research is driven by the Parsonian notion of the primary task. Each system or subsystem has a primary duty to perform the task for which it was created. For the private corporation, the primary task is that of accruing profit. It is the primary task which unites the organization as a whole. Also, for Rice the organismic open systems analogy is combined with the view of the organization as a unitary social system. The social system is a positive force contributing to the accomplishment of the primary task. Technology, on the other hand, is a force which imposes constraints upon the range of organizational arrangements, but within which choice is possible. The crucial variable is organizational design or, more correctly, the design of a mode of work organization which meets the demands of technology and the needs of individuals: a design which produces a consensual and productive organization. The concept of an open sociotechnical system is employed with this in mind. The relationship between the various subsystems which make up the case gains their significance from this basic perspective on management and organization.

Contingency theory

Whereas the sociotechnical systems approach formed one of the major perspectives on management during the 1950s and 1960s, during the 1970s a kindred form of analysis, known as *contingency theory*, became the dominant approach for reconciling open-systems concepts at a number of organizational levels.

Contingency theory asserts that to be effective an organization needs to develop appropriate matches between its internal organization and the demands of its environment. In developing a set of propositions for achieving these matches, contingency theory draws upon empirical research into, for example, leadership style, work motivation, job satisfaction, technology and organization structure. As an example of the contingency approach, one of the earliest and purest statements comes in research documented by Paul Lawrence and Jay Lorsch in their book *Organization and Environment*, published in 1967.

Lawrence and Lorsch developed a study of the those variables most contingent upon the relationship between the organization's internal structure and the demands of its external environment. The research seeks to discover the forms of organization best suited to achieving success in a range of market and economic conditions. Adopting the open-systems perspective, the research views the organization as a set of interrelated parts influenced by the wider society. One of the main objectives is to identify patterns for the functioning of systems in different environments. To this end, their analysis turns on implications arising from two particular aspects of systems functioning. The first is the principle that as systems become larger they have to be *differentiated* into parts, the functioning of which has to be *integrated* if the system is to operate successfully. Second, they contend that a central function of any system is its adaptation to the demands of the wider environment. Lawrence and Lorsch argue that a complex organization, as a system which is internally differentiated, must attain a satisfactory level of integration if it is to adapt to the demands of the wider environment. The most effective organizations will be those which achieve levels of integration and differentiation compatible with environmental demands.

At one extreme, Lawrence and Lorsch show that for dynamic and diverse sectors, such as the plastics industry, effective organizations are those whose structures are highly differentiated and highly integrated. On the other hand, in environments which are more stable and less diverse, like the container industry, effective organizations are those whose structures are much less highly differentiated; the difference between these organizational forms is similar to the difference Burns and Stalker (1961) noted between organic and mechanistic structures.

It is often suggested that the importance of contingency theory lies in its ability to reconcile the antagonistic traditions of Taylorism and human relations – which both promote universal solutions to organizational problems, but which cite vastly different prescriptions (Miles, 1980). In contrast, contingency theory stresses that, depending upon the nature of the environment, business success can be achieved through adopting, on the one hand, highly structured, authoritarian and bureaucratic procedures or, on the other hand, flexible, participative and organic ones. Contingency theory emphasizes that management is context-dependent, and that management principles must be concordant with the type of contingent factors being encountered. What managers do in practice depends upon a given set of circumstances: the nature of managerial work depends on the nature of the situation (Fiedler, 1967).

Managerial roles

In more recent times, the positivism of open-systems research has been complemented by a range of ideographic perspectives on management. These have been based both on participative research in organizations and on high-profile consultancy exercises. We have seen an increase in observational studies of management and also a return to specifying universal principles of administration. A notable example of the former is research on *managerial roles* by Henry Mintzberg: an example of the latter is the celebrated *search for corporate excellence* conducted by members of the management consulting firm McKinsey. Both developments are related to a third topic of recent management interest – *corporate culture*.

The work of Henry Mintzberg is central to an analysis of management and the nature of managerial work (Mintzberg, 1973). As such, an appreciation of Mintzberg's research will be presented and specifically a review of the tenets of his *managerial roles* approach.

Mintzberg's approach is to observe what managers actually do and from these observations conclude what the main managerial activities are. From a detailed study of five chief executives in a range of organizations, Mintzberg came to the conclusion that senior managers do not act out the classical description of their functions, that is, planning, organizing, commanding, coordinating and controlling. Instead he found a series of 10 roles, these being subcategorized into three main categories of interpersonal roles, informational roles and decision roles.

Interpersonal roles

The three *interpersonal* roles stem from the manager's formal authority. The first interpersonal role is the *figurehead* role. This mainly involves the manager participating in ceremonial duties, such as entertaining local dignitaries and major customers or attending the weddings of employees. While these duties may seem unimportant, they are expected, for they demonstrate that management cares about its employees, customers and others who deserve recognition.

The *leadership* role involves directing and coordinating the actions of subordinates in order to accomplish organizational goals. The leadership role involves both formal staffing activities, such as hiring, promoting and firing, and informal motivational activities. The aim of the latter is to ensure that the needs of the organization are consistent with the job-related needs of the employees.

The *liaison* role involves dealing with people other than subordinates or supervisors: people such as clients, suppliers, government officials, board members, etc. In enacting the liaison role, the manager gathers information from the environment which can affect the organization's success. The liaison role helps to build the manager's information system and is closely related to the monitor informational role.

Informational roles

Through interpersonal roles, managers build a network of contacts which help them to receive and transmit information. Managers obtain and process this information by enacting three *informational* roles.

The first informational role is that of *monitor*, in which the manager scans the environment for information which may affect the department or organization's effectiveness. In performing the role of monitor the manager should become the best-informed person in his or her part of the organization.

In playing the *disseminator* role, the manager distributes information to subordinates. Often this information is passed to subordinates as privileged information.

Finally, as a *spokesperson*, the manager transmits information to others in the capacity as a corporate official.

Decision roles

The *decisional* roles are perhaps more important than the interpersonal and informational roles, because through them the manager commits the organization to action. A manager can enact four different roles as decision-maker.

As an *entrepreneur*, the manager seeks to improve the organization's effectiveness by developing new ideas and initiating new projects. This may often involve a change in strategic direction for the organization.

In enacting the role of *disturbance handler*, managers react to situations beyond their immediate control, such as strikes, broken contracts, supplier bankruptcies, etc. Managers handle such disturbancies by learning the appropriate 'recipes' for strategic action, which are based on combinations of operational, financial and human resources strategies.

As *resource allocator*, the manager is responsible for deciding who will get resources and how much they will get. This role involves budgeting for money, equipment, personnel and time.

Finally, linked to the role of resource allocator is that of the *negotiator*. In this role, managers bargain with others to obtain advantages for their department or company.

Although widely cited in the management literature, Mintzberg's research has been criticized on several accounts. Firstly, his conclusions are based on data collected from only five executives. The question arises of whether this sample is too small to support Mintzberg's sweeping conclusions.

Second, many of the activities Mintzberg identifies are, in fact, examples of classical functions of planning, organizing, staffing, leading and controlling (Koontz and Weirich, 1988). For example, resource allocation is related to planning; the entrepreneurial role is also an element of planning; the interpersonal roles are mainly instances of leading; and the informational roles can be fitted into a number of functional areas.

And third, there appear to be several areas of omission. It is difficult to spot references to important managerial activities such as structuring organization, selecting and appraising managers, and determining major strategies.

It can be argued, however, that observing what managers do, and assembling data on managerial work, is of considerable value. Initially, it is important for the greater development of management theory and training. Subsequently, it allows managers to know how their actions compare with the actions of effective counterparts.

The search for managerial excellence

Our final contribution to the history of management thought is that style of analysis associated with the consulting firm of McKinsey, and in particular the development of the McKinsey 7-S framework for management analysis.

This framework is important because it has formed the basis for three influential books on management: *The Art of Japanese Management* by Richard Pascale and Anthony Athos (1981), *Managing on the Edge* by Richard Pascale (1990), and *In Search of Excellence* by Tom Peters and Bob Waterman (1982).* These books use the 7-S framework to identify key aspects of the management system and to show the interrelatedness of management variables. In brief, the McKinsey 7-Ss stand for:

1 *Strategy* – systematic action and allocation of resources to achieve company goals.

2 *Structure* – organization structure and authority relationships.
3 *Systems* – procedures and processes such as information systems, manufacturing processes, budgeting and control processes.
4 *Style* – the way management behaves and collectively spends its time to achieve organizational goals.
5 *Staff* – the people in the organization and their socialization into the corporate culture.
6 *Skills* – the distinctive capabilities of the enterprise.
7 *Shared values* – the values and philosophies shared by members of the organization.

Graphically the McKinsey model is presented in the form of a six-pointed star with a central locus. The star points are all linearly interconnected with the locus and with each other. The first six Ss thus form satellites around the seventh S, *shared values*, which is the linchpin of the framework. By using the term shared values (also sometimes called superordinate goals), the McKinsey writers emphasize the central role of *culture* in work organizations. Special attention is given to the link between personal and organizational values in the search for corporate excellence.

The 7-S model has been used extensively by McKinsey's consultants in analysing companies in a wide range of industrial and service sectors. The framework has also been used with considerable success in business schools such as Harvard and Stanford. A simple and easy-to-remember framework, it has played a key role in emphasizing the importance of developing strong corporate cultures if we are to achieve business success.

The key work based on the model is Peters and Waterman's book, *In Search of Excellence*. This book is a paradigm of the so-called excellence school of management thought, an approach that attempts to highlight good western management practice in an era dominated by Japanese business success (Ouchi, 1981; Oliver and Wilkinson, 1992).

Peters and Waterman researched 43 successful American companies, including International

---

* A Peters and Waterman-type analysis in the UK context is found in *The Winning Streak* (1986) by W. Goldsmith and D. Clutterbuck (Penguin, Harmondsworth). Also in the UK, much recent attention has been given to the series of company profiles by the former ICI chief executive Sir John Harvey Jones. This series of consultancy-type investigations into corporate style and effectiveness has been presented on television and in book form under the title *Troubleshooter* volumes 1 and 2 (1988, 1992) (BBC Publications, London). A further, and extremely important, volume which must be mentioned in this vein is *The Change Masters* (1983) by Rosabeth Moss Kanter (Counterpoint, Boston MA). Often nicknamed the thinking person's *In Search of Excellence*, the main theme of *The Change Masters* is similarly that of describing American corporations that have stimulated internal entrepreneurship and subsequently become market leaders.

Business Machines (IBM), Procter and Gamble, Minnesota Mining and Manufacturing (3M), Texas Instruments and Dana. In their analysis, they identified eight common characteristics, or principles, of these successfully managed corporations. Briefly, these are:

1 *Bias for action.* Successful managers have a preference for doing something, rather than cycling a problem through analysis and committee reports. At Procter and Gamble, new product ideas must be condensed to one page or less.
2 *Simple form, lean staff.* Small plants are generally more productive than large ones. The key is small groups producing higher-quality goods or providing more personalized services. Small organizations avoid excessive overhead and large numbers of staff employees. Hewlett-Packard and Digital Equipment managers say there should be no more than 300–400 people per plant.
3 *Close to the customer.* The importance of listening to customer ideas and complaints. The textile manufacturer Milliken receives more than 50% of its product innovations from customers.
4 *Productivity through people.* The people who do the work must be involved in decisions and excercise at least some control over the work. At the Edison plant of the Ford Motor Company, senior management put a button at each worker's station on an assembly line, and employees can push the button to shut down the line if they consider that work up to that point does not meet quality standards.
5 *Autonomy and entrepreneurship.* Managers must be encouraged to be entrepreneurs and compete against each other. To encourage competition between divisions, at Johnson and Johnson, 3M and Hewlett-Packard divisional managers are given a free hand to create new markets.
6 *Value-driven.* The company must not allow conflicting values to weaken its primary emphasis. Managers must set one priority and try to do that one thing well; for example, customer service at IBM, new product development at Hewlett-Packard, and product quality at Procter and Gamble.
7 *Stick to the knitting.* A successful company defines its strength – for example, marketing, new-product innovation, low-cost manufacturing – then builds on it. The rule is: 'never acquire a business you don't know how to run'.
8 *Simultaneous loose – tight properties.* If a few variables are tightly controlled – for example, costs and revenues – management may allow lee-way in day-to-day operations.

Peters and Waterman claim that corporations that recognize and act on these characteristics perform better than those that do not use them. The message of *In Search of Excellence* is that successful companies have a competetive edge over other companies by paying more attention to people – employees and customers – and by sticking to the skills and values that they know best.

Part 2: The managerial society

Having provided a history of management thought, we now offer a brief sociological analysis of the rise of professional management in modern societies. We examine theories and concepts used to interpret the increasing significance of the management function in contemporary organizations and discuss the related theses of the industrial society, the separation of ownership from control, the managerial revolution, and the technostructure (Poole *et al.*, 1981; Reed, 1990). Through this analysis, we demonstrate how wider social and economic forces impinge on the development of management functions.

The industrial society

Of the many theories that have been developed to account for the growth of management in the 20th century, the *industrial society thesis* has been the most celebrated. Among the key writers who advance this thesis are Raymond Aron (1961), Ralf Dahrendorf (1959), J.K. Galbraith (1967), Harbison and Myers (1959), and Clark Kerr and colleagues (1962). These writers profess that during the present century the role of managers – in both developed and developing nations – has become more critical. The argument is made that:

> as industrialization proceeds, the number of persons in management increases both absolutely and relatively in the economy. This is the inevitable consequence of larger capital outlay, the pace of innovation, the use of more modern machinery and processes, the growth of markets, and the increasing complexity of the advancing industrial societies (Kerr *et al.*, 1962).

An *industrial society* is defined simply as 'a society in which large scale industry . . . is the characteristic form of production' (Aron, 1961). The economies of modern industrial societies are characterized by the separation of the enterprise from the family, a new technological division of labour, an accumulation of capital, rational calculation and a concentration of workers in the enterprise.

Writers on the industrial society attach particular importance to the role of managers (Harbison and Myers, 1959; Kerr et al., 1962). Those who occupy the top-authority positions in large-scale enterprises are of key concern, for it is they who are the organization builders. Managers, it is claimed, should be analysed in four important respects:

1 as an economic resource;
2 as a class into which access is limited;
3 as an internal authority system;
4 as a rule-making authority over the managed (Kerr et al., 1962).

As an *economic resource*, the defining characteristics of modern managers are sought in terms of management representing a form of capital which is indispensable for successful industrial development. For Kerr et al., managerial resources in the labour force inevitably increase because a greater number of highly trained personnel are required as an enterprise becomes larger and more complex; the growth of markets implies more complex enterprises; capital and management intensity are coterminous phenomena; external problems occasioned by exigencies of the political and social environment require specialized staff; and the use of high-level human resources expands commensurately with an increasing pace of innovation. Although managerial resources have historically emanated from diverse social groupings, e.g. artisans, merchant capitalists, dynastic élites, senior civil servants, under industrialism it becomes increasingly important to produce indigenous managers of high calibre.

In accounting for the rise of managers, Kerr et al. also focus on issues of *social class and social mobility*. They argue that not only does upward social mobility into managerial grades gradually come to reflect technical ability, experience, education, knowledge of the organization, and an ability to impress people who make decisions, but also that managers are able through time to dispense with extant ruling élites, especially 'proprietary capitalists, family patriarchs [and] political commissars' (Kerr et al., 1962).

The *internal authority system* and *rule-making processes* are also major areas of concern. For Kerr et al., the system of authority governs both the direction of an organization and the coordination of internal authority. Faced with the dynamic of organizational growth and complexity, and thus with pressures to decentralize, managers attempt to convert the structure of control into a system of rule-making authority – a legitimate form of domination. As Kerr and colleagues noted:

> a primary concern for management, in its relationship to workers, is to establish, to make legitimate, and to maintain its authority. The logic of industrialization impels management to covet the role of rule-maker. It seeks control over any of the factors which must be co-ordinated in the planning – production – selling process. The specialization of functions which industrialization demands also requires that the workplace accepts tasks whose nature, time and method of accomplishment are to be determined by management in its role of planner and order giver (Kerr et al., 1962).

The study by Kerr et al. provides a productive theoretical basis for the analysis of modern managers, notably in that the rise rather than the eclipse is explained. Under industrialism the major implicit reward for the modern manager comes from organization building – the construction of complex administrative and productive enterprises. We see also the prediction of the replacement of earlier ruling groups by a new managerial class and the notion that meritocratic criteria for promotion and selection will be progressively instituted. The growing role of the state is another important factor: it not only serves to increase the number of managers, but also acts as a pressure for the proliferation of rule-making procedures. Finally, as the dominant actors of the future are considered to be managers, the issue of ownership is considered to be of declining significance: under pluralistic industrialism organizational control is the primary activity.

The separation of ownership from control

No issue is so closely associated with the industrial society thesis than the argument of the divorce of ownership from control. The rise of managerialism assumes that a separation of ownership and control has occurred in all large-scale organizations of the modern world (Berle, 1960). It is argued that the ownership of productive capital is no longer such a signal feature of social structure, for it is the control of organizations which is of critical concern. The position is well put by Berle, who states;

> the rise of the corporate system, with attendant separation of ownership from management due to concentration of industry in the corporate form, was the first great twentieth century change. In three decades it led to a rise of autonomous corporation management. The second tendency, pooling of savings, voluntary or forced, in fiduciary institutions now is steadily separating the owner (if the stockholder can properly be called an 'owner') from his residual ultimate power – that of voting for management. In effect, this is gradually removing power of selecting boards of directors and managements from these managements themselves as self perpetuating oligarchies, to a different and rising group of interests – pension trustees, mutual fund managers and (less importantly) insurance company managements (Berle, 1960).

There are, however, variations of the managerialist thesis, and these lead to radically different implications for corporate strategy and the locus of power in contemporary enterprises. Berle's concept of managerialism is founded on the thesis of a separation of ownership from control, the implications of which are conceived in nonsectional terms. Berle wishes that, in future, freed from shareholder control, managers will become responsible arbiters of the public good – they will constitute a 'neutral management élite' which will seek a balance amongst the stakeholders in an organization in order to ensure satisfaction for all who have legitimate claims on the resources of the enterprise. In this view, the legitimate corporation will not only facilitate a more equitable distribution of rewards and promote more advanced human relations policies, but also will pay more attention to public and societal issues than has been evident in the behaviour of earlier entrepreneurial corporate leaders.

The managerial revolution

In contrast, James Burnham's (1941) influential treatise on managerialism, *The Managerial Revolution*, develops what is usually referred to as its sectional variant. Like Berle, Burnham acknowledges the consequences of large-scale industry,

bureaucratization, the separation of ownership from control, the power of new managers, and their rise to a position of ascendency in modern communities. However, he draws radically different conclusions. Burnham argues that the consequences of the rise of the manager are not the beginnings of a neutral management élite, but rather a managerially dominated society – and ultimately a managerially dominated world – in which both socialism and democratic capitalism will be replaced by a new managerial society. Further, whereas Berle is primarily interested in the growth of managers in private-enterprise economies, Burnham is mainly concerned with state enterprise and predicted the rise of a new ruling class, consequential upon increasing government intervention in industry and the economy, since this provides the primary basis for managerial control of the means of production in the first place. For Burnham, the corporate state will become an enduring feature of all industrial societies. State ownership of the means of production will lead to the emergence of a powerful stratum of new managers, and because managers perform indispensable functions and have access to the means of production, they will inevitably exercise power in their own interests (Nichols, 1969).

The technostructure

However, even among those who generally endorse the thesis of the separation of ownership, there remain key problems concerning the precise locus and distribution of power in the modern corporation. While both Berle and Burnham largely focus on decision-making at the top of the enterprise, commentators such as Galbraith identify a broader group – the so-called *technostructure* – as being dominant in this respect.

In *The New Industrial State*, Galbraith (1967) indeed admits that there is a steady accumulation of evidence on the shift of power from owners to managers within the modern large corporation. He argues, however, that the managerialists only include in their analyses 'a small proportion of those who, as participants, contribute information to group decisions'. As such, they fail to embrace 'all those who bring specialised knowledge, talent or experience' to the formulation and implementation of strategic and day-to-day policies.

This argument in many ways anticipates later discussions on the possibility of a new working class of scientific and technical employees: a class which would usurp the very functions of management which the employee – manager had wrested away from the ownership class (Mallet, 1975).

Part 3: Perspectives on management

We complete this chapter by describing some analytical perspectives which inform the study of management. Specifically we discuss the functional, action and radical perspectives in management theory.

The functional perspective

The functional perspective sees management as a neutral technology used to realize legitimate social goals within the framework of formal organization. From this perspective, management is a control system designed to attain productive efficiency through the coordination of human actions. At the heart of the approach is the assumption that corporations are media which transform individual goals into collective goals in order to achieve superior levels of productive output. Management is portrayed as the social machinery which allows this transformation to take place.

Management is also characterized as a structural phenomenon: it is shaped into various forms along various dimensions, such as the degree of internal functional differentiation, the degree of centralized decison-making or the extensiveness of explicit rules and procedures (Reed, 1990a). Indeed, the configuration of structural elements represents the analytical focus for the functional approach to management. Devoid of structure, the notion of management as a medium of functional coordination and control is bereft of theoretical power.

As the functional perspective focuses on the structural nature of management, so it takes recourse to a *systems* analysis of organizational behaviour. Emphasis is placed on the structural forces which produce social order and ensure effective control over human interaction. In this framework, corporations are organic entities which must satisfy the functional demands placed upon them by their environment. Management structures are evaluated in terms of the contribution they make to the reproduction of the system as a whole.

In contrast, system *change* results from the failure of the management structure to adapt to developments in the organization's environment. If there is imbalance or disequilibrium between the component parts of the structure, this induces tension and strain within the system, the result being suboptimal performance of system parts. The main practical implication of systems analysis of organization is to identify those areas in which strain is occurring and to assist managers in taking action to restore an appropriate balance between internal structures and external demands.

The internal dynamic of the functional approach is thus the need to secure the effectiveness of structural form by ensuring that any dysfunctional consequences of organizational change are identified and resolved. This necessitates analysis of the demands which environmental contingencies such as size, technology, product and market place upon the organization, and the degree to which these are satisfied by existing methods for ensuring internal coordination and control. The main criterion for judging the adequacy of the structural form is the goodness of fit between the organization's internal control and the shifting nature of its environmental demands.

The action perspective

The second major perspective is that of the *action* approach. From this perspective, management is construed as a voluntaristic social process. We see a rejection of the rational, static and deterministic view of management associated with the functional perspective, and instead the image of management as purposive social activity. In this perspective, managers do not simply respond to the environment (or better, context) – they actively shape and define it.

The action perspective draws upon that style of organizational analysis associated with David Silverman's work (Silverman, 1970; Silverman and Jones, 1975), especially his notion of the 'action frame of reference'. This notion portrays management structures as continually negotiated networks of social interaction. Formal control systems, such as rules and regulations, chains of command and measurement techniques constitute an objective background which is reworked and redefined through the everyday actions engaged by competent organization members; that is, personnel who successfully interpret the *meaning* of work through understanding implicit and shared assumptions about its contextual enactment. On being defined as *interactional processes*, management systems are continually reproduced and reconstructed by those associated with them. Rather than being a determining factor of social interaction, management is, instead, a product of the way it is interpreted by participants who hold tenure within the organization.

Research in the action perspective often focuses upon the power sources available to the manager and how these are deployed. The aim is to document the way the manager strategically mobilizes power bases in order to manipulate control over decision-making processes. The ability to define the decision-making agenda is a function of the manager's skill in minimizing dependence on others within the limits presented by the situation. The form of political opportunities available and the skills required to exploit the potential for control constitute key foci for research enquiry.

In recent years the action perspective has been important in bringing about a re-evaluation of the principles underpinning the dominant model of management as a series of rational and functional control systems. The action perspective has highlighted the role of managers as political actors who purposefully shape the environment in an instrumental way, often with disregard to the formal goals of the corporation. Organizational practices are continually redefined and reworked in line with political negotiations. In contrast to the technical rationality of the functional perspective, it is political pluralism which is the key point of reference.

This negotiated order view of management sees power relations as fluid and unstable structures which are liable to degenerate as the balance of power between the plurality of of interests that constitutes the organization's political system fragments and changes (Reed, 1990b). Although the hierarchical nature of power relations is given some recognition, its explanatory significance is downplayed in favour of a view of power that focuses on the negotiating processes through which corporate order is established and transformed. This sensitivity to the subtle political processes through which corporate change is negotiated influences the realization of more effective forms of managerial control: obstacles to preferred outcomes are identified and strategies for their removal defined and enacted.

Research on management from the action perspective dates back to the early 1950s. An early work from this perspective was Melville Dalton's book *Men Who Manage* (1959), which analyses the changing loci of power and influence within management structures and how this impacts upon organizational adaption.

Further research in this area has focused upon the role of strategic choice as a notion for describing the considerable voluntarism evident in the decision activities of senior managers. The strategic choice thesis has highlighted the power of dominant coalitions to ensure the design and implementation of preferred organizational systems.

The radical perspective

From the radical or Marxist perspective, management systems are the instruments through which the interests of the bourgeois ruling class are advanced and protected. Management is both a control device which operates to meet the *economic* demands of the capitalist mode of production and an *ideological* medium which serves to obscure capitalist structural realities. The economic goal that management has to realize is sufficient control over the production process to ensure the extraction of surplus value and thus profit. The ideological goal it has to realize is the maintenance of the subordination of labour within the production process so that any potential for resistance is minimized.

The radical view of management links the everyday work of managers to the wider social relations of capitalist production. This perspective highlights the explanatory role of political conflicts between management and other social groups for an understanding of the superstructure of corporate life. In so doing, however, it contends that these internal processes are analytically subordinate to the deep structure (or base) of capitalist production relations.

Indeed, managers and management structures are considered to be direct products of the capitalist socioeconomic system. Managers are agents for an economic philosophy which requires that labour is controlled in such a way that it furthers the interests of a class to which it would otherwise be opposed. This class provides the institutional means through which this process can be realized, in the form of material blandishments, ideological appeals and management systems which contain labour resistance and incorporate it within a cultural framework which mystifies the structural realities of capitalism.

In recent years, researchers from this perspective have directed their interests towards the internal contradictions contained within management control systems. The contradictions which beset management systems stimulate waves of organizational changes, the goal of these being the eradication of tensions within the authority structure. However, researchers contend that, rather than eradicate such tensions, change attempts succeed only in exacerbating the problems they were meant to solve. The prime contradiction is the simultaneous demand for control over and cooperation from labour, and the parallel implementation of structural and ideological mechanisms which ensure that these goals are negated simultaneously (Reed, 1990a).

The influence of the radical perspective on the sociology of management has been felt most in that series of theoretical analyses and empirical studies emerging in the wake of Braverman's landmark attempt at a Marxist analysis of work organization and the labour process (Braverman, 1974). For management research, the significance of this work is in marking a shift away from functionalist analysis towards a dialectical approach, and the contradictions in management control it has revealed. This has resulted in less emphasis being placed upon an abstract appreciation of the structural imperatives which impose themselves on capitalist forms of work organization, and more emphasis upon management as a mechanism which mediates between external economic constraints and internal organizational systems. It is argued that this mechanism consists of ideas, techniques, methods and practices related to the effective control of work that necessarily contain contradictory recipes for action which produce unanticipated outcomes (Reed, 1990b).

However, this model has been complicated by a recognition of the forms of labour resistance which are mobilized in response to the implementation of new control systems. The growing acceptance that the link between capital accumulation and transformations of the labour process is an indirect one has provided the stimulus for a reworking of a radical model of management which is more voluntaristic than the one suggested by Braverman (1974).

Conclusions

The aim of this section has been to offer an introduction to theories of management and organization. Initially we outlined a history of management and managerial work: we analysed contributions from the scientific, classical, human relations, open systems, contingency and corporate excellence approaches. It was argued that the study of management has moved from the specification of universal laws to principles which are sensitive to the uniqueness of administrative situations.

We then went on to develop a more sociological approach to the role of management within modern society. We outlined a thesis based on the notions of the industrial society, the separation of ownership from control, the managerial revolution, and the technostructure. We described the rise of managerialism within the 20th century and its central role in the development of the modern industrial state. Finally, we considered three analytical frameworks used to interpret the subject of management and organization – the functionalist, action and radical. We outlined the distinctive insights that each brings to the study of management.

References

Argyris, C. (1964) *Integrating the Individual and the Organization*. John Wiley, New York.

Aron, R. (1961) *18 Lectures on Industrial Society*. Weidenfeld and Nicholson, London.

Barnard, C.I. (1938) *The Functions of the Executive*. Harvard University Press, Cambridge, MA.

Bennis, W. (1966) *Changing Organizations*. McGraw-Hill, New York.

Berle, A. (1960) *Power Without Property: A New Development in American Political Economy*. Sidgwick & Jackson, London.

Blake, R. and Mouton, J. (1964) *The Managerial Grid*. Gulf Publishing, Houston, TX.

Boulding, K. General systems theory: the skeleton of science. *Management Science* **3**, 197–208.

Braverman, H. (1974) *Labor and Monopoly Capital*. Monthly Review Press, New York.

Burnham, J. (1941) *The Managerial Revolution*. Day, New York.

Burns, T. and Stalker, G. (1961) *The Management of Innovation*. Tavistock, London.

Burrell, G. and Morgan, G. (1979) *Sociological Paradigms and Organizational Analysis.* Heinemann, London.

Clegg, S. and Dunkerley, D. (1980) *Organizations, Class and Control.* Routledge and Kegan Paul, London.

Dahrendorf, R. (1959) *Class and Class Conflict in Industrial Society.* Routledge and Kegan Paul, London.

Dalton, M. (1959) *Men who Manage.* John Wiley, New York.

Drucker, P. (1949) *TVA and the Grass Roots.* University of California Press, Berkeley, CA.

Durkheim, E. (1893) *De la Division du travil Social* (The Division of Labour). F. Alcan, Paris.

Emery, F. and Trist, E. (1960) Socio-technical systems. In: *Proceedings of 6th Annual International Meeting of the Institute of Management Sciences.* Pergamon Press, London. p. 94.

Fayol, H. (1949) *General and Industrial Administration.* Pitman, London.

Fiedler, F. (1967) *A Theory of Leadership Effectiveness.* McGraw-Hill, New York.

Galbraith, J. K. (1967) *The New Industrial State.* Penguin, Harmondsworth.

Gulick, L. and Urwick, L. (eds) (1937) *Papers on the Science of Administration.* Institute of Public Administration, New York.

Harbison, F. and Myers, C. (1959) *Management in the Industrial World: An International Analysis.* McGraw-Hill, New York.

Hertzberg, F. (1958) *The Motivation to Work.* John Wiley, New York.

Homans, G. (1958) *The World of Work: Industrial Society and Human Relations.* Prentice-Hall, Englewood Cliffs, NJ.

Johnson, J., Kast, F. and Rosenweig, J. (1963) *The Theory and Management of Systems.* McGraw-Hill, New York.

Katz, D. and Kahn, R. (1950) *The Human Group.* Harcourt, Brace and World, New York.

Katz, D. and Kahn, R. (1966) *The Social Psychology of Organizations.* Wiley, New York.

Kerr, C., Dunlop, J., Harbison, F. and Myers, C. (1962) *Industrialism and Industrial Man.* Heinemann, London.

Koontz, H. and O'Donnell, C. (1976) *Management: A Systems and Contingency Analysis of Managerial Functions.* McGraw-Hill, New York.

Koontz, H. and Weirich, H. (1988) *Management.* McGraw-Hill, New York.

Leavitt, H. (1958) *Managerial Psychology.* University of Chicago Press, Chicago, IL.

Lepawsky, A. (1949) *Administration.* Alfred A. Knopf, New York.

Lewin, K. (1951) *Field Theory in Social Science.* Harper, New York.

Likert, R. (1961) *New Patterns of Management.* McGraw-Hill, New York.

McGregor, D. (1964) *Managerial Behaviour.* McGraw-Hill, New York.

Mallet, S. (1975) *The New Working Class.* Spokesman, Nottingham.

Maslow, A. (1960) *The Human Side of Enterprise.* McGraw-Hill, New York.

Mayntz, R. (1964) The study of organizations. *Current Sociology* **13**, 94–156.

Mayo, E. (1933) *The Human Problems of an Industrial Civilisation.* Macmillan, New York.

Miles, R. (1980) *Macro Organizational Behaviour.* Goodyear, Santa Monica, CA.

Mintzberg, H. (1973) *The Nature of Managerial Work.* Harper & Row, New York.

Mooney, J. D. (1947) *The Principles of Organization.* Harper & Row, New York.

Nichols, T. (1969) *Ownership, Control and Ideology.* Allen and Unwin, London.

Pareto, V. (1916) *Trattato di Sociologia generale* (2nd edn 1923) Florence. English translation published as *The Mind and Society: A Treatise on General Sociology* (1935) Harcourt, Brace, New York.

Parsons, T. (1951) *The Social System.* Free Press, New York.

Parsons, T. (1956) A sociological approach to the study of organizations. *Administrative Science Quarterly* **1**, 63–85, 225–239.

Parsons, T. (1960) *Structure and Process in Modern Societies.* Free Press, New York.

Pascale, R. (1990) *Managing on the Edge.* Simon and Schuster, New York.

Pascale, R. T. and Athos, A. G. (1981) *The Art of Japanese Management.* Warner Books, New York.

Peters, T. J. and Waterman, R. H. (1982) *In Search of Excellence.* Harper & Row, New York.

Poole, M., Mansfield, R., Blyton, P. and Frost, P. (1981) *Managers in Focus.* Gower, Aldershot.

Reed, M. (1985) *Redirections in Organizational Analysis.* Tavistock, London.

Reed, M. (1990a) *The Sociology of Management.* Harvester Wheatsheaf, Brighton.

Reed, M. (1990b) *The Sociology of Management.* Harvester Wheatsheaf, Brighton.

Rice, A. K. (1958) *Productivity and Social Organization: The Ahmedabad Experiment.* Tavistock, London.

Roethlisberger, F. J. and Dickson, W. J. (1939) *Management and the Worker*. Harvard University Press, Cambridge, MA.

Rose, M. (1975) *Industrial Behaviour: Theoretical Developments Since Taylor*. Penguin, Harmondsworth.

Sayles, L. (1959) *Individual Behaviour and Group Achievement*. Oxford University Press, Oxford.

Selznick, P. (1966) *The Social Psychology of Organizations*. John Wiley, New York.

Silverman, D. (1970) *The Theory of Organizations*. Heinemann, London.

Silverman, D. and Jones, J. (1975) *Organizational Work*. Collier Macmillan, London.

Stogdill, R. (1961) *Leadership and Organization: A Behavioural Science Approach*. McGraw-Hill, New York.

Trist, E. and Bamforth, K. (1955) Some social and psychological consequences of the long-wall method of coal getting. *Human Relations* **4**, 1–38.

Trist, E., Higgin, G., Murray, H. and Pollock, A. (1963) *Organizational Choice*. Tavistock, London.

von Bertalanffy, L. (1961) General systems theory: a new approach to the unity of science. *Human Biology* **23**, 303–361.

Wright Bakke, E. (1950) *Bonds of Organization*. Harper & Row, New York.

Index